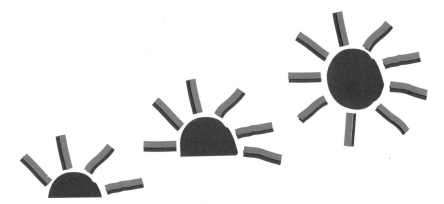

# Bright Futures

## Guidelines for Health Supervision of Infants, Children, and Adolescents

Morris Green, M.D., Editor

Sponsored by
Maternal and Child Health Bureau
Health Resources and Services Administration
Public Health Service
U.S. Department of Health and Human Services

Medicaid Bureau
Health Care Financing Administration
U.S. Department of Health and Human Services

Published by
National Center for Education in Maternal and Child Health
Arlington, Virginia

**Cite as**

Green M. (Ed.). 1994. Bright Futures: **Guidelines for Health Supervision of Infants, Children, and Adolescents.** Arlington, VA: National Center for Education in Maternal and Child Health.

The mission of NCEMCH is to promote and improve the health, education, and well-being of children and families by providing a national focus for the collection, development, and dissemination of information and educational materials on maternal and child health; and collaborating with public agencies, voluntary and professional organizations, research and training programs, policy centers, and others to advance education and program and policy development. Established in 1982 at Georgetown University, the National Center for Education in Maternal and Child Health is part of the Graduate Public Policy Program. NCEMCH is funded primarily by the Maternal and Child Health Bureau, U.S. Department of Health and Human Services.

Library of Congress Catalog Card Number 94-68903
ISBN 1-57285-009-4

**Published by**
National Center for Education in Maternal and Child Health
2000 15th Street North, Suite 701
Arlington, VA 22201-2617
(703) 524-7802 • (703) 524-9335 fax
Internet: ncemch01@gumedlib.dml.georgetown.edu

**Additional copies of this publication are available for $20 from**
National Maternal and Child Health Clearinghouse
2070 Chain Bridge Road, Suite 450
Vienna, VA 22182
(703) 821-8955 • (703) 821-2098 fax

This publication has been produced by the National Center for Education in Maternal and Child Health under its cooperative agreement (MCU-117007) with the Maternal and Child Health Bureau, Health Resources and Services Administration, Public Health Service, U.S. Department of Health and Human Services.

# Table of Contents

**Infancy: 0–12 Months** `1`

**Early Childhood: 1–5 Years** `79`

# The Challenge of Bright Futures

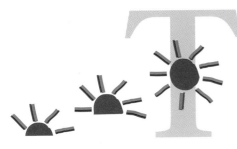

The world of America's children and families has changed rapidly and extensively during the 20th century. As we prepare for the beginning of a new century, it is now appropriate to take stock of the progress we have made and the distance we still have to travel. For many children and their families, each new day is an opportunity for further self-realization, enhancement of good health, and promotion of self-esteem.

For millions of others, however, the future holds little promise; their health status is poor, the risks to their health are many, and the prospects for them to successfully overcome these problems are limited. These children, and all our nation's children, deserve the attention, the encouragement, and the intervention of care providers from many disciplines to ensure that they develop the healthy bodies, minds, emotions, and attitudes to prepare them to be competent and contributing adults.

Health supervision policies and practices have not kept up with the pervasive changes that have occurred in the family, the community, and society. It has become evident that a "new health supervision" is urgently needed to confront the "new morbidities" that challenge today's children and families.

The goal of Bright Futures is to respond to the current and emerging preventive and health promotion needs of infants, children, and adolescents. To meet the complex challenge of developing new health supervision guidelines, the expertise and informed opinions of a large number of health professionals and consumers were elicited. These guidelines, based on their wise and creative suggestions, are an exciting response to the needs of the times, a vision for the future and, more importantly, a direction for child health supervision well into the 21st century.

The next step will be to promote the implementation of Bright Futures in the great variety of settings and arrangements that provide opportunities for health supervision throughout this country. It is also important to further an in-depth exploration of the science of prevention and health promotion and engage health professionals, educators, and families in this venture. It is time to walk into that bright future.

*Morris Green, M.D.*

# Acknowledgments

The Bright Futures project has been a four-year journey during which scores of dedicated, caring people have explored the nature of health supervision and its impact on the health and well-being of children. As with so many child health issues, the journey began with the unqualified support of the Maternal and Child Health Bureau (MCHB) of the Health Resources and Services Administration (HRSA). For six decades, MCHB has asked questions and sought information critical to making health practices responsive to the changing needs of our nation's children. Launched during the tenure of MCHB's former director, Vince L. Hutchins, M.D., the Bright Futures project received enthusiastic support from Audrey H. Nora, M.D., current director of MCHB, and Ciro V. Sumaya, M.D., administrator of HRSA. Woodie Kessel, M.D., and David Heppel, M.D., division directors, provided leadership, guidance, expert counsel, and commitment from MCHB during every phase of this project. In addition, William Hiscock, former chief of Special Initiatives at the Medicaid Bureau of the Health Care Financing Administration, had the foresight to involve his agency in supporting this project. J. David Greenberg, M.B.A., has been instrumental in providing the Medicaid perspective.

The board of directors and expert panels made enormous contributions of time and expertise to focus the project, research the issues, and formulate the recommendations. Renowned for their prior accomplishments, the panel chairs—Barry S. Zuckerman, M.D., Infancy Panel; George G. Sterne, M.D., Early Childhood Panel; Judith S. Palfrey, M.D., Middle Childhood Panel; and Elizabeth McAnarney, M.D., Adolescence Panel—skillfully shaped and guided the work of their panels.

With a grant from MCHB, the National Center for Education in Maternal and Child Health (NCEMCH), Georgetown University, under the leadership of Rochelle Mayer, Ed.D., director, provided continuous and dedicated staff support to the project. Pamela Mangu, M.A., and Meri McCoy-Thompson, M.A.L.D, project directors, assisted the chair at every turn and supervised the development of the Bright Futures guidelines. They and their colleagues served as liaisons to the expert panels and as writers, editors, artists, designers, desktop publishers, and printing and production managers. We are especially grateful to Robin Landis, M.A., former design director of NCEMCH, for creating the original design concepts for the book.

Also under a grant from MCHB, the Center for Health Policy Research of the George Washington University, under the leadership of Peter Budetti, M.D., director, and Michele Solloway, Ph.D., senior research scientist, focused upon the organization, delivery, and cost-effectiveness of services and produced important background materials to put the project in proper perspective.

# Organizations That Support Bright Futures

- Ambulatory Pediatric Association

- American Academy of Child and Adolescent Psychiatry

- American Academy of Pediatric Dentistry

- American Academy of Pediatrics

- American College of Nurse-Midwives

- American Dietetic Association

- American Medical Association

- American Medical Women's Association

- American Nurses Association

- Association of Maternal and Child Health Programs

- Association of State and Territorial Health Officials

- Child Welfare League of America, Inc.

- March of Dimes Birth Defects Foundation

- National Association of Pediatric Nurse Associates and Practitioners

- National Association of School Nurses, Inc.

- National Association of Social Workers

- National Early Childhood Technical Assistance System (NEC*TAS)

- National Organization of Nurse Practitioner Faculties

- Society of Pediatric Nurses

- The National PTA

- Zero to Three

# Participants in Bright Futures

## Board of Directors

**Morris Green, M.D., Chair**
Perry W. Lesh Professor of Pediatrics, James Whitcomb Riley Hospital for Children, Indiana University School of Medicine

**Polly Arango**
Parent, Family Voices

**Richard Behrman, M.D.**
Managing Director, Center for The Future of Children, David and Lucile Packard Foundation

**John Bogert, D.D.S.**
Executive Director, American Academy of Pediatric Dentistry

**Otis Bowen, M.D.**
Former Secretary of the Department of Health and Human Services, Former Governor of Indiana

**Robert Brodell, M.D.**
Chairman, American Academy of Pediatrics Task Force on Preventive Health Services, Children's Medical Group, Cumberland, Maryland

**Larry Culpepper, M.D., M.P.H.**
Director of Research and Professor of Family Medicine, Memorial Hospital of Rhode Island/Brown University

**Juanita Fleming, R.N., Ph.D.**
Professor of Nursing and Special Assistant to the President for Academic Affairs, University of Kentucky

**Robert Haggerty, M.D.**
Professor of Pediatrics Emeritus, University of Rochester Medical Center

**Birt Harvey, M.D.**
Professor of Pediatrics, Stanford University School of Medicine, Past President, American Academy of Pediatrics

**Jennifer Howse, Ph.D.**
President, March of Dimes Birth Defects Foundation

**Michael Jellinek, M.D.**
Chief of Child Psychiatry Service, Massachusetts General Hospital

**H. Raymond Klein, D.D.S.**
President, American Academy of Pediatric Dentistry, Private Dental Practice, Florida

**David S. Liederman**
Executive Director, Child Welfare League of America

**Richard Nelson, M.D.**
Past President, Association of Maternal and Child Health Programs, Professor of Pediatrics, University of Iowa

**Roselyn Payne Epps, M.D., M.P.H., M.A.**
Expert, Public Health Applications Research Branch, National Cancer Institute, National Institutes of Health, Professor of Pediatrics and Child Health, Howard University College of Medicine

**Howard Pearson, M.D.**
Past President, American Academy of Pediatrics, Professor of Pediatrics, Yale University School of Medicine

**Julius Richmond, M.D.**
Professor of Health Policy Emeritus, Harvard Medical School

**Joe M. Sanders, Jr., M.D.**
Executive Director, American Academy of Pediatrics

**Daniel Shea, M.D.**
Past President, American Academy of Pediatrics

**Vernon Smith, Ph.D.**
Director, Medical Services Administration, Michigan Department of Social Services

**James Strain, M.D.**
Immediate Past Executive Director, American Academy of Pediatrics, Clinical Professor of Pediatrics, University of Colorado, Denver

**David Sundwall, M.D.**
President, American Clinical Laboratories Association

**James Williams, M.Ed.**
Executive Director, National Education Association, Health Information Network

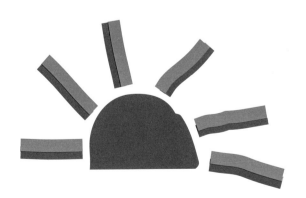

## Infancy Panel

**Barry S. Zuckerman, M.D., Chair**
Boston City Hospital

**Kathryn E. Barnard, R.N., Ph.D.**
University of Washington

**Patrick Casey, M.D.**
Arkansas Children's Hospital

**Evelyn Davis, M.D.**
Harlem Hospital

**Howard Dubowitz, M.D., M.S.**
University of Maryland School of Medicine

**Neal Halfon, M.D., M.P.H.**
University of California, Los Angeles

**Barbara Jo Howard, M.D.**
Duke University Medical Center

**Kathi Kemper, M.D., M.P.H.**
Swedish Medical Center, University of Washington

**Sanford R. Kimmel, M.D.**
Medical College of Ohio

**Howard S. King, M.D., M.P.H.**
Private Practice, Massachusetts

**Arthur Nowak, D.M.D.**
University of Iowa Colleges of Dentistry and Medicine

**Lucy Osborn, M.D.**
University of Utah Medical Center

**Kathryn K. Peppe, R.N., M.S.N.**
Ohio Department of Public Health

**Craig T. Ramey, Ph.D.**
University of Alabama at Birmingham

**Wilma J. Smith, R.N., P.N.P.**
Multnomah County Health Department, Portland, Oregon

## Early Childhood Panel

**George G. Sterne, M.D., Chair**
Private Practice, Louisiana

**Gil Buchanan, M.D.**
Arkansas Pediatric Clinic

**Albert Chang, M.D., M.P.H.**
San Diego State University

**Iris Marie Graville, R.N., M.N.**
Whatcom County Health Department, Washington

**David Johnsen, D.D.S.**
Case Western Reserve University School of Dentistry

**Barbara M. Korsch, M.D.**
Children's Hospital of Los Angeles

**Bruce Meyer, M.D.**
Administrative Medical Director, Columbus Children's Hospital, Private Practice, Ohio

**Lucy Osborn, M.D.**
University of Utah Medical Center

**Ellyn Satter, R.D., A.C.S.W.**
Family Therapy Center of Madison, Wisconsin

**Jack P. Shonkoff, M.D.**
University of Massachusetts Medical Center

## Middle Childhood Panel

**Judith S. Palfrey, M.D., Chair**
Children's Hospital, Boston

**Elaine Brainerd, R.N., M.A., C.S.N.**
State Department of Education, Connecticut

**Christopher DeGraw, M.D., M.P.H.**
Center for Health Policy Research, Washington, DC

**Paul H. Dworkin, M.D.**
St. Francis Hospital and Medical Center, Connecticut

**Leonard S. Krassner, M.D.**
Choate Rosemary Hall, Connecticut

**Erlinda Martinez**
Picacho Middle School, New Mexico

**Dennis McTigue, D.D.S., M.S.**
Ohio State University College of Dentistry

**Philip R. Nader, M.D.**
University of California, San Diego

**Edward L. Schor, M.D.**
New England Medical Center, Boston

## Adolescence Panel

**Elizabeth McAnarney, M.D., Chair**
University of Rochester Medical Center

**Robin K. Beach, M.D., M.P.H.**
Denver Department of Health and Hospitals

**Paul Casamassimo, D.D.S.**
Children's Hospital, Columbus, Ohio

**Arthur B. Elster, M.D.**
American Medical Association

**Renee R. Jenkins, M.D.**
Howard University College of Medicine

**Donald P. Orr, M.D.**
James Whitcomb Riley Hospital for Children, Indiana University School of Medicine

**Sue Panzarine, Ph.D., R.N.**
University of Missouri at St. Louis

**Mary Story, Ph.D., R.D.**
University of Minnesota

## Liaisons and Staff

**Carol Adams, M.A.**
Editorial Director,
NCEMCH

**Peter Budetti, M.D., J.D.**
Director, Center for Health
Policy Research, The George
Washington University

**Suzanne Connaughton,
M.P.H.**
Senior Health Policy Analyst,
American Academy of
Pediatrics

**Felix de la Cruz, M.D., M.P.H.**
Chief of Mental Retardation
and Developmental Disabilities
Branch, National Institute of
Child Health and Human
Development, NIH

**Susana Eloy**
Conference Coordinator,
NCEMCH

**Herbert L. Green, Jr., M.P.H.**
Chair, Cost and Effectiveness
Work Group, Center for Health
Policy Research, The George
Washington University

**Oliver Green**
Graphic Designer,
NCEMCH

**J. David Greenberg, M.B.A.**
Senior Health Insurance
Specialist, Office of Planning
and Special Initiatives,
Medicaid Bureau, HCFA

**David Heppel, M.D.**
Director, Division of Maternal,
Infant, Child and Adolescent
Health, Maternal and Child
Health Bureau, HRSA

**Ina Heyman**
Public Affairs Specialist,
Maternal and Child Health
Bureau, HRSA

**William Hiscock**
Former Chief, Medicaid Special
Program Initiatives Staff,
Medicaid Bureau, HCFA

**Katrina Holt, M.S., R.D.**
Adolescence Panel Liaison,
NCEMCH

**Vince Hutchins, M.D., M.P.H.**
Former Director, Maternal and
Child Health Bureau, HRSA

**Woodie Kessel, M.D., M.P.H.**
Director, Division of Systems,
Education and Science,
Maternal and Child Health
Bureau, HRSA

**Robin Landis, M.A.**
Former Design Director,
NCEMCH

**Pamela B. Mangu, M.A.**
Project Director,
Early Childhood Panel Liaison,
NCEMCH

**Rochelle Mayer, Ed.D.**
Director,
NCEMCH

**Christine Nye**
Former Director, Medicaid
Bureau, HCFA

**Meri McCoy-Thompson,
M.A.L.D.**
Project Director,
Infancy Panel Liaison,
NCEMCH

**Merle McPherson, M.D.**
Director, Division of Services
for Children with Special
Health Needs, Maternal and
Child Health Bureau, HRSA

**Audrey H. Nora, M.D., M.P.H.**
Director, Maternal and Child
Health Bureau, HRSA

**Jerome Paulson, M.D.**
Chair, Organization and
Delivery Work Group,
Department of Health Sciences,
The George Washington
University Medical Center

**Sally Richardson**
Director, Medicaid Bureau,
HCFA

**Christopher Rigaux**
Director of Communications,
NCEMCH

**Rebecca L. Selengut**
Project Associate,
NCEMCH

**Paula Sheahan**
Middle Childhood
Panel Liaison,
NCEMCH

**Elmer Smith**
Office of Planning and Special
Initiatives, Medicaid Bureau,
HCFA

**Michele Solloway, Ph.D.**
Senior Research Scientist,
Center for Health Policy
Research, The George
Washington University

**Nancy Witty, M.A.**
Project Consultant

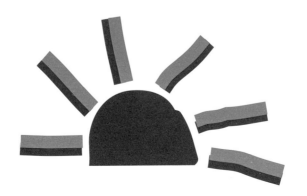

# Foreword

At the beginning of the 20th century, infectious disease caused most of the morbidity and mortality in children. Health supervision of children consisted of little more than a cursory examination to detect contagious diseases.[1] The first public health revolution promoted immunizations and pasteurization, improved nutrition and sanitation, and succeeded in reducing the childhood mortality rate by 25 times.

Although there has been great success in reducing contagious disease, children today face new issues. Over the past several decades, major economic, social, and demographic changes have significantly affected American families. These changes include a worrisome decline in the time parents spend with their children, less direct contact between children and their grandparents and extended family members, increased geographic mobility, a shortage of quality child care services, a reduction in neighborhood cohesiveness and social supports, and a widespread restructuring of family relationships.

Today one out of four infants and toddlers and one older child in five lives in poverty. The population of children in low-income families has increased by 2.5 million in the past decade, and includes more than 44 percent of black children, almost 40 percent of Hispanic children, and 16 percent of white children.[2] Frequently ill-clothed and marginally housed, these children are plagued by hunger, poor nutrition, violence, and neglect. They are frustrated and often angered by the lack of options they see for the future.

More than 25 percent of the nation's children (a percentage that has doubled in the last decade) now live in single-parent households, usually with their mothers.[3] Many children grow up in step, blended, sequential, homeless, or foster families. Divorce affects more than 1 million children each year, and an equal number of infants are born to unmarried mothers.[4] Single parents as well as families with two working parents experience task overload and role strain. Almost 11 million mothers with preschool youngsters work outside the home.[5]

These societal changes have brought with them changes in the chief causes of morbidity and mortality among children and adolescents. New health supervision guidelines are needed to prevent the "new morbidities." Injuries are now the leading cause of death for children over one year of age. Conservatively estimated, 12–15 percent of American children have mental and emotional disorders.[6,7] Among 15 year olds, one in seven smokes, one in three has consumed alcohol excessively, one in five has smoked marijuana daily, and one in four girls and one in three boys are sexually active.

Developmental problems, educational failure, low reading comprehension, immoderate risk taking, lack of supervision, and school dropout are almost commonplace in some neighborhoods. Reports of child abuse and neglect have increased by 40 percent since 1985. The population of children with special health needs due to illness or disability has also grown.

Health professionals, concerned about the detrimental effect these changes have had on children and families, have been searching for ways to respond. In 1979, Surgeon General Julius Richmond initiated the second public health revolution when he published *Healthy People: The Surgeon General's Report on Health Promotion and Disease Prevention*.[8] The report's emphasis on health promotion and disease prevention highlights the need for strategies beyond simply treating contagious disease. The problems families face today demand a more comprehensive approach—one that actively promotes health and prevents disease before it occurs. *Bright Futures: Guidelines for Health Supervision of Infants, Children, and Adolescents* seeks to answer the challenging question of how those who care for children can be more effective in disease prevention and health promotion. The recommendations offered by *Bright Futures*—consonant with the principles included in the Children's Health Charter on the following page—portend major changes in the delivery of preventive and health-promoting services, and in the education of health professionals.

1. Cone TE Jr. 1979. *History of Pediatrics*. Boston, MA: Little Brown and Company.

2. U.S. Department of Health and Human Services, Public Health Service, Health Resources and Services Administration, Maternal and Child Health Bureau. 1994. *Child Health USA '93* (DHHS Pub. No. HRSA-MCH-94-1). Washington, DC: U.S. Government Printing Office.

3. Bureau of the Census. 1990. Marital status and living arrangements: March 1989. In *Current Population Reports* (Series P-20, No. 445, p. 3). Washington, DC: U.S. Government Printing Office.

4. U.S. Congress, Select Committee on Children, Youth and Families. 1989. *U.S. Children and Their Families: Current Conditions and Recent Trends* (pp. 58–59). Washington, DC: U.S. Government Printing Office.

5. Bureau of Labor Statistics. 1990. *March 1990 Current Population Survey* (table 48). Unpublished data.

6. U.S. Congress, Office of Technology Assessment. 1986. *Children's Mental Health: Problems and Services—A Background Paper* (p. 4). Washington, DC: U.S. Government Printing Office.

7. Institute of Medicine. 1989. *Research on Children and Adolescents with Mental, Behavioral and Developmental Disorders: Mobilizing a National Initiative* (pp. 1, 32–33). Washington, DC: National Academy Press.

8. U.S. Department of Health, Education and Welfare. 1979. *Healthy People: The Surgeon General's Report on Health Promotion and Disease Prevention*. Washington, DC: U.S. Government Printing Office.

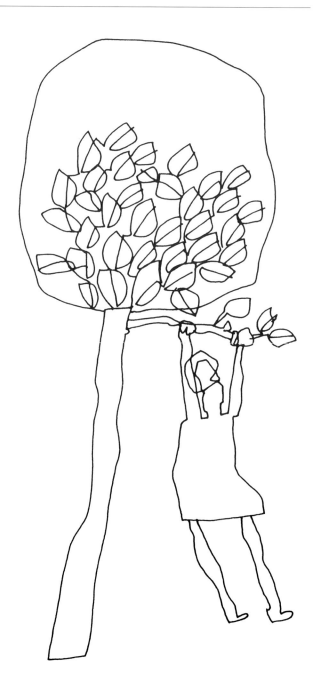

# Bright Futures Children's Health Charter

Throughout this century, principles developed by advocates for children have been the foundation for initiatives to improve children's lives. Bright Futures participants have adopted these principles in order to guide their work and meet the unique needs of children and families into the 21st century.

Every child deserves to be born well, to be physically fit, and to achieve
self-responsibility for good health habits.

•

Every child and adolescent deserves ready access
to coordinated and comprehensive preventive, health-promoting, therapeutic,
and rehabilitative medical, mental health, and dental care. Such care is best provided
through a continuing relationship with a primary health professional or team,
and ready access to secondary and tertiary levels of care.

•

Every child and adolescent deserves a nurturing family
and supportive relationships with other significant persons who provide security,
positive role models, warmth, love, and unconditional acceptance.
A child's health begins with the health of his parents.

•

Every child and adolescent deserves to grow and develop
in a physically and psychologically safe home and school environment
free of undue risk of injury, abuse, violence, or exposure to environmental toxins.

•

Every child and adolescent deserves satisfactory housing, good nutrition,
a quality education, an adequate family income, a supportive social network,
and access to community resources.

•

Every child deserves quality child care
when her parents are working outside the home.

•

Every child and adolescent deserves the opportunity to develop ways to cope
with stressful life experiences.

•

Every child and adolescent deserves the opportunity to be prepared for parenthood.

•

Every child and adolescent deserves the opportunity to develop positive values
and become a responsible citizen in his community.

•

Every child and adolescent deserves to experience joy, have high self-esteem,
have friends, acquire a sense of efficacy, and believe that she can succeed in life.
She should help the next generation develop the motivation and habits
necessary for similar achievement.

# Preface

The Bright Futures project was sponsored by the Maternal and Child Health Bureau of the U.S. Public Health Service and the Medicaid Bureau of the Health Care Financing Administration. It represents a significant advancement in formulating expert guidance for providing health services to children and their families. More than 100 distinguished professionals, representing a wide range of child health and related perspectives, served on four expert panels and the board of directors. These professionals were charged with the mission of developing health supervision guidelines responsive to the current and emerging disease prevention and health promotion needs of infants, children, and adolescents.

## Historical perspective

The Bright Futures project can best be understood in the historical context of child health programs such as Title V (Maternal and Child Health Services Block Grant) and Title XIX (Medicaid) of the Social Security Act. For many decades, both programs have been at the forefront of promoting and funding important child health promotion and treatment initiatives.

First authorized by legislation in 1935, Title V programs have been and remain valuable resources for improving infant and child health. They provide perinatal and primary child health care services and comprehensive services for children with special health needs in 59 states and jurisdictions. Through a federal grant program they support leadership training for maternal and child health program personnel, expand knowledge through applied research projects, and foster the development of comprehensive, family-centered, community-based systems for delivering services.

The Medicaid program, enacted in 1965, was amended in 1967 to better serve the health needs of eligible children through the Early and Periodic Screening, Diagnostic and Treatment (EPSDT) program. EPSDT is a preventive and comprehensive health program for Medicaid-eligible individuals under age 21. The EPSDT program encourages and assists eligible children and their families in obtaining periodic screening, dental, vision, and hearing services, as well as medically necessary follow-up care.

Over the last decade, other federal and state initiatives have focused on some of the special needs addressed by *Bright Futures*. The Individuals with Disabilities Education Act, the Ryan White Comprehensive AIDS Resources Emergency Act, and a multitude of innovative state approaches to outreach and service delivery all represent targeted efforts to improve child health. More recently, the Vaccines for Children program—enacted to provide federally funded vaccines for immunizing low-income and uninsured children—presents a new opportunity for collaborative federal, state, and local efforts to protect the health of children.

## The new health supervision

The process of creating a vision for appropriate health supervision required an inclusive perspective. Health supervision consists of those measures that help promote health, prevent mortality and morbidity, and enhance subsequent development and maturation. Physical well-being, mental health, cognitive development, the new morbidities, and social efficacy are affected by socioeconomic considerations, behavioral factors, family and cultural variables, environment, education, access to health care, and availability and quality of community resources. *Bright Futures* acknowledges the impact of these contextual forces, while emphasizing the role health professionals can play.

Effective delivery of health services to children may involve coordinating services among a broad array of provider disciplines (e.g., pediatricians, family and general practitioners, physician assistants, nurse practitioners, nurses, dentists) and settings (e.g., private offices, public clinics, schools). In addition, effective service delivery works best in a family context where supports and services can be integrated to respond to a broad range of family needs. Nutrition, financial assistance for needy families, and special plans for children with disabilities and other special needs are all examples of the types of financial aid, social supports, and educational services that are needed for the goals of Bright Futures to be achieved.

## Creating *Bright Futures*

To realize the expert vision for health supervision, four multidisciplinary panels were convened to discuss health supervision issues for the developmental periods of infancy, early childhood, middle childhood, and adolescence. After a review of the literature and extensive dialogue, the panels drafted the *Bright Futures* guidelines based on their review of the science and on expert opinion and consensus.

The expert panels based their work on the belief that health supervision is:

- A longitudinal process that promotes a partnership and shared agenda between the health professional, the child, and the family.

- Personalized to fit the individual.

- Contextual—i.e., views the child in the context of the family and the community.

- Supportive of the child's self-esteem, sense of competence, and mastery.

- Based on a health diagnosis.

- Focused on the strengths as well as on the problems and issues of the family and community.

- Part of a seamless system that includes community-based health, education, and human services.

- Complementary to health promotion and disease prevention efforts in the family, the school, the community, and the media.

After the guidelines were drafted, they were sent to 950 health professionals (e.g., pediatricians, family physicians, child psychiatrists, dentists, nurses, nurse practitioners, nutritionists, public health professionals, social workers, parents, and policymakers) for review and comment. National experts and organizational officials serving on the board of directors also provided guidance and suggestions.

Members of the expert panels and the reviewers also gave references in support of specific guidelines, as well as other publications offering helpful supplementary material. These have been included in the general bibliography and in the endnotes and bibliographies at the end of each developmental section.

## Need for more research

The Bright Futures panels recommend that health supervision research be promoted more vigorously than it has been in the past. A literature review of more than 900 journal articles and books revealed that there are a limited number of definitive scientific supporting studies, even for the biomedical aspects of disease prevention and health promotion. Even fewer studies examine the outcomes of interventions that included both psychosocial and biomedical aspects of health supervision.

While there is a lack of well-designed studies proving efficacy and efficiency, there is empirical knowledge that attests to the value of specific guidelines and health promotion and disease prevention efforts. This is a critical area for further exploration and investment. The current literature and expert opinion indicate that the interventions recommended in *Bright Futures* will lead to desired outcomes.

Definitive health supervision research is critical, notwithstanding the difficulties inherent in such efforts, including the very large samples required; the many intervening variables; the expectation of relatively small, short-term differences in outcomes between groups; and the necessity for long-term follow-up.

## Implementing *Bright Futures*

The *Bright Futures* recommendations were developed as goals to be pursued in the interest of better child health. The specificity of these recommendations should prove useful to those working toward a brighter future for our nation's children—child health professionals and ancillary staff, public and private insurers, health departments, community health centers, schools, child development programs, parents, educators, leaders of managed care organizations, and many others. The recommendations support the *Healthy People 2000* national health promotion and disease prevention objectives related to mothers, infants, children, and adolescents.

The guidelines, however, are not intended to serve as the standard of health care per se. Variations of these guidelines that respond to individual differences and circumstances are appropriate. In the case of public agencies or programs at federal, state, and local levels, other considerations—such as specific legislative requirements, resource limitations, or court orders—may affect the degree to which the *Bright Futures* content and periodicity recommendations can be fully implemented.

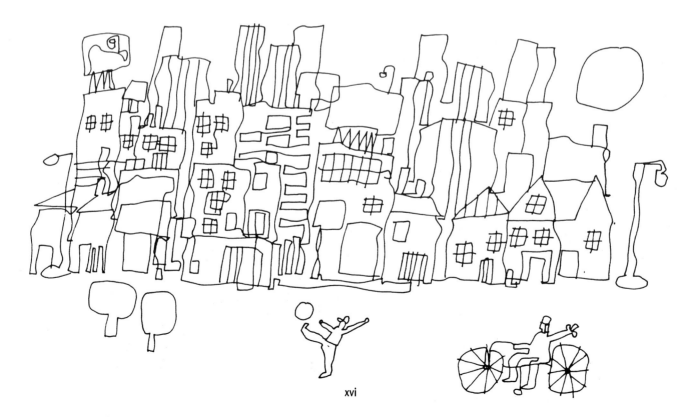

# Introduction

How can health professionals and others who care for children, adolescents, and families be more effective in health promotion and disease prevention, especially in relation to behavior, development, and function? If the current burden of preventable morbidity, mortality, dysfunction, and disability is to be significantly lessened and good health behaviors fostered, health supervision must become more comprehensive and intensive.

The potential for effective health promotion is far greater with children, adolescents, and their parents or other caregivers than with any other population group. Health supervision visits offer the health professional the opportunity to monitor physical health, development, and parent-child relationships. They also provide excellent opportunities to enhance the competence, confidence, and active participation of children, adolescents, and families. Ideally, they have the capacity to optimize functioning, enhance well-being, clarify misconceptions, and promote the realization of potential.

Effective health supervision is often challenging and complex. The linear model of prevention, in which the intervention prevents the problem, may work well in the case of the measles vaccine providing immunity to measles. However, the linear model is inadequate in relation to most of the developmental, social, psychological, behavioral, and educational problems so prevalent in the United States today. Just as clinicians know that minimal or subtherapeutic doses of antibiotics or anticonvulsants do not work, they recognize that minimal "doses" of health supervision are ineffective. Policies for improving health supervision have economic implications; they are cost-effective and prudent investments in the development of socially productive citizens. More importantly, these policies have humanitarian, ethical, and moral roots. The implementation of preventive and health-promoting interventions in the breadth, intensity, depth, and duration suggested in *Bright Futures* is a long-overdue strategy.

## A contextual approach

Since health, educational, and social issues are strongly interrelated, they cannot be assessed in isolation from each other. The health professional must use a contextual approach and be sensitive to the world of the child. Comprehensive, family-centered, and community-based health supervision requires that the child or adolescent be viewed in the context of his or her family and community and that health care be integrated with other human services.

Health supervision may require many types of intervention. Community supports and resources can be provided for infants not progressing well developmentally or at risk for abuse or neglect; screening for risks during health supervision visits may be followed by counseling in the primary care setting or by referral for more intensive care; dysfunctional parents (e.g., depressed mothers, alcoholic fathers) may be referred for treatment; and strengths identified in the child or family may be reinforced. Health supervision also helps educate children and families about the efficient use of health care and other community services.

## Partnership between families and health professionals

Families are big, small, extended, nuclear, or multigenerational, with one parent, two parents, or grandparents. They live under one roof or many. A family can be as temporary as a few weeks, or as permanent as forever. We become part of a family by birth, adoption, or marriage, or through a desire for mutual support. As family members, we nurture, protect, and influence each other. Families are dynamic and are cultures unto themselves, with different values and unique ways of realizing dreams. Each family has strengths and qualities that flow from individual members and from the family as a unit. Families create neighborhoods and communities, becoming the source of our rich cultural and spiritual diversity.

The *Bright Futures* guidelines are based on the belief that health supervision requires a partnership between health professionals and families—the core of any good health care system. Family experiences mold one's expectations of what it means to be healthy. The day-to-day practices of families have a profound effect on individual well-being. Families are the primary caregivers in any health care system; they are often the first to recognize that a health problem exists. With support, families can provide services in their home that, in a hospital or institutional setting, would be very expensive. This holds true for all families, including those who have children with special health needs. The essential task of a health care system is to reinforce the role of the family as educator, promoter of good health, and caregiver.[1]

Most parents are heavily invested in learning how they can contribute to their children's growth, development, adaptation, and functioning. Health supervision can facilitate this learning. Important health supervision goals include enhancing families' strengths, addressing their problems and vulnerabilities, promoting resiliency, building parental competence and confidence, and helping families share in the responsibility for preventing illness or disability and promoting health.

Older children and adolescents should also be partners in health supervision as they mature, and should assume increasing responsibility for their own health.

## Longitudinal health supervision

Health is a prospective enterprise. What happens during infancy may not result in positive or negative outcomes until adolescence or even adulthood. Therefore, health supervision must be viewed as a longitudinal process—one that occurs over time. As the health professional or team becomes familiar with individual children or adolescents, the partnership between the family and the health professional can become a therapeutic alliance. Health professionals gain a better understanding of the needs and priorities of the children and their families, and the families are more likely to accept and adopt the professionals' expert knowledge. This therapeutic alliance is especially important for children who are at risk due to family, social, economic, or environmental factors, or who have special health needs.

Longitudinal health supervision allows interventions to be introduced at multiple points in time. Since health risks and needs can change over a period of weeks or months, they need to be addressed in a timely fashion. Families who establish an effective relationship with a primary health care provider use services more appropriately and save on health care costs.

The benefits of continuing care are best ensured by a "medical home" offering health services that are accessible, continuous, comprehensive, family centered, coordinated, and compassionate. Many children and adolescents do not have such a medical home. Managed care may improve continuity of care and provide access to a medical home, although frequent changes in providers may work against this goal. Families may also lack access to health supervision because of financial or language barriers, geographic mobility, or other inability to use available services.

Because there is no systematic follow-up or tracking system in most communities, an unknown but large number of children and adolescents receive only sporadic or no preventive care. In an effort to achieve a complete record of care, some communities now provide parents with a personal health record or "medical passport," in which data, such as those on a child's immunizations or development, are entered at each health supervision visit.

## Individualization

It is well known that excellent care of families is always highly personal. Interventions are more likely to be effective when tailored to individual needs. To date, most preventive and health-promoting interventions have not been sufficiently individualized; many have relied on the traditional public health approach of focusing more on at-risk populations than on individual children or adolescents. Effective health supervision requires attention to individuals and families as well as disease prevention and health promotion at the community level.

The heterogeneity of the U.S. population has increased dramatically in recent years. As a result, there is an immense need for increased awareness of the diversity of communities, families, and children. There are individual differences in culture, ethnicity, language, socioeconomic status, special health needs, educational background, and other personal characteristics. The *Bright Futures* expert panels sought to craft guidelines sensitive to these differences. More work needs to be

done, however, to ensure that health supervision is accessible to all infants, children, adolescents, and their families. This goal could be facilitated through provider education curricula and increased linkages between community leaders and health professionals.

## Health diagnosis

Although the term *diagnosis* usually relates to pathology (i.e., evaluation of biomedical or psychosocial symptoms and disease), a similar diagnostic approach applies to the child or adolescent seen primarily for health supervision. In the case of disease, diagnosis is a necessary prelude to proper therapeutic intervention; in the case of health, diagnosis determines the selection of appropriate preventive and health-promoting interventions, whether medical, dental, nutritional, or psychosocial. In both health and disease, the more comprehensive and precise the diagnosis, the more targeted and potentially effective the intervention.

For the health professional, components of the diagnostic process for health supervision include the interview, developmental and educational surveillance, observation of parent-child interactions, physical examination, screening procedures, and assessment of strengths and issues. Individualization of health supervision requires that the health professional have adequate data about the family. Baseline information should include household composition, the parents' and siblings' health, the family's nutritional practices, the employment status of the parent(s), and recent major changes in the family. The health professional also needs information about the family's community, including resources such as child care centers, preschools, schools, churches, and other organizations.

Families also take part in the diagnostic process. They can complete a child and family medical history form at the first health supervision visit and update it period-ically. To prepare for each subsequent visit, parents, older children, and adolescents may be encouraged to write down the questions, concerns, observations, and achievements they would like to discuss with the physician, nurse, nurse practitioner, or other member of the health supervision team. A questionnaire or checklist can also be completed at home or administered in the reception room. This survey instrument may include a list of symptoms or problems (both biomedical and psychosocial) relevant to the age group concerned, especially those common in the specific community.

The success of health supervision is largely determined by the extent to which the agendas of the parent, child, or adolescent are addressed and adaptable to advice and change. Families may ask questions, express concerns, and share information about such matters as family violence, marital discord, alcoholism, or depression more freely if the visit is conducted in a private setting.

Further health supervision research and training are needed to enhance professionals' understanding of children's vulnerabilities and risks, and of the circum-stances that cause risks to be contained or expressed as pathology.

## Partnership with the community

Successful interventions often require efforts that extend beyond what can be provided in any one setting or through any one discipline. Health supervision can be provided in many settings, often with collaboration between a variety of organizations and disciplines.

Integrated preventive and health-promoting services may be delivered in a physician's office, a community health clinic, a home, a school, a child care center, a shelter, a correctional institution, or some other commu-nity facility. Whatever the setting, the family and the child need a medical home that provides a continuing relationship with an accessible physician, nurse, nurse practitioner, dentist, or team. The team may include a public health nurse, a home visitor, a social worker, a nutritionist, an early childhood educator, or a child care worker.

In some instances, group health supervision sessions that complement individual visits can serve as a way of conveying information while offering families mutual support and reinforcement. Parents may benefit from hearing the answers to questions asked by others and gain a greater appreciation of the wide range of normal behavior and development. Group sessions for older children and adolescents are another approach facilitating peer support.

## Integration of health care with other human services

To be fully effective, health supervision must be part of a seamless system, integrated with other health and human services such as secondary and tertiary care, dental care, child care centers, early intervention programs, mental health centers, diagnostic and evalua-tion programs, schools, family support centers, food and nutrition referral resources, public health departments, outreach services, and others.

Unfortunately, in many communities such services may be nonexistent or underdeveloped. Those that do exist often lack integration and coordination. Access to these services may be limited due to financial, educational, or psychological reasons, or as a result of transportation or language barriers. Regrettably, many of the families whose children could benefit the most do not bring them in for help, are unable to deal with the bureaucracy involved, or believe that the services provided are not relevant to their needs. It is crucial that these barriers be addressed and steps taken to broaden services to people and communities that have had inadequate care.

Many health supervision services are appropriately delivered to the individual child and family, but others should be population or community focused. Health promotion requires a supportive and healthy environment, including the availability of community resources such as child care centers, early childhood and parent-child programs, mental health services, secondary and tertiary medical resources, adequate housing, employment and recreational opportunities, and quality schools. Health and family life curricula in the schools and information conveyed through the media strengthen health supervision and encourage family responsibility and functioning.

## Periodicity

The *Bright Futures* recommendations for how often children require health supervision by health professionals are based on the tenets of child and family development. The specific frequency and timing of health supervision were developed to target prevalent issues and opportunities to enhance strengths at key developmental stages. For pragmatic reasons, units of care are expressed as visits, which utilize a normative approach that is intended to be appropriate for most children and families while respecting and encouraging individual adaptation to promote health.[2]

The schedule suggests the amount of care needed by infants, children, and adolescents judged not to be at

undue risk. However, health supervision should always be tailored to meet individual needs. The vulnerabilities and areas of potential for each child should continuously be assessed to determine if more health supervision or intervention is necessary—an assessment which should occur in a primary continuing relationship between a child, family, and health professional. If mortality and significant morbidity are to be prevented and developmental potential realized, children and adolescents at greater risk need not only an augmented schedule of care, but an intensity of care not unlike that required for complex medical conditions.

Moreover, special populations such as those of children and adolescents with chronic illness or disability, in foster care, living in chaotic households, or assessed as being at high risk—medically, developmentally, or socially—will require more health supervision or interventions. Special care or supplementary health supervision may also be needed during critical periods of family transition or discontinuity such as divorce, remarriage, death, parental mental or physical illness, moving, unemployment, school entrance, adoption, or foster care placement. The augmented schedule of care should be determined according to each family's needs.

## Evidence for effectiveness of health supervision

Three recent reports have attempted to assess the scientific evidence for the effectiveness of some aspects of health supervision across the age spectrum. These include a report of the U.S. Preventive Services Task Force (USPSTF); the Office of Technology Assessment (OTA) report *Healthy Children: Investing in the Future*; and *Guidelines for Adolescent Preventive Services (GAPS), Recommendations and Rationale*, a report published by the American Medical Association.

The U.S. Preventive Services Task Force rated the effectiveness of preventive care for conditions such as breast cancer, hypertension, and thyroid disease. The USPSTF report, however, did not fully examine all preventive interventions nor those particularly applicable to children. It did not, for example, evaluate child health supervision. Nonetheless, special consideration was given to high-risk groups, in that some interventions were recommended for these groups although the evidence for their effectiveness was not compelling. The rationale used was that the absence of evidence did not necessarily imply a lack of effectiveness, and that persons at high risk were likely to gain the most if the interventions were of benefit.

The OTA report focused primarily on medical interventions and did not review the evidence supporting prevention of disability and emotional disorders, continuing care for children with chronic illness, or health promotion. Moreover, the report used the term "no evidence" for interventions that had not been studied as well as for interventions that had been the subject of research that concluded them ineffective. The GAPS report provided an extensive evaluation of literature relevant to adolescent health and preventive interventions, and helped form the basis of discussion for the work of the Bright Futures Adolescent Panel.

*Bright Futures* begins where many studies left off, further informing and enriching the health supervision knowledge base through a more comprehensive review of the science. Measuring the outcomes of health supervision interventions is challenging and necessary. The *Bright Futures* guidelines are consistent with the view that promoting the overall health of children requires a broader definition of health—one that includes psychosocial, educational, familial, and community influences; drugs/alcohol and sexuality education; nutrition; and injury prevention. Most of these factors were not taken into consideration in previous scientific studies.

More research clearly needs to be done to prove the effectiveness of health supervision interventions. Over the past several years a wealth of new information published in journals and books has informed our collective knowledge of health supervision. The bibliographies at the end of each section of these guidelines and in the appendices present up-to-date sources on research related to the methods and effectiveness of health supervision. Explanatory endnotes appear at the end of each developmental section as well. A companion publication is also available, citing the more than 1,000 journal articles and books used to inform the discussions of the expert panels through the process of developing the *Bright Futures* guidelines and specifically commissioned papers.

The current disturbing trends in the health of infants, children, and adolescents provide a clear imperative to increase our knowledge and our efforts in disease prevention and health promotion. Further supportive work needs to be conducted throughout the many sites where health supervision occurs, as more and more providers and families embrace the therapeutic, medical, and developmental advantages to promoting the health and well-being of children and families.

1. New Mexico Children's Continuum. 1990. *Family Voices: A National Coalition Speaking for Children with Special Health Needs.* Albuquerque, NM: New Mexico Children's Continuum.

2. Federal Medicaid law requires states to set their own periodicity schedules for screening, dental, vision, and hearing services for their Medicaid EPSDT programs, after consultation with recognized medical and dental organizations involved in child health care. States must also provide Medicaid-eligible children with these services at intervals more frequent than those specified in their EPSDT periodicity schedules, if medically necessary.

# Organization of Health Supervision Guidelines

The health supervision guidelines are organized into four sections: infancy, early childhood, middle childhood, and adolescence. Each developmental section includes elements that provide an overview of the issues for that age period:

- Theme chapter

- Chart of achievements, tasks, and outcomes

- Family preparation for health supervision

- Strengths of the child, family, and community

- Issues of the child, family, and community

- Health supervision summary

Each section also describes the health supervision care for that developmental period. The components of health supervision are presented as a package of services for each visit. Intended to promote optimal outcomes at each age, the following topics are covered:

- Snapshot of the child and family

- Health supervision interview

- Developmental surveillance and milestones or developmental surveillance and school performance

- Observation of parent-child interaction

- Physical examination

- Additional screening procedures

- Immunizations

- Anticipatory guidance for the family

Although the components of health supervision are discussed separately in these guidelines, in actual practice they are integrated so as to respond flexibly to the needs of individual families. For example, some aspects of anticipatory guidance are provided in response to questions asked by the parent or child during the interview or physical examination. Obviously, not all the questions or topics listed in these guidelines can or need to be addressed. Rather, to individualize health supervision, the health professional should selectively choose trigger questions and elements from the anticipatory guidance sections that are the most appropriate, using clinical judgment to decide what is timely and relevant to a particular child and family.

## Developmental Sections

### Theme chapter

The study of child development serves as the basic science for much of health supervision, especially health promotion, just as the biological sciences provide justification for the preventive and therapeutic interventions in disease. To provide a brief orientation to child development, a theme chapter prefaces each of the four sections of the guidelines. It describes common issues and developmental changes for the age period.

### Developmental chart

Each section of the guidelines includes a chart of keywords that characterize some of the achievements, tasks for the family, and health supervision outcomes for the specific developmental period. This chart summarizes some of the critical aspects of health supervision that are described more fully in the visits.

At each health supervision visit, the health professional needs to reassess the achievements of the infant, child, or adolescent since the last visit. Monitoring the developmental status of the child and family is a crucial part of developmental surveillance and the formulation of a health diagnosis.

Health professionals should also provide guidance to the family on the anticipated tasks for the age period. This anticipatory guidance should be individualized for each child.

The health supervision outcomes represent both short- and long-term goals for health supervision during each age period and a means by which its benefits may later be measured.

## Family preparation for health supervision

Each developmental section includes suggestions for helping the parent and the child or adolescent prepare for health supervision visits, an essential component of the process. Such an investment supports a partnership in which the health professional and the parent, child, or adolescent share responsibility.

Along with an appointment reminder, tools such as psychosocial and developmental screening instruments, an initial or interval history form, and an injury prevention survey may be mailed to the parent and child or adolescent for completion prior to the visit. Questions about the parents' health habits—e.g., smoking or seat belt use—may be included. If there is a language or literacy barrier, it would be helpful for a staff member to assist the family on site (although resources currently are not available to provide this service in most settings). The family should also be asked to bring along school report cards, school health examination forms, and the personal health record of the child or adolescent.

## Strengths and issues of the child, family, and community

Part of determining the health diagnosis of an infant, child, or adolescent involves assessing the strengths and issues for a specific child, family, and community. Some of the more common strengths and issues are listed in each section. Although they are listed separately for the child, the family, and the community, they are of course interrelated and interdependent.

The lists of strengths can help health professionals remind families of their assets as they adapt to the various stages of development. The lists of issues can facilitate a case-finding strategy. As used in these guidelines, the term *issues* refers to those concerns, problems, and stressors that may be present in a specific child, family, or community. Although health supervision is not intended to be primarily problem oriented, these issues may be priority items on the agenda of the parent, child, or adolescent.

Some problems can be addressed adequately during the time scheduled for a health supervision visit. When the problem is more complex, however, a decision must be made on whether to address it immediately and reschedule the health supervision visit, arrange another time to manage the problem, or refer the child for secondary or tertiary care. Detecting problems early allows therapeutic interventions to be introduced in a timely fashion, enhancing the goal of secondary prevention.

# Health Supervision Visits

## Snapshot of the child and family

Each visit is introduced by a snapshot that represents some of the common processes and issues at each age. These snapshots provide glimpses into the development of children and families, but they are not meant to serve as standards of measurement.

## Health supervision interview

The health supervision interview offers the health professional the opportunity to both obtain diagnostic data and forge a partnership with the family. The nature and phrasing of trigger questions can contribute to both of these goals. The most successful visits are those in which the interview is shaped primarily by issues raised by the parent and child, with their expectations, questions, and concerns addressed.

Ideally, both parents should participate; however, this is often not possible. When the child's primary caregiver is an individual other than a parent, such as a grandmother, that person should participate in the interview. Beginning with the middle childhood years, the child or adolescent should be included in the interview. Talking with older children and adolescents alone contributes to creating a therapeutic alliance and encourages their self-responsibility for health.

A good health supervision interview is a focused conversation between the health professional and the family. Since parents, children, or adolescents do not know exactly what information the professional needs, open-ended questions are helpful in starting the conversation: "How are you today?" "How are things going at home?" While some families are comfortable sharing concerns and asking questions, others are not, especially before a trusting relationship has been established. Parents who fear being viewed as inadequate may hesitate to disclose problems or concerns; others tend to be passive and expect that they will be asked whatever the health professional needs to know; and still others seem unaware of the impact that family stressors and important life events have on their children.

Some parents and families may need trigger questions to direct the information they provide. Useful questions may be general or they may focus on a specific age concern (e.g., "How is your child sleeping?"). Other questions depend on the age of the child, the information obtained from the parent, or observations made by the health professional. Trigger questions should be modified to meet the health professional's style and individualized for the family and community.

Developing a relationship with the child during the interview is also crucial. The health professional's personal warmth, empathy, and ability to elicit trust and admiration are major professional strengths. Friendliness from the health professional will place most children at ease, although some may be reserved initially. Trigger questions may include the following: "How do you like school?" "What are some of the things you're very good at?" "Do you have a best friend?" Health professionals may play with toddlers and preschoolers during the interview as a means of getting acquainted. Blocks, a ball, crayons, a pad of paper, picture books, a stuffed animal, a hand puppet, or a doll and bottle are useful facilitators.

With older children or adolescents, the invitation to "tell me about some of the things that you are proud of" provides verbal recognition of their strengths and conveys unconditional acceptance. Adolescents are more likely to discuss their thoughts and feelings if confidentiality is assured and if the provider makes a conscious effort to be open and supportive. They should be informed at the outset about the ground rules—i.e., that they are free to discuss the details of the interview with their parents, but that the health professional will not do so unless he or she believes that the parents need to be informed to protect the child's health or safety.

Active listening is important. Parents, children, and adolescents who have significant problems or concerns are likely to ask them directly or tangentially at some time during the visit.

Since a child's family and parents are highly influential role models, an interest in the parents' health, development, and behavior is an appropriate part of health supervision. The health supervision visit offers a good opportunity to introduce or reinforce health-promoting messages for parents (e.g., regular physical activity, use of seat belts, healthy eating, and avoidance or discontinuation of smoking and drug use).

## Developmental surveillance and milestones or developmental surveillance and school performance

Through developmental surveillance, health professionals and families observe the emergence of abilities in children over time. The process is longitudinal and collaborative, as the family and the health professional both note the progress of the child and share concerns. The status of infants and young children can generally be assessed from the developmentally appropriate trigger questions, developmental questionnaires completed by the parent, and observations throughout the visit, including those that occur during the physical examination. For older children and adolescents, academic performance may be appraised through a review of report cards, school achievement records, and performance on psychoeducational tests when indicated.

If the child is not progressing through milestones as expected, developmental surveillance should become more vigilant. Careful monitoring is generally the next step, with parental responsibilities well defined and expectations for follow-up clearly articulated. Formal developmental examinations are recommended when surveillance suggests a delay or abnormality, especially when the opportunity for continuing observation is not anticipated. Since no formal developmental screen is perfect, developmental surveillance requires some tolerance for ambiguity.

## Observation of parent-child interaction

The interview and the physical examination provide opportunities for behavioral observations that help identify strengths, issues, and potential risk factors for the child and family. One may note, for example, whether parents respond reciprocally to their baby; whether parents have the ability to set limits for a toddler; whether parents of a school-age child contribute to the child's self-esteem; and whether parents of an adolescent seem to encourage independence. Observation may also suggest the presence of depression or another emotional disorder in a parent or child.

## Physical examination

In addition to active listening and observation, a complete physical examination at each visit is recommended. Rather than presenting the specific details of the general physical examination for each visit, these guidelines include a focus on those aspects most relevant at various ages. In addition to detecting physical and developmental abnormalities, the physical examination can reassure parents and adolescents. Since parents, children, and adolescents may talk more readily during or after the physical examination, additional questions or concerns may be raised at those times.

## Additional screening procedures

The health supervision visit (the interview, the physical examination, the observation of the child and family, and the psychosocial, educational, and developmental surveillance) is a basic screening procedure. Additional screening procedures—including vision, hearing, and metabolic screening—are included to identify areas that may warrant further assessment and intervention. Both vision and hearing screening depend to some extent on the ability of the child to cooperate. For children under three, the health professional should note whether the child can track and respond to visual stimuli. The recommended tests for vision screening of older children, along with criteria for referral, are discussed in the appendix. After the newborn hearing screening, health professionals can use clinical voice screening such as clapping, talking, or making other noise to determine if there is a hearing problem that needs formal testing. Even if the screening does not reveal deficiencies, all children should have a routine audiological test before school entry. Moreover, all children above the age of one should be referred to a dentist. A blood lead test must be used to screen Medicaid-eligible children for lead poisoning (see appendix E, page 264). Many screening tools may change as more is understood, and newer approaches should be adopted over time. Some children and adolescents are at special risk for some conditions and thus need additional or more frequent procedures. Each visit is intended, in large part, to be a screening process for problems, vulnerabilities, strengths, and evidence of health.

## Immunizations

Immunizations are an essential part of health supervision. For families with new babies, the immunization schedule also helps reinforce and ensure regular health supervision visits. Every contact with the family, including acute care visits, provides an opportunity to ensure that the child's or adolescent's immunization status is up to date. The schedule included in the *Bright Futures* guidelines for administering immunizations needs to be updated periodically to conform to current recommendations. Federal law requires that state Medicaid programs use the most current immunization schedule of the Advisory Committee on Immunization Practices (ACIP). The January 1994 schedule is included in appendix D, page 263. Refer to the latest recommendations of the ACIP for additional guidance relating to administration of this schedule.

## Anticipatory guidance

Anticipatory guidance provides the family with information on what to expect in the child's current and next developmental phase. It is most helpful to families if the health professional views it as a personal tutorial rather than a lecture. Finding out what families already know and are doing will enable the health professional to target the anticipatory guidance, use the available time to clear up misconceptions, introduce new information, and reinforce what the family is doing well.

Anticipatory guidance topics to be considered for each visit include: healthy habits, prevention of illness and injury, nutrition, oral health, sexuality, social development, family relationships, parental health, community interactions, self-responsibility, and school/vocational achievement. Since not all of these can be adequately discussed during time-limited visits, supplementary educational handouts and videotapes for parents and older children are recommended for home study. The anticipatory guidance in the *Bright*

*Futures* guidelines presents tasks for the parent or child to accomplish.

Anticipatory guidance should also be supplemented and complemented by school health education curricula, parent education programs, and information conveyed through the media. If the health professional is aware of what the child's school is teaching on issues such as good nutritional practices, sexuality, injury prevention, conflict resolution, and avoidance of smoking and substance abuse, he or she can reinforce similar themes with the child. Such reiteration of health promotion messages by a trusted health professional can be highly effective. Group health supervision visits for parents, older children, and adolescents are another effective means of providing health education and anticipatory guidance.

## Health supervision summary

The health professional's findings and recommendations may be summarized briefly at the end of the visit. Specific health and developmental achievements and strengths should be identified and the family and child commended. Many families appreciate and benefit from a written summary of the visit, including weight, height, instructions, dietary changes, other suggestions, and referrals.

For children and families not assessed as being at risk, an appointment should be made for the next regularly scheduled health supervision visit. However, the health professional should state that if there are major changes in health before the next scheduled visit, or if family stressors such as divorce, remarriage, death, or parental illness arise, a contingency visit may be arranged. Additional visits beyond those shown in the health supervision periodicity table should be scheduled as appropriate.

Some families will benefit from referral to community resources such as home visitor programs, food sources, child care centers, preschool programs, and early intervention or developmental stimulation programs. Older children and adolescents may be encouraged to join recreational programs or 4-H Clubs, or be provided with a tutor. Parents may be referred to parenting classes, support groups, marriage counselors, substance abuse programs, family support centers, or mental health professionals, or for medical consultation.

Public health and social service providers may assist in providing the complementary and supplementary services required. The health professional should establish lines of referral and working relationships with community resources before the need to refer arises. The health professional should seek to provide services that are family centered, culturally competent, comprehensive, and incorporated into a community-based system of care. Since dysfunctional families may not seek needed services, follow-up with the resource after referral helps ensure that the child and family actually receive care.

The health professional can also help Medicaid and other insurers assess health supervision efforts and improve access by regularly reporting health supervision encounters using established claims and reporting procedures.

*Editor's note:* In order to avoid the awkwardness of "he or she," and yet describe children of both genders, "he" and "she" are used in alternate visits throughout this book.

# Bright Futures Highlights

- Health supervision consists of those measures that help promote health, prevent mortality and morbidity, and enhance subsequent development and maturation.

- Health supervision goals include enhancing families' strengths, addressing families' problems, promoting resiliency, building parental competence, and helping families share in the responsibility for preventing illness or disability and promoting health.

- Health supervision requires a partnership between health professionals and families.

- Health supervision is shaped primarily by issues raised by the parent and child, with their expectations, questions, and concerns addressed.

- Health supervision involves assessing the strengths and issues for a specific child, family, and community.

- Health supervision includes the interview, the physical examination, observation of the child and family, and psychosocial, educational, and developmental surveillance. Additional screening procedures—including vision, hearing, and metabolic screening—are also included to identify areas that may warrant further assessment and intervention.

- Health supervision that employs specific preventive and health-promoting interventions leads to improved outcomes. These social, developmental, and health outcomes occur along a continuum, varying in their timing from child to child and family to family.

- Since health risks and needs can change over a period of weeks or months, they need to be reassessed periodically.

- The benefits of continuing health supervision are best ensured by a medical home offering health services that are accessible, continuous, comprehensive, family-centered, coordinated, compassionate, and integrated into a system of care.

- Health supervision can be provided in many settings, often with collaboration between a variety of organizations and disciplines.

- Health supervision helps educate children and families about the efficient use of health care and other community services.

- Child development serves as the basic science for much of health supervision, especially health promotion.

- Special populations such as those with chronic illness or disability will require more health supervision.

- Supplemental health supervision may also be needed during periods of family transition or stress.

# Bright Futures Health Supervision Outcomes

Central to the concept of health supervision is the belief that specific preventive and health-promoting interventions lead to desired outcomes. The social, developmental, and health outcomes summarized below contribute to the overall health and well-being of infants, children, adolescents, and families. These outcomes occur along a continuum, varying in their timing from child to child and family to family.

Independence
Sense of morality
Sense of identity
Self-esteem
Self-efficacy and mastery
Reduction of high-risk behavior
Educational/vocational success
Social competence
Self-responsibility
Personal safety
Success in school
Good health habits
Prevention of secondary disability and dysfunction
Promotion of developmental potential
Prevention of behavior problems
Injury prevention
Early autonomy
Optimal nutrition
Parental effectiveness
Immunizations
Promotion of family strengths
Adaptation
Parental preparation
Therapeutic alliance

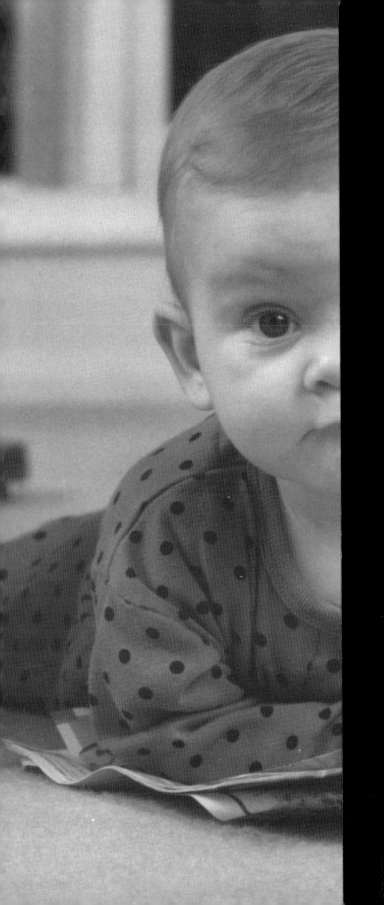

# 0–12 Months
# Infancy

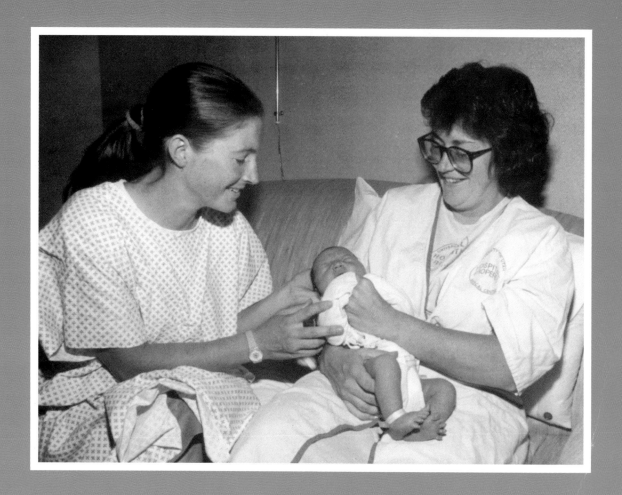

*Children are our future.*
*They will not have a bright future unless they receive*
*the preventive health care they need.*

—Betty Bumpers
Every Child By Two, Immunization Advocacy Coalition

# Infancy

Foundations for the health, development, and social relationships of the child are established during pregnancy and the first year of life. The strong bond the parents feel with the baby even before birth blossoms during infancy into a profound attachment. The infant's relationships and experiences provide the sense of basic trust needed for him to venture on to toddler autonomy. Health supervision is especially crucial during infancy.

The relationship between the family and the health professional can be most intense in the first year, as the parents learn how to care for their child and to trust and communicate with their health care providers. The goal for health professionals is to progressively increase the parents' knowledge and independence regarding the physical, intellectual, and emotional care of their child, as well as to facilitate their personal growth as parents and the family's development as a cohesive unit. This partnership plays a large role in determining the effectiveness of health supervision.

The most dramatic growth of the child's life—physical, cognitive, social, and emotional—occurs during infancy. By one year of age, the infant triples his birthweight, adds almost 50 percent to his length, and achieves most of his brain growth. The healthy baby has received initial immunizations against diphtheria, pertussis, tetanus, polio, Hemophilus influenza type B, and hepatitis B. Adequacy of nutrition, growth, and development are monitored.

## Prenatal period

Pregnancy is a time of initial family adaptation, the success of which may predict later parental coping.

During the prenatal period, a time when families need and are open to support, contact between health professionals and families allows a relationship to begin to develop. Such a relationship is especially helpful in the event of problems at delivery or with the newborn.

Education is particularly powerful at this time. A prenatal visit is an opportunity to advise prospective parents on many prenatal issues, including the effectiveness of prenatal care, smoking cessation (if this has not been accomplished prior to conception), avoidance of alcohol and drug use, appropriate weight gain, preparation for childbirth, and the presence of the father during delivery. It is also time to discuss the immediate postpartum issues, such as early physical contact, rooming-in, breastfeeding, circumcision, sibling preparation, use of car seats, and planning for care for the mother and infant after birth. The process of meeting health supervision goals—education, early detection, disease prevention, and a trusting relationship between the health professional and the family—begins prenatally.

## Birth

The healthy infant is born full term, with an appropriate weight and free of infection, severe trauma, or congenital disabilities. Even with healthy newborns, long-term outcomes are improved when health professionals advocate for close and early physical contact, breastfeeding, and rooming-in, and when they demonstrate the newborn's abilities for the family. The parents should also be educated regarding infant susceptibility to injury (e.g., shaken baby syndrome).

## Self-regulation

Born with unstable physical functions such as temperature control, breathing, and swallowing, the infant develops smoother functioning over time. Randomly alternating periods of sleep and alertness, easily influenced by the environment, develop into a regular diurnal pattern of waking and sleeping. Over the first year, the infant develops ways of coping with his strong feelings, learns to console himself, and expands his ability to choose a task and sustain his focus on it over several minutes. There may be huge individual differences in self-regulatory abilities; low-birthweight babies, infants who are small for gestational age, those of diabetic mothers, and those born to drug-addicted mothers are at particular risk for problems with regulation.

Health professionals can contribute by teaching parents how to help their infant modulate his states. A major component of infant health supervision consists of counseling regarding temperament, colic, temper tantrums, sleep disturbances, and discipline. This is an important anticipatory guidance issue, especially for parents of sensitive or difficult infants. The goodness of fit between parent and infant helps determine whether infant behaviors become problematic.

## Physical

Brain and body grow rapidly in the first year. Deficient growth can be a sign of chronic illnesses, nutritional deficiencies, or an inadequate parent-child relationship. One problem is that some parents may not give their child enough attention during feeding, which can contribute to failure to thrive. On the other hand, some infants are difficult to feed, and feeding does not always come naturally to parents. Working out these difficulties is complicated; parents often measure their own competence by their ability to feed their child and promote growth. Feeding can be central to the parent-child relationship. Health supervision should encourage parents in their efforts, especially since most newly breastfeeding mothers require affirmation and support to successfully breastfeed their infants.

From birth to the end of the first year, a huge change in infant gross motor skills occurs. As tone, strength, and coordination improve sequentially from head to heel, the baby attains head control, rolls, sits, crawls, pulls to stand, cruises, and may even walk by one year of age. Abnormal gross motor milestones or patterns of muscle use should be detected and evaluated, and early intervention should be considered.

Hand-eye coordination also changes dramatically during infancy. It progresses from reflexive grasping to voluntary grasp and release, midline play, transferring, shaping of the hand to the object, inferior then superior pincer grasps, and use of the fingers to point, self-feed, and even mark with a crayon by one year of age. Babies need opportunities to play with toys and food to advance these important fine motor skills.

Teeth, which erupt in the infant's first year at highly variable ages, should be protected by fluoride before as well as after their eruption. Oral hygiene begins with cleaning teeth, prohibiting bottles in bed, and avoiding frequent exposure to foods that promote tooth decay.

Concepts related to the prevention of illness and injury should be reinforced frequently by the health professional. Since most infants experience at least one minor illness in the first year, parents have the opportunity to learn about signs of illness and how to deal with them.

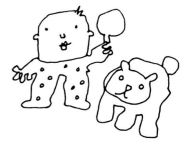

## Cognitive/linguistic

Newborns have color vision and can see in three dimensions and track visually. Close-up, they even show a preference for the pattern of human faces. Visual acuity progresses rapidly to near adult levels by the time infants are six months of age. At birth, newborns already hear as well as adults do, but they may have difficulty showing their responses. The hearing of all newborns should be tested as part of health supervision, and hearing and vision should be screened regularly and whenever caregivers express concern.

Infants can distinguish their mother's voice by three months of age, and they understand a tone of voice or words with gestures by the time they are one year old. They copy facial expressions from birth, use the emotional expressions of others to interpret events, and both understand and use gestures by eight months. By eight weeks babies coo, and by one year they babble and speak a few single words. There is a large normal range for the acquisition of these prelinguistic skills, with progress beyond babbling dependent on the language stimulation a child receives. Health professionals should educate parents about the importance of language stimulation, including singing songs to infants and children, reading to them, and conversing with them.

Developmental surveillance, screening questions, and assessments are important. Formal assessment is indicated if there are signs of developmental delay.

## Social/emotional

Through the endless repetition of having their parents respond to their needs (e.g., being fed when hungry), babies come to trust and love their parents. By three months of age, infants interact distinctly with different people. By eight months, their emotions are influenced by signals from others, and they show anxiety with strangers. Their social awareness advances from a tendency to cry when they hear crying to attempts to offer food, initiate games, and even take turns by one year of age. As autonomy emerges, babies begin to bite, pinch, and grab to get what they want. Health professionals should tell parents to anticipate these infant behaviors and advise on appropriate nonpunitive discipline.

The reciprocal interaction between parent and infant is central to the infant's physical, cognitive, social, and emotional development, as well as to his self-regulation abilities. The infant brings his strengths to this interaction, in terms of temperamental style, physical attractiveness, health integrity, and vigor. The ability of the parents to respond well is determined by their life stresses, their past experiences with children, and their own experiences of being nurtured in childhood. Their perceptions of the infant can also color the interaction. These perceptions derive from their own expectations, needs, and desires, as well as from the projection of other people's characteristics onto the child.

Infant emotional tone may be affected by the emotional health of the caregiver. Depression is common in many mothers of infants and can seriously impair the baby's emotional and even physical well-being. Parental substance abuse, with or without emotional illness, can have similar effects. Health supervision for the child must, therefore, include monitoring the emotional health of primary and alternate caregivers.

## Family and community

A mother's feeling of comfort with working outside the home or being at home, and the father's emotional support of the mother, can have a positive effect on an infant's emotional development. Since more than half of infants' mothers work full time outside the home, much of developmental stimulation is delegated to others. High-quality child care nurtures infants as well as parental care does, but it requires responsive, loving caregiving by a few consistent adults. Advising parents in their choice of child care options is an important role for health professionals.

Fathers are important caregivers and educators for their infants. Their participation in infant care is enhanced if they are present at delivery, have early infant contact, and learn about the newborn's abilities. Emotional support between the parents has a strong effect on adaptation to parenting.

Adolescent mothers may have particular difficulty adapting to parenting. They may move in and out of the home and share care with the maternal grandmother. They often lack parenting skills as well as resources such as transportation to appointments related to health care. They may need more health supervision visits to negotiate their new responsibilities.

Other stressors for families include cultural, ethnic, educational, or religious differences. Community problems may include violence, inadequate housing, poverty, and unemployment. The effect of these problems on infants, other than through direct physical harm or malnutrition, depends on the adequacy of parental coping.

Friends, relatives, and community organizations can support parents by providing advice, encouragement, praise, and respite. Adequately supported parents are better able to be responsive, gentle, and consistent with their infants. Health supervision should include assessing the parents' support and, if necessary, helping them get into a social support network.

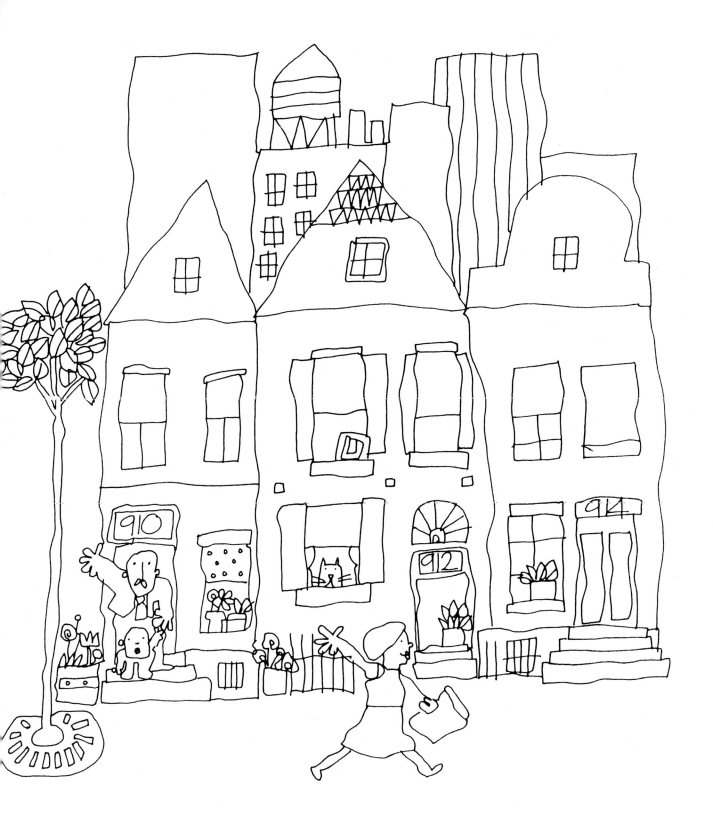

7

# INFANCY DEVELOPMENTAL CHART

Health professionals should assess the achievements of the infant and provide guidance to the family on anticipated tasks.
The effects are demonstrated by health supervision outcomes.

## ACHIEVEMENTS DURING INFANCY

Good physical health and growth

Regular sleep pattern

Self-quieting behavior

Sense of trust

Family adaptation to infant

Mutual attachment between infant and parents

Healthy sibling interactions

Partnership between family and health professional

## TASKS FOR THE FAMILY

Meet infant's nutritional needs

Establish regular eating and sleeping schedule

Prevent baby bottle tooth decay

Prevent injuries and abuse

Obtain appropriate immunizations

Promote normal development

Promote warm, nurturing parent-infant relationship

Promote responsiveness and social competence

Encourage vocal interactions with parents, siblings, and others

Encourage play with toys, siblings, parents, and others

Encourage exploration of the environment

## HEALTH SUPERVISION OUTCOMES

Formation of therapeutic alliance

Preparation of parents for new role

Optimal nutrition

Satisfactory growth and development

Injury prevention

Immunizations

Promotion of developmental potential

Prevention of behavioral problems

Promotion of family strengths

Enhancement of parental effectiveness

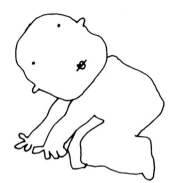

# FAMILY PREPARATION FOR INFANCY HEALTH SUPERVISION

Instructions to be provided to the family by the health professional.

Be prepared to give updates on the following at your next visit:

Illnesses and infectious diseases

Injuries

Visits to other health facilities or providers

Use of the emergency department

Hospitalizations or surgeries

Immunizations

Food and drug allergies

Eating habits

Medications

Supplementary fluoride and vitamins

Chronic health conditions

Update your infant's personal health record.

Be prepared to provide the following information on your family:

Health of and location of each significant family member

Genetic disorders

Depression or other mental health problems in the immediate or extended family

Alcoholism or other substance abuse (including use of tobacco) in the immediate or extended family

Family transitions (e.g., birth, death, marriage, divorce, loss of income, move, frequently absent parent, incarceration, change in child care arrangements)

Home environment/pets/neighborhood

Hazardous exposures (e.g., violence, lead, asbestos, tuberculosis)

Plans for future pregnancies or prevention of pregnancy

Information about your baby if you are not the biological parent (i.e., if you are an adoptive or foster parent)

Prepare and bring in questions, concerns, and observations about issues such as:

Your infant's development (sleep, feeding, bowel movements, activity level, overall temperament, self-comforting techniques such as thumb sucking or use of pacifier, achievements)

Your assessment of your own well-being and support from friends and family

Your attitudes about discipline

Talk to the infant's other caregivers and family members about any issues they might want you to raise with the health professional.

Bring in the Individualized Family Service Plan (IFSP) if the infant has special needs.

Complete and bring in any special questionnaires or self-evaluation forms provided by the health professional (e.g., questionnaires regarding practices that promote family health and safety).

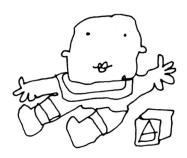

9

# STRENGTHS DURING INFANCY

Health professionals should remind families of their strengths during the health supervision visit.
Strengths and issues for infant, family, and community are interrelated and interdependent.

## INFANT

Is born wanted by parents

Has good physical health and nutritional status

Grows normally

Has normal feeding, bowel, sleep patterns

Has positive, cheerful, friendly temperament

Feels parents' unconditional love

Responds to parents and others

Is attached to parents and trusts them

Smiles, vocalizes

Is adaptable

Has some self-comforting behaviors

Explores environment actively

Plays with toys

Achieves developmental milestones

## FAMILY

Meets basic needs (food, shelter, clothing, health care)

Provides a safe, childproof environment (smoke detectors, car seats)

Enjoys and feels attached to infant

Responds to infant's developmental needs

Responds to and encourages infant's interactive behaviors

Offers emotional support and comfort when needed

Encourages exploration

Uses appropriate disciplinary measures

Parents are physically and mentally healthy

Parents have a strong relationship with each other and opportunities to nurture their relationship

Parents share care of infant

Siblings are interested in and involved with infant in age-appropriate ways

Has support of extended family and others

Parents pursue additional education or career advancement

## COMMUNITY

Provides support to new parents (parenting classes, support groups)

Provides educational opportunities for parents

Provides support for families with special needs (WIC, early intervention programs, community outreach)

Provides affordable, high-quality child care

Provides an environment free of hazards (violence, pollution, lead, asbestos, radiation)

Ensures that neighborhoods are safe

Provides affordable housing and public transportation

Develops integrated systems of health care

Fluoridates drinking water

Promotes community interactions (neighborhood watch programs, support groups, community centers)

Promotes positive ethnic/cultural milieu

# ISSUES DURING INFANCY

Health professionals should address issues—problems, stressors, and concerns—that families raise during health supervision. Strengths and issues for infant, family, and community are interrelated and interdependent.

## INFANT

Prematurity

Congenital disabilities

Feeding problems, food intolerances

Sleep problems

Sleeping with bottle

Baby bottle tooth decay

Fussing, crying, colic, irritability

Infections, illnesses

Constipation, diarrhea

Failure to thrive

Iron deficiency anemia

Chronic illness

Developmental delay

## FAMILY

Dysfunctional parents or other family members (depressed, mentally ill, abusive, disinterested, overly critical, overprotective, incarcerated)

Marital problems

Domestic violence (verbal, physical, or sexual abuse)

Frequently absent parent

Rotating "parents" (parents' girlfriends or boyfriends)

Inadequate child care arrangements

Family health problems (illness, chronic illness or disability)

Substance use (alcohol, drugs, tobacco)

Financial insecurity/homelessness

Family transitions (move, births, divorce, remarriage, incarceration, death)

Lack of knowledge about infant development

Lack of parenting skills or parental self-esteem, especially for adolescent parent

Sleep deprivation

Intrusive family members

Lack of social support/help with newborn and siblings

Neglect or rejection of child

## COMMUNITY

Poverty

Inadequate housing

Environmental hazards (e.g., lead)

Unsafe neighborhood

Community violence

Poor opportunities for employment

Lack of affordable, high-quality child care

Lack of programs for families with special needs (WIC, early intervention)

Lack of social support

Isolation in a rural community

Lack of educational programs and social services for adolescent parents

Lack of social, educational, cultural, and recreational opportunities

Discrimination and prejudice

Lack of access to medical/dental services

Inadequate public services (transportation, garbage removal, lighting, repair of public facilities, police and fire protection)

Inadequate fluoride levels in community drinking water

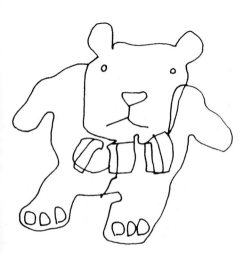

11

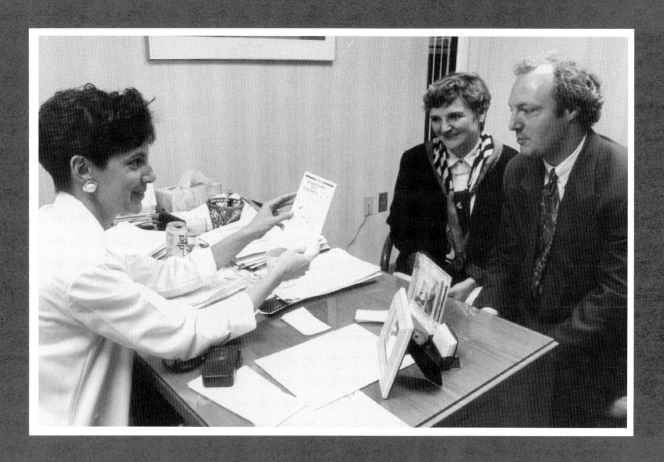

*The main purpose of the prenatal visit is
to initiate and set the tone for the working relationship
between the family and the health professional.*

# Prenatal Visit

The health supervision partnership between the family and the health professional begins with the prenatal visit. The main purpose of the prenatal visit is to initiate and set the tone for the working relationship between the family and the health professional. The parents have been awaiting the birth of the baby for many months, but if they are first-time parents, they have no real understanding of what parenthood will mean for them. The prenatal health supervision visit can be another step that prepares them for their new role. In their conversation with the health professional, they will have their questions answered and receive their first anticipatory guidance.

While they are obtaining useful information, the parents are also learning about the process of health supervision. If the health professional listens actively to them and discusses with empathy the issues they raise, they will begin to trust their own intuition and their ability to make decisions.

Even before the baby is born, most parents have expectations—conscious or unconscious—about their child. If the child is very active in utero, the parents might expect an active baby. They may think the child will be blond like the mother or musical like the father. They may worry that the uncle's heart problems will be inherited. Parents also often have strong feelings about having a boy or girl. Talking through these expectations with the parents allows the health professional to share their excitement and help sort out their concerns. The discussion can demonstrate for the parents that a therapeutic relationship is a powerful tool for promoting the health of their children.

Health professionals should make the extra effort to reach out to fathers during this time, in order to emphasize how important the fathers will be in the health supervision of their children. If the family situation permits, health professionals should encourage both parents to attend the prenatal health supervision visit and future visits.

# HEALTH SUPERVISION INTERVIEW

## TRIGGER QUESTIONS

To be used selectively by the health professional. Discuss any issues or concerns of the family.

**What questions do you have for me today?**

**How has your pregnancy gone? What has been the most exciting aspect?**

**How are your preparations for your baby going?**
**Who will help you when you come home with your baby?**

**Do you have other children? Have you talked with them about your pregnancy?**
**Who will look after them while you are in the hospital?**

**Many expectant parents have concerns about the baby or themselves. Do you have any concerns?**

**Have you had any physical or emotional problems during the pregnancy?**

**How do you plan to feed your baby? Breastfeeding? Formula? Why?**

**What have you decided to do about circumcision if your baby is a boy?**

**Was this a good time for you to be pregnant? How does your family feel about it?**

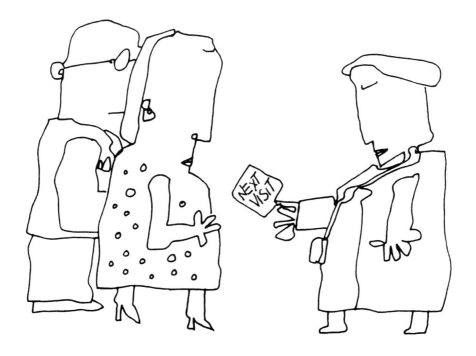

How do you think the baby will change your lives?

How were things for you when you were growing up?

Do you plan to raise your baby the way you were raised or somewhat differently?
What would you change?

Are you concerned that your child will inherit any diseases or other characteristics that run in the family?

Do you smoke? Do you drink? Have you taken any drugs? Does your partner take drugs?

During this pregnancy, have you had any sexually transmitted diseases,
exposure to the herpes virus, or an abnormal pap smear?

Do you plan to return to work? To school? Have you thought about child care arrangements?
(Advise parents to start looking for child care.)

Are you concerned about being able to afford food or supplies for your baby?

If the mother is alone:
Does your partner ever lose his temper, throw things, threaten you, or hurt you?

# ANTICIPATORY GUIDANCE FOR THE FAMILY

The prenatal health supervision visit offers the best opportunity to promote breastfeeding among those parents who have not yet decided on a feeding method, and to reinforce the preference for breastfeeding among parents who have already made this choice. The health professional should encourage breastfeeding and discuss the parents' knowledge and expectations about breastfeeding. Nipple care should be addressed.

## Promotion of healthy habits

Obtain an infant car seat in which to transport your newborn home.

Ensure that your crib is safe. The slats should be no more than 2 3/8" apart, and the mattress should be firm and fit snugly into the crib. Do not put the baby to sleep on a soft surface such as a waterbed, couch, or pillow.

Do not use baby walkers at any age. Tell family members not to give one as a gift.

Install smoke detectors if not already in place and make sure they work properly.

Set hot water heater thermostat at less than 120 °F.

Make the home and car nonsmoking zones, with all smoking done outside. Protect your baby's health by attending a smoking cessation program. Stop using drugs or alcohol.

Learn infant cardiopulmonary resuscitation (CPR).

Ask the health professional any questions you have about breastfeeding.

If you are bottlefeeding: To avoid developing a habit that will harm your infant's teeth, do not put her to bed with a bottle or prop it in her mouth. Hold the baby in a semisitting position to feed her.

Obtain a dental checkup and treatment before the birth of the baby.

Keep your prenatal appointments.

Attend childbirth classes.

## Promotion of constructive family relationships and parental health

With the new baby, expect changes in your family relationships. Having a new baby in the family is often stressful. Plan on helping each other take care of the infant.

Let go of less important tasks and functions for the first month or two.

Prepare older siblings for the new baby.

Anticipate that there may be times when you feel tired, overwhelmed, inadequate, or depressed. Many women feel the baby blues for a short period.

Develop a support system, whether with friends or family members or through community programs.

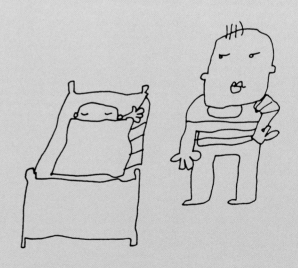

# CLOSING THE VISIT

Provide information on Family Preparation for Infancy Health Supervision so that families will be prepared for future health supervision visits.

Offer other materials for the parents to review at home, including literature or videotapes on child safety, childproofing the home, and breastfeeding.

Provide resources to support breastfeeding: handouts, videotapes, books, or telephone numbers of community resources such as breastfeeding question lines, lactation consultants, or La Leche League.

Discuss plans for assessing the baby in the hospital.

If the family needs financial assistance to help pay for health care expenses, refer them to the state Medicaid programs or other state medical assistance programs.

If the family is eligible for WIC, help them enroll.

Suggest community resources that help with financial concerns, parental inexperience, inadequate housing, absence of social supports, limited food resources, lack of transportation, and need for car seats.

Provide parents with information about parenting classes or support groups.

Discuss how the family should access health care (e.g., your medical practice or clinic hours, help available after hours, telephone advice, when to use the emergency department, how to call an ambulance).

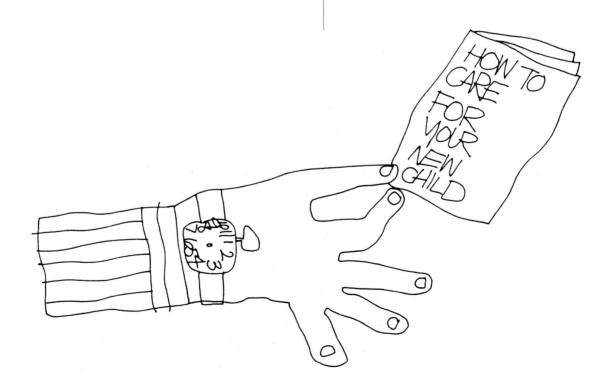

17

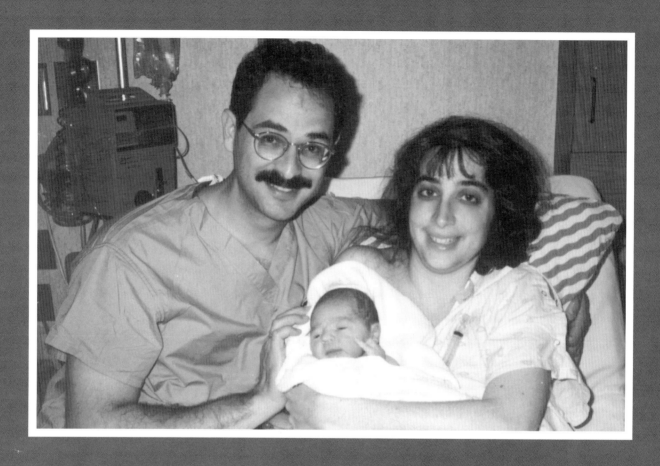

*Assuming that all has gone well,
the first question parents will ask is,
"Is our baby perfect?"*

# Newborn Visit

New parents may be overwhelmed with excitement and fatigue. Parents must cope with hospital staff coming in and out of the room and with initiating the feeding process, choosing a name, deciding on circumcision if the baby is a boy, and receiving phone calls and visits from friends. Ideally, the parents have been seen by the health professional for a prenatal visit and a health supervision partnership has been initiated. Assuming that all has gone well, the first question parents will ask is, "Is our baby perfect?" Once they hear that their baby is normal, they just want to get on with the task of beginning feeding, getting their baby on a good schedule, recovering their feelings of well-being, and going home.

Parents of babies who are premature or born with a disability are usually extremely stressed. The care of these parents should be as intensive as that of the infant, especially for mothers who are very young or in suboptimal health, or have limited coping abilities. The first step for the health professional is to explain the baby's condition honestly and sensitively. In the case of a long-term disability, the interpretation is never accomplished in one visit but in small steps over time, according to the readiness of parents. The health professional should emphasize the child's normal characteristics as much as possible. The next step is for the parents to participate in their baby's care as much as they can.

The birth of a baby with a disability often precipitates family and personal crises and underscores the need for the health professional to be a specialist in providing care to both parents and children. There are few times when support is more necessary, sophisticated care more appropriate, and the presence of a prepared professional more compelling. A partnership between the family and the physician, nurse, and other care providers can be forged during this time of special vulnerability and receptivity. Health professionals who examine the newborn in front of the parents, refer to the baby by name, convey some of the infant's temperament, and talk to and smile at the baby will facilitate both the parents' attachment to the baby and the development of a health supervision partnership with the family.

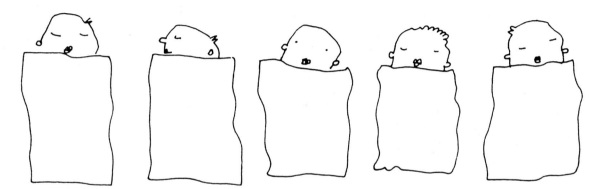

# HEALTH SUPERVISION INTERVIEW

## TRIGGER QUESTIONS

To be used selectively by the health professional. Discuss any issues or concerns of the family.

**Congratulations on your new baby!**
**Theresa is doing well and weighs 7 pounds and 10 ounces today.**

**Have things gone as you expected?**

**How are you feeling? How did the delivery go?**

**What do you think of Michael?**

**What do your other children think about the new baby?**

**What are some of your questions?**

**What are your questions about feeding?**

**Is everything set for you to take your baby home?**

**Who will help you when you get home?**

**Do you have a car seat to use when you take Joel home?**

**When you have questions about the baby, whom do you expect to ask?**

**What's the most important thing in the world to you right now?**

**How do you think Madeline will enrich your lives?**

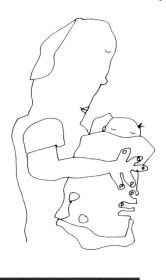
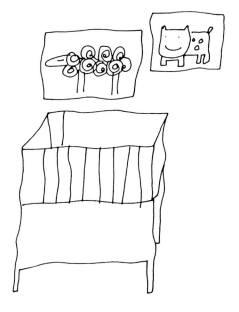

# Observation of Parent-Infant Interaction

Do the parents respond to the baby's needs?

Are they comfortable when feeding, holding, or caring for the baby?

Do they have visitors or any other signs of a support system?

Does the baby attach and suck well when breastfeeding?

# Physical Examination

If possible, the health professional should examine the infant in front of the parents so that they can ask questions and the health professional can comment on the physical findings.

As part of the complete physical examination, the following should be noted:

  Length, weight, head circumference

  Cranial molding, cephalohematoma, or caput-succedeum

  Red reflex, subconjunctival hemorrhages, puffy eyes

  Patent nares

  Palate

  Cardiac murmurs

  Breast engorgement

  Femoral pulses

  Peripheral cyanosis

  Jaundice

  Abdominal masses or distention

  Genitalia

Clavicle fractures, developmental hip dysplasia, foot abnormalities

Moro reflex, muscle tone, symmetrical movements

Skin mottling, toxic erythema, hemangiomas, nevi, mongolian spots, birthmarks

Ability of infant to fix and follow a human face and respond to human voice, and other newborn abilities

# ANTICIPATORY GUIDANCE FOR THE FAMILY

In addition to providing anticipatory guidance, many health professionals give families handouts
at an appropriate reading level or a videotape that they can review or study at home.[1]

## Promotion of healthy habits

### Injury and illness prevention

Use an infant car seat that is properly secured at all times.

Ensure that the baby's crib is safe. The slats should be no more
than $2^3/_8$" apart, and the mattress should be firm and fit
snugly into the crib. Keep the sides of the crib raised. Do not
put the baby to sleep on a soft surface such as a waterbed,
couch, or pillow.

Put the baby to sleep on his back or side.

Set hot water heater thermostat at less than 120 °F.

Test the water temperature with your wrist to make sure it is
not hot before bathing the baby.

Never leave the baby alone or with a young sibling or pet.

Do not leave him alone in a tub of water or on high places
such as changing tables, beds, sofas, or chairs. Always keep
one hand on the baby.

Keep the baby's environment free of smoke. Make the home
and car nonsmoking zones.

Do not drink hot liquids or smoke while holding the baby.

Avoid overexposure to the sun.

Recognize early signs of illness:

> Fever
>
> Failure to eat
>
> Vomiting
>
> Diarrhea
>
> Dehydration
>
> Unusual irritability, lethargy
>
> Jaundice, skin rash

Know what to do in case of emergency:

> When to call the health care professional
>
> When to go to which emergency department
>
> Ask your child care provider what happens when an
> emergency occurs in the child care setting

## Nutrition

Review successful breastfeeding practices with the health professional: How to hold the baby and get him to latch on properly; feeding on cue 8–12 times a day for the first four to six weeks; and feeding until the infant seems content.

Review your care with the health professional: Obtaining plenty of rest; drinking plenty of fluids; relieving breast engorgement; caring for nipples; and eating properly. Receive follow-up support from the health professional by telephone, home visit, nurse visit, or early office visit.

Newborn breastfed babies should have six to eight wet diapers per day, as well as several "mustardy" stools per day.

Give the breastfeeding infant 400 I.U.'s of vitamin D daily if he is deeply pigmented or does not receive enough sunlight.

If you are bottlefeeding: Ask the health professional about type of formula, preparation, feeding techniques, and equipment. Hold baby in semisitting position to feed. Do not use a microwave oven to heat formula.

To avoid developing a habit that will harm your infant's teeth, do not put him to bed with a bottle or prop it in his mouth.

## Infant care

Discuss any questions or concerns you have about:

Cord care

Circumcision care; noncircumcised infant care

Skin and nail care: bathing, soaps, lotions, diaper area preparations, detergent

Vaginal discharge or bleeding

Crying

Sneezing and hiccups

Burping, spitting up

Thumbsucking and pacifiers

Change from meconium to transitional stools

Normal sleep patterns; sleeping arrangements

Amount of clothing needed; exposure to hot or cold temperatures

Use of thermometer (in infants, a rectal temperature of 38.0 °C/100.5 °F or higher is considered a fever)

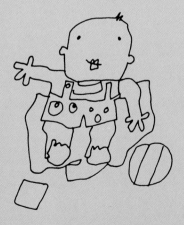

## Promotion of parent-infant interaction that is mutually satisfying and enjoyable

Learn about the baby's temperament and how it affects the way he relates to the world.

Try to console the infant, but recognize that the infant may not always be consolable regardless of what you do. Discuss this with the health professional.

Nurture the baby by holding, cuddling, and rocking him, and by talking and singing to him.

## Promotion of constructive family relationships and parental health

Encourage your partner to attend the health supervision visits.

Try to rest when the baby is sleeping.

Realize that there may be times when you feel tired, overwhelmed, inadequate, or depressed.

Accept support from your partner, family members, and friends.

Discuss with the health professional how to deal with unwanted advice from family and friends.

Discuss sibling reactions with the health professional.

For mother returning to work: Begin to make plans for child care.

Address your own oral health needs.

# CLOSING THE VISIT

Prepare the family for the next health supervision visit.

Point out the infant's strengths and appropriately commend the parents on their growing comfort with the new baby.

Provide resources to support breastfeeding: handouts, videotapes, books, or telephone numbers of community resources such as breastfeeding question lines, lactation consultants, or La Leche League.

If the family needs financial assistance to help pay for health care expenses, refer them to the state Medicaid programs or other state medical assistance programs. If the family is eligible for WIC, help them enroll.

Suggest community resources that help with financial concerns, parental inexperience, inadequate housing, absence of social supports, limited food resources, lack of transportation, and need for car seats.

Inquire about the number of rooms in the family's home, the number of people living there, and the adequacy of heating in cold weather.

Arrange a time to call the family in 24–72 hours.

Schedule another health supervision visit within the next week.

Discuss how the family should access health care (e.g., your medical practice or clinic hours, help available after hours, telephone advice, when to use the emergency department, how to call an ambulance).

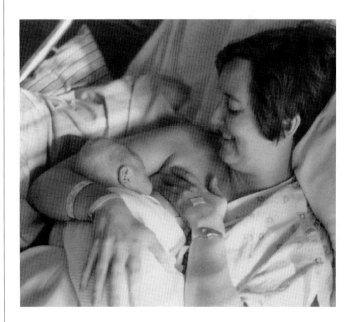

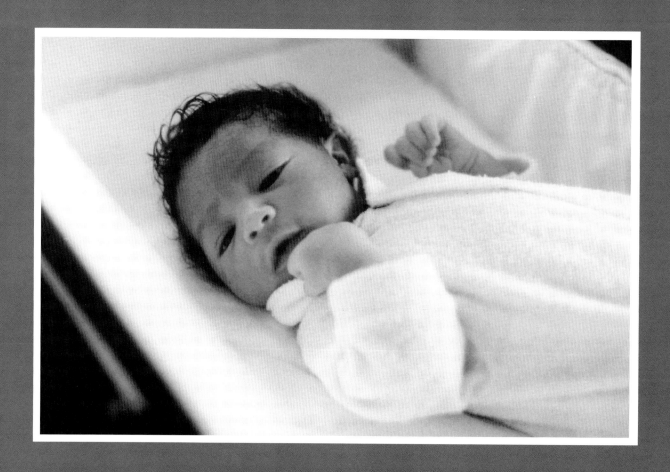

*The health professional should call the mother
the first day after discharge and also schedule an office visit
within three days.*

# First Week

Since mothers are now often discharged within 24 hours of childbirth, families need more intensive health supervision than in the past. A health professional should call the mother the first day after discharge and schedule an office visit within three days. A home visit by a nurse (if possible) is important as well, especially if the mother intends to breastfeed the baby. If the mother is discharged more than 48 hours after childbirth, the first office visit may occur within four days of discharge.

The first week of a baby's life requires major adjustments on the part of her parents, who are often exhausted and overwhelmed by caring for their new baby. Mothers are trying to heal their bodies and care for the newborn at the same time. Their initial elation may give way to frustration at the high level of the newborn's demands or to the baby blues. At the same time, excitement about the new baby can carry parents through this adjustment period and help them cope with their lack of sleep and the constant pressure to attend to the baby's needs. Most parents will have to use trial and error to discover the behaviors that comfort their baby. Families who experience perinatal problems or congenital disabilities have special needs.

Even at this stage, parents can take advantage of the baby's limited waking time to communicate with and play with her. Parents who cuddle the infant and sing and vocalize to her will help establish the parent-infant relationship.

Within the next week after the visit, a newborn regains the weight she lost after delivery. Breastfeeding the infant every few hours in response to her cues will usually ensure that she gets enough to eat, as reflected by a steady weight gain, six or more wet diapers a day, and daily stools. Occasionally, a breastfed infant does not act hungry even though she is receiving insufficient calories. Mothers who are breastfeeding should make sure that they receive the nutrition and sleep they need, so that they do not overtax themselves while supplying milk to the baby. A health professional or lactation counselor can provide information and support to prevent or minimize sore nipples, breast infections, and improper latching-on.

If a baby who receives formula is not gaining weight or wetting her diaper six to eight times per day, parents and health professionals can discuss the quantity and frequency of feeding.

To avoid being overwhelmed, parents need to conserve their energy and rest when the baby sleeps. Extended family members or friends who assist with daily chores can be very helpful. New parents need a supportive person that they trust to listen to their concerns, but they also need privacy to become a family and fashion their own solutions.

27

# HEALTH SUPERVISION INTERVIEW

## TRIGGER QUESTIONS

To be used selectively by the health professional. Discuss any issues or concerns of the family.

**How are you?**

**How is Kemi doing?**

**Are you enjoying Bruce?**

**What questions or concerns do you have at this time?**

**Who helps you with Carlota?**

**How would you describe Jennifer's personality?**

**Is Jesse easy or difficult to console?**

**Has Heidi been fussy? What have you found that seems to work?**

**Can you tell when Matthias wants to eat? Go to sleep?**

**How is feeding going?**
If infant is breastfed: **How often and for how long do you breastfeed?**
**Do you have any concerns about breastfeeding?**
If infant is bottlefed: **How many ounces are consumed per feeding, and what is the total for 24 hours?**
**Do you have any concerns about feeding?**

**Are you getting enough rest?**

**Have you been feeling tired or blue?**

**Is transportation a problem for you? Do you have enough money for food?**

**Are you planning to return to work or school?**
**Have you begun to think about possible child care arrangements?**

**How are your other children doing?**

# Developmental Surveillance and Milestones

Responds to sound by blinking, crying, quieting, changing respiration, or showing a startle response

Fixates on human face and follows with eyes

Responds to parent's face and voice

Has flexed posture

Moves all extremities

# Observation of Parent-Infant Interaction

Does the parent appear depressed, tearful, angry, anxious, fatigued, overwhelmed, or uncomfortable? If both parents are present, do they share caring for and holding the infant during the visit? Do they both provide information? Do they appear able to read and respond to the infant's cues? Are they comfortable with the baby?

# Physical Examination

The physical examination permits the health professional to detect abnormal findings and to model for the parent how to respond to the baby's cues, console the baby by talking, and show interest in the baby.

Measure and plot on a standard chart the head circumference, length, weight, and weight for length. Share the information with the parent.

As part of the complete physical examination, the following should be noted:

Red reflex

Strabismus

## ADDITIONAL SCREENING PROCEDURES

Metabolic and hemoglobinopathy screening as required by the state
(If not performed on newborn in hospital)

Hearing screening
(Prior to three months of age)

## IMMUNIZATIONS

Hepatitis B Virus (HBV) Vaccine          #1
(If it was not administered in the hospital)

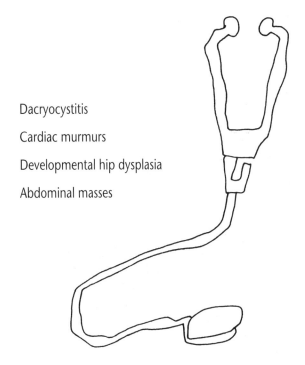

Dacryocystitis

Cardiac murmurs

Developmental hip dysplasia

Abdominal masses

# ANTICIPATORY GUIDANCE FOR THE FAMILY

In addition to providing anticipatory guidance, many health professionals give families handouts
at an appropriate reading level or a videotape that they can review or study at home.[1]

## Promotion of healthy habits

### Injury and illness prevention

Use an infant car seat that is properly secured at all times.

Ensure that the baby's crib is safe. The slats should be no more than 2 3/8" apart, and the mattress should be firm and fit snugly into the crib. Keep the sides of the crib raised. Do not put the baby to sleep on a soft surface such as a waterbed, couch, or pillow.

Put the baby to sleep on her back or side.

Set hot water heater thermostat at less than 120 °F.

Test the water temperature with your wrist to make sure it is not hot before bathing the baby.

Never leave the baby alone or with a young sibling or pet.

Do not leave her alone in a tub of water or on high places such as changing tables, beds, sofas, or chairs. Always keep one hand on the baby.

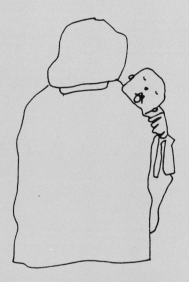

Continue to keep the baby's environment free of smoke. Keep the home and car nonsmoking zones.

Install smoke detectors if not already in place and make sure they work properly.

Do not drink hot liquids or smoke while holding the baby.

Avoid overexposure to the sun.

Recognize early signs of illness:

>    Fever
>
>    Failure to eat
>
>    Vomiting
>
>    Diarrhea
>
>    Dehydration
>
>    Unusual irritability, lethargy
>
>    Jaundice, skin rash

Know what to do in case of emergency:

>    When to call the health professional
>
>    When to go to which emergency department

## Nutrition

Ensure that the infant is gaining enough weight.

If you are breastfeeding: Ensure that breastfeeding is of appropriate frequency and duration. Ensure that you have an appropriate diet. Discuss with the health professional any problems you are having with breastfeeding.

Give the breastfeeding infant 400 I.U.'s of vitamin D daily if she is deeply pigmented or does not receive enough sunlight.

If you are bottlefeeding: Ensure that the infant receives an appropriate amount of iron-fortified formula at the appropriate frequency. Hold the baby in a semisitting position to feed her. Do not use a microwave oven to heat formula.

Do not give the infant honey until after her first birthday to prevent infant botulism.

## Oral health

To avoid developing a habit that will harm your infant's teeth, do not put her to bed with a bottle or prop it in her mouth.

## Infant care

Discuss any questions or concerns you have about:

> Cord care
>
> Circumcision care; noncircumcised infant care
>
> Skin and nail care: bathing, soaps, lotions, diaper area preparations, detergent
>
> Colic/crying
>
> Sneezing and hiccups, spitting up
>
> Thumbsucking and pacifiers
>
> Normal sleep patterns; sleeping arrangements
>
> Bowel movements
>
> Amount of clothing needed; exposure to hot or cold temperatures
>
> Use of thermometer (in infants, a rectal temperature of 38.0 °C/100.5 °F or higher is considered a fever)

31

## Promotion of parent-infant interaction that is mutually enjoyable and satisfying

Learn about the baby's temperament and how it affects the way she relates to the world.

Try to console the infant, but recognize that she may not always be consolable regardless of what you do. Many infants have a daily fussy period in the late afternoon or evening. Crying may increase during the next month, including a possible peak of approximately three hours per day at six weeks of age. Discuss any concerns with the health professional.

Nurture the baby by holding, cuddling, and rocking her, and by talking and singing to her.

Spend time playing with and talking to the baby during her quiet, alert states.

## Promotion of constructive family relationships and parental health

Try to rest and take time for yourself.

Realize that there may be times when you feel tired, overwhelmed, inadequate, or depressed.

Spend some individual time with your partner.

Accept support from your partner, family members, and friends.

Discuss with the health professional how to deal with unwanted advice from family and friends.

Encourage your partner to participate in care of your infant.

Continue to provide attention to the other children in the family, appropriately engaging them in the care of the baby.

Discuss family planning with your partner.

Schedule a postpartum checkup.

## Promotion of community interactions

If you need financial assistance to help pay for health care expenses, ask about resources or for referrals to the state Medicaid programs or other state medical assistance programs.

Ask about resources or referrals for food (e.g., WIC), housing, or transportation if needed.

Learn about and consider attending parent education classes and/or parent-child play groups.

Maintain or expand ties to your community through social, religious, cultural, volunteer, and recreational organizations.

For mother returning to work: Discuss child care referral agencies or similar community services with the health professional. Discuss how to continue breastfeeding.

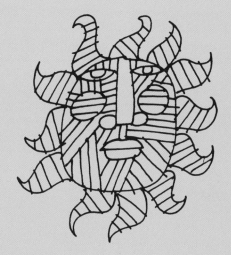

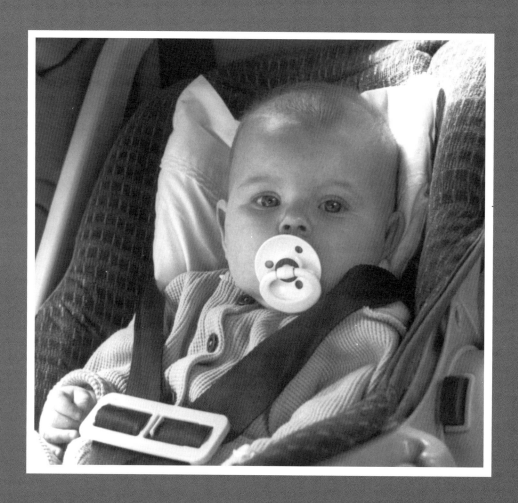

*Parents should know basic rules of injury prevention, such as using an infant car seat, keeping one hand on the baby when he is on a high surface, and never leaving the infant alone with young children or pets.*

# One Month Visit

By the time the infant is one month old, his parents have mastered their early adaptation to him, and parents and baby are attuned to each other. Now able to interpret their infant's cry, the parents have learned that he can be comforted in a variety of ways, such as through touch, a voice, or a smile. They know when to pick him up and when to feel confident that the crying will soon stop. They enjoy feeling close to the baby and are comfortable talking to him and holding, cuddling, and rocking him.

The infant responds to his parents' overtures. The baby fixes on a face or an object, following it with his eyes, and he responds to his parents' voices. He shows some ability to console himself, possibly by putting his fingers or hands in his mouth.

Sensitive parents also recognize the early indicators of their infant's individual temperament. They know how to avoid overstimulating the baby and how to calm him down. They also understand that infants vary in their need for feeding, in terms of frequency and amount.

Physically, the baby displays good muscle tone, deep tendon reflexes, and primitive reflexes. His weight, height, and head circumference continue to increase along his expected growth curve. Stooling interval and consistency vary, and many healthy babies strain and turn red when having a bowel movement. Constipation is signaled by a hard stool, although babies fed exclusively through breastfeeding usually do not become constipated.

Some babies develop the classic symptoms of colic, including pulling their legs into their abdomen. It is more common, however, for babies just to have a fussy period at the end of the day, when they cry to "sort themselves out."

In spite of their new responsibilities and periods of increased stress, parents should have gained enough confidence in the first month to be able to enjoy their baby. Intermittent periods of anxiety, depression, and feelings of inadequacy are normal. It will help if each parent spends time alone away from the baby, and if the parents spend time together as well as with relatives or other important supportive figures. Parents with other children should attempt to give individual attention to each sibling.

It is important that parents know to seek medical help if the infant does not look right, has a fever or diarrhea, refuses to feed, vomits excessively, sleeps too much, or is irritable. In addition, parents should know basic rules of injury prevention, such as using an infant car seat, keeping one hand on the baby when he is on a high surface, and never leaving the infant alone with young children or pets.

# HEALTH SUPERVISION INTERVIEW

## TRIGGER QUESTIONS

To be used selectively by the health professional. Discuss any issues or concerns of the family.

**How are you?**

**How are you feeling these days?**

**How is José doing?**

**What do you enjoy most about Cameron?**

**What questions or concerns do you have at this time?**

**Have there been any major changes in your family since you came home from the hospital?**

**Who helps you with Alicia?**

**How would you describe Jessica's personality?**

**Is Monika easy or difficult to console?**

**What have you found that seems to work during Mark's fussy periods?**

**Can you tell when Kim wants to eat? Go to sleep?**

**How is feeding going?**
If infant is breastfed: **How often and for how long do you breastfeed?**
**Do you have any concerns about breastfeeding?**
If infant is bottlefed: **How many ounces are consumed per feeding, and what is the total for 24 hours?**

**Are you getting enough rest?**

**Have you been feeling tired or blue?**

**Have you and your partner had some time for yourselves? Are you using baby sitters?**

**How are the other children doing?**

**What do you do when problems seem to be getting to you? To whom do you turn at times like that?**

**What disciplinary measures are you considering?**

**Is transportation a problem for you? Do you have enough money for food?**

**Are you planning to return to work or school?**
**Have you begun to look into possible child care arrangements?**

## Developmental Surveillance and Milestones

Responds to sound by blinking, crying, quieting, changing respiration or showing a startle response

Fixates on human face and follows with eyes

Responds to parent's face and voice

Lifts head momentarily when in prone position

Has flexed posture

Moves all extremities

Can sleep for three or four hours at a time; can stay awake for one hour or longer

When crying, can be consoled most of the time by being spoken to or held

## Observation of Parent-Infant Interaction

Does the parent appear depressed, tearful, angry, anxious, fatigued, overwhelmed, or uncomfortable? If both parents are present, do they share caring for and holding the infant during the visit? Do they both provide information? Do they appear able to read and respond to the infant's cues? Are they comfortable with the baby?

## Physical Examination

The physical examination permits the health professional to detect abnormal findings and to model for the parent how to respond to the baby's cues, console the baby by talking, and show interest in the baby.

Measure and plot on a standard chart the head circumference, length, weight, and weight for length. Share the information with the parent.

### ADDITIONAL SCREENING PROCEDURES

Hearing screening
(Prior to three months of age)

Assessment of risk of high-dose lead exposure[2]

### IMMUNIZATIONS

Hepatitis B Virus (HBV) Vaccine     #1
(If it was not administered previously)

As part of the complete physical examination, the following should be noted:

Red reflex

Dacryostenosis

Dacryocystitis

Cardiac murmurs

Developmental hip dysplasia

Abdominal masses

Thrush

Cradle cap

Diaper dermatitis

Evidence of neglect or abuse

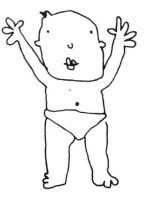

# ANTICIPATORY GUIDANCE FOR THE FAMILY

In addition to providing anticipatory guidance, many health professionals give families handouts at an appropriate reading level or a videotape that they can review or study at home.[1]

## Promotion of healthy habits

### Injury and illness prevention

Continue to use an infant car seat that is properly secured at all times.

Continue to put the baby to sleep on his back or side.

Continue to test the water temperature with your wrist to make sure it is not hot before bathing the baby.

Never leave the baby alone or with a young sibling or pet.

Do not leave him alone in a tub of water or on high places such as changing tables, beds, sofas, or chairs. Always keep one hand on the baby.

Continue to keep the baby's environment free of smoke. Keep the home and car nonsmoking zones.

Install smoke detectors if not already in place and make sure they work properly.

Avoid overexposure to the sun.

Do not drink hot liquids or smoke while holding the baby.

Keep toys with small parts or other small or sharp objects out of reach.

Recognize early signs of illness:

Fever

Failure to eat

Vomiting

Diarrhea

Dehydration

Unusual irritability, lethargy

Skin rash

Review emergency procedures:

When to call the health professional

When to go to which emergency department

## Nutrition

Ensure that the infant is gaining enough weight.

If you are breastfeeding: Ensure that breastfeeding is of appropriate frequency and duration. Ensure that you have an appropriate diet. Discuss with the health professional any problems you are having with breastfeeding.

Give the breastfeeding infant 400 I.U.'s of vitamin D daily if he is deeply pigmented or does not receive enough sunlight.

If you are bottlefeeding: Ensure that the infant receives an appropriate amount of iron-fortified formula at the appropriate frequency. Hold the baby in a semisitting position to feed him. Do not use a microwave oven to heat formula.

Delay the introduction of solid foods until the infant is four to six months of age. Do not put cereal in a bottle.

Do not give the infant honey until after his first birthday to prevent infant botulism.

## Oral health

To avoid developing a habit that will harm your infant's teeth, do not put him to bed with a bottle or prop it in his mouth.

## Infant care

Discuss any questions or concerns you have about:

Skin and nail care: bathing, soaps, lotions, diaper area preparations, detergent

Colic/crying

Thumbsucking and pacifiers

Normal sleep patterns; sleeping arrangements

Bowel movements

Thermometer use

## Promotion of parent-infant interaction that is mutually enjoyable and satisfying

Learn about the baby's temperament and how it affects the way he relates to the world.

Try to console the infant, but recognize that he may not always be consolable regardless of what you do. Crying may increase during the next few weeks, including a possible peak of approximately three hours per day at six weeks of age. Discuss any concerns with the health professional.

Nurture the baby by holding, cuddling, and rocking him, and by talking and singing to him.

Spend time playing with and talking to the baby during his quiet, alert states.

## Promotion of constructive family relationships and parental health

Continue to try to rest and take time for yourself.

Spend some individual time with your partner.

Keep in contact with friends and family members. Avoid social isolation.

Encourage your partner to participate in the care of your infant.

Continue to provide attention to the other children in the family, appropriately engaging them in the care of the baby.

Discuss family planning with your partner.

Have your postpartum checkup. Interpartum care and preconceptional risk assessment should be part of the obstetrical counseling provided to all parents, especially those of low birthweight infants. If you decide to have another baby, he will be healthier if there is adequate spacing between your pregnancies, if you maintain an appropriate maternal weight for height, and if you avoid smoking.

## Promotion of community interactions

If you need financial assistance to help pay for health care expenses, ask about resources or for referrals to the state Medicaid programs or other state medical assistance programs.

Ask about resources or referrals for food (e.g., WIC), housing, or transportation if needed.

Learn about and consider attending parent education classes and/or parent-child play groups.

Maintain or expand ties to your community through social, religious, cultural, volunteer, and recreational organizations or resources.

For mother returning to work: Discuss child care referral agencies or similar community services with the health professional. Discuss how to continue breastfeeding. It is also useful to discuss potential role tensions before returning to work.

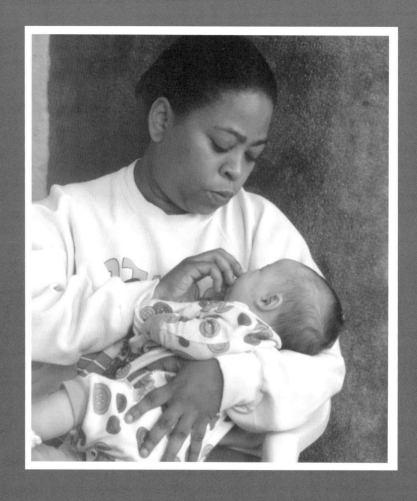

*The infant's responses to her parents provide*
*important feedback when they cuddle her or talk and sing to her.*

# Two Month Visit

By two months after birth, parents and their baby are communicating with each other. Parents can gain the infant's attention, and she responds to their cues. The baby looks into her parents' eyes, breaks into a big smile, coos, and vocalizes reciprocally. She is attentive to the parents' voices and reacts with enjoyment to pleasant visual, auditory, and tactile stimuli. The infant's responses to her parents provide important feedback when they cuddle her or talk and sing to her.

The baby has established a regular feeding and sleeping schedule. The schedule for the bottlefed baby repeats approximately every three to four hours; the feedings may be more frequent for the breastfed baby. Feeding intervals may now be less frequent at night. The baby will not need solid foods until she is four to six months old, and parents should wait until that point to introduce cereal. Adding cereal to her bottle will not make her sleep through the night. The baby can hold her head erect while being held for brief periods of time. Her weight, height, and head circumference continue to increase along her predicted growth curve.

Parents may still need to take naps. They should have settled into their new roles, learning how to divide the tasks of caring for the infant and each other. Just as they have settled into these roles, however, many parents must negotiate new ones. Those returning to work need to make plans regarding future caregiving arrangements. Concerns about leaving the child may conflict with the need to support the family or pursue career goals. Separation often brings on guilt feelings that need to be resolved.

High-quality, affordable child care is a concern at this stage since caregivers should provide developmental stimulation as well as physical care. Although many families rely on relatives or friends to care for their children, such caregivers do not always have the necessary skills. Child care courses are often offered through community hospitals or organizations such as the American Red Cross.

Ideally, parents plan time together. If the parent is single, time may be spent on outside interests and relationships. It is also important that other siblings in the family have some time alone with their parents for activities they enjoy. To alleviate feelings of being left out, responsible siblings can be encouraged to participate in the care of the infant.

Mothers should have had a postpartum checkup by this time. They should have discussed family planning arrangements and lifetime reproductive plans with their partner and the health professional.

# HEALTH SUPERVISION INTERVIEW

## TRIGGER QUESTIONS

To be used selectively by the health professional. Discuss any issues or concerns of the family.

**How are you?**

**How have things been going in your family?**

**How is Jamil doing?**

**What do you and your partner enjoy most about Kaitlin?**

**What questions or concerns do you have about Keisha?**

**Have there been any unexpected stresses, crises, or illnesses in your family since your last visit?**

**Who helps you with Ron?**

**How would you describe Zoe's personality? How does she respond to you?**

**Is it easy or hard to know what Leon wants?**

**How is Kyra sleeping? Are you getting enough rest?**

**Does Jan have a regular schedule now?**

If infant is breastfed: **How often and for how long do you breastfeed?**
**Do you have any concerns about breastfeeding?**
If infant is bottlefed: **How many ounces are consumed per feeding, and what is the total for 24 hours?**

**Do you think Ahmed hears all right? Sees all right?**

**Have you been out of the house without the baby, either with your partner or a friend or on your own?**

**Do you have the opportunity to spend time with other parents and babies?**

**How are your other children?**

**Are you returning to work or school? What plans have you made for child care?**

**Have you had a postpartum checkup?**
**Did you discuss family planning arrangements at this checkup? With your partner?**

**Do you have a gun at home? Do you keep it locked up?**
**Where do you keep the ammunition?**

# Developmental Surveillance and Milestones

Coos and vocalizes reciprocally

Is attentive to voices

Shows interest in visual and auditory stimuli

Smiles responsively

Shows pleasure in interactions with adults, especially primary caregivers

In prone position, lifts head, neck, and upper chest with support on forearms

Some head control in upright position

# Observation of Parent-Infant Interaction

Are the parent and infant interested in and responsive to each other (e.g., gazing, talking, holding, cuddling, and smiling)? Does the parent appear depressed, tearful, angry, anxious, fatigued, overwhelmed, or uncomfortable? Is the parent aware of the infant's distress and effective in comforting her? Does the parent give any signs of disagreement with or lack of support from partner? Does the parent generally appear comfortable?

# Physical Examination

Measure and plot on a standard chart the head circumference, length, weight, and weight for length. Share the information with the parent.

## IMMUNIZATIONS

Hemophilus Influenza Type b (Hib) Vaccine[3]     #1

Diphtheria, Tetanus, Pertussis (DTP) Vaccine     #1
(Hib and DTP can be combined.)[3]

Oral Poliovirus (OPV) Vaccine     #1

Hepatitis B Virus (HBV) Vaccine     #2
(To be administered at age 1–2 months)

Describe side effects of immunizations and when to call about them.

As part of the complete physical examination, the following should be noted:

Red reflex

Strabismus (eyes should be aligned by this time)

Developmental hip dysplasia

Torticollis

Metatarsus adductus

Cardiac murmurs

Neurologic problems

Abdominal masses

Evidence of neglect or abuse

# ANTICIPATORY GUIDANCE FOR THE FAMILY

In addition to providing anticipatory guidance, many health professionals give families handouts
at an appropriate reading level or a videotape that they can review or study at home.[1]

## Promotion of healthy habits

### Injury and illness prevention

Continue to use an infant car seat that is properly secured
at all times.

Continue to put the baby to sleep on her back or side.

Continue to test the water temperature with your wrist to
make sure it is not hot before bathing the baby.

Never leave the baby alone or with a young sibling or pet.

Do not leave her alone in a tub of water or on high places
such as changing tables, beds, sofas, or chairs. Always keep
one hand on the baby.

Continue to keep the baby's environment free of smoke.
Keep the home and car nonsmoking zones.

Install smoke detectors if not already in place and make sure
they work properly.

Do not drink hot liquids or smoke while holding the baby.

Avoid overexposure to the sun.

Keep toys with small parts or other small or sharp objects
out of reach.

Recognize early signs of illness:

> Fever

> Failure to eat

> Vomiting

> Diarrhea

> Dehydration

> Unusual irritability, lethargy

> Skin rash

Review emergency procedures:

> When to call the health care professional

> When to go to which emergency department

Ask your child care provider what happens when an
emergency occurs in the child care setting.

## Nutrition

Ensure that the infant is gaining enough weight.

If you are breastfeeding: Ensure that breastfeeding is of appropriate frequency and duration. Discuss with the health professional any problems you are having with breastfeeding.

Give the breastfeeding infant 400 I.U.'s of vitamin D daily if she is deeply pigmented or does not receive enough sunlight.

If you are bottlefeeding: Ensure that the infant receives an appropriate amount of iron-fortified formula at the appropriate frequency. Hold the baby in a semisitting position to feed her. Do not use a microwave oven to heat formula.

Delay the introduction of solid foods until the infant is four to six months of age. Do not put cereal in a bottle.

Do not give the infant honey until after her first birthday to prevent infant botulism.

## Oral health

To avoid developing a habit that will harm your infant's teeth, do not put her to bed with a bottle or prop it in her mouth.

## Infant care

Discuss any questions or concerns you have about:

- Skin and nail care: bathing, soaps, lotions, diaper area preparations, detergent
- Colic/crying
- Thumbsucking and pacifiers
- Normal sleep patterns; sleeping arrangements
- Bowel movements
- Thermometer use

## Promotion of parent-infant interaction that is mutually enjoyable and satisfying

Discuss with the health professional the baby's temperament and how you are dealing with it.

Nurture the baby by holding, cuddling, and rocking her, and by talking and singing to her.

Encourage the baby's vocalizations. Talk to her during dressing, bathing, feeding, playing, walking, and driving.

Read to the baby. Play music.

Establish a bedtime routine and other habits to discourage night awakening.

Stimulate your child with age-appropriate toys.

## Promotion of constructive family relationships and parental health

Take some time for yourself and spend some individual time with your partner.

Keep in contact with friends and family members. Avoid social isolation.

Encourage your partner to participate in the care of the infant.

Continue to meet the needs of other children in the family, appropriately engaging them in the care of the baby.

Discuss family planning with your partner. If you decide to have another baby, it will be healthier if there is adequate spacing between your pregnancies, if you maintain an appropriate maternal weight for height, and if you avoid smoking.

## Promotion of community interactions

If you need financial assistance to help pay for health care expenses, ask about resources or for referrals to the state Medicaid programs or other state medical assistance programs.

Ask about resources or referrals for food (e.g., WIC), housing, or transportation if needed.

Learn about and consider attending parent education classes and/or parent-child play groups.

Maintain or expand ties to your community through social, religious, cultural, volunteer, and recreational organizations or resources.

For mother returning to work: Discuss child care arrangements with your health professional, including how to continue breastfeeding. It is also useful to discuss potential role tensions before returning to work.

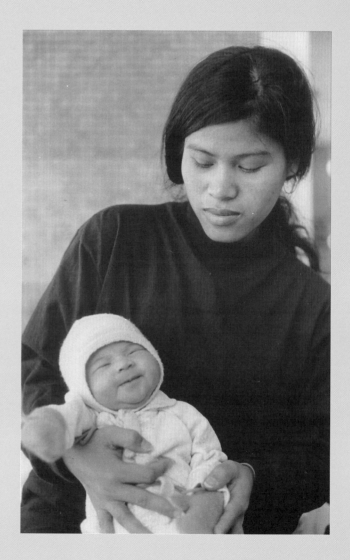

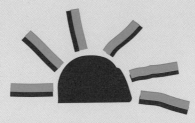

# Only I Can Care for Him

*While the initial general questions do not reveal problems or concerns, Ms. Conforti does admit that she and her husband have not been out by themselves since Tony was born.*

During the two month health supervision visit, Dr. Meyer notices Ms. Conforti's vigilance as she hovers over her baby, Tony, during the physical examination. Though all parents are concerned about their infant, Ms. Conforti seems especially anxious. She has called frequently about "colds" and has brought Tony in for five sick visits. While the initial general questions do not reveal problems or concerns, Ms. Conforti does admit that she and her husband have not been out by themselves since Tony was born. On further questioning, Ms. Conforti states that she has not been away from her baby since his birth. "I just don't feel comfortable leaving my baby with a baby sitter or even with my husband. I'm afraid that whoever I leave Tony with might not know what to do if there's a problem." She acknowledges that she feels worried all the time.

Dr. Meyer remembers that Ms. Conforti had some vaginal bleeding during pregnancy and that Tony was born three weeks early. Dr. Meyer discusses Ms. Conforti's anxious feelings with her. "While you did have vaginal bleeding and Tony was born small, he is now a perfectly healthy child," Dr. Meyer says. "Tony suffered no consequences from any of these problems." He shows her Tony's growth curve, reviews the physical examination with her, and assures her that many parents worry if there was a problem during pregnancy or their child was born premature. At the end of the visit, he suggests, "Ms. Conforti, why don't you bring Tony in for a follow-up visit in two weeks with your husband so we can talk more about your concerns and how you and your husband can best support one another?"

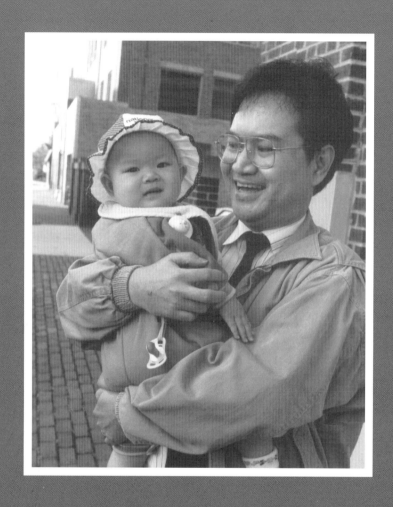

*Most employed mothers will have returned to work
by the time their infant is four months old,
and it is important that child care arrangements work
for the baby and the parents.*

# Four Month Visit

The relationship between parents and their four-month-old infant is pleasurable and fun. The baby's ability to smile, coo, and laugh encourages his parents to talk and play with him. Clear and predictable cues provided by the infant are met by appropriate and predictable responses from his parents and promote mutual trust. During this period, the infant masters early motor, language, and social skills by interacting with those who care for him.

Responding to the sights and sounds around him, the four-month-old baby raises his body from the prone position with his hands and holds his head steady. Often, he may be so interested in his world that he refuses to settle down to eat. He pulls off the breast or bottle after just a few sucks to check out what else is happening in the room. Parents may need to feed him in a quiet, darkened room for the next few weeks.

Over the next two months, the baby will be ready to start eating solid foods. If he sits well when supported, holds his head up, and seems to be hungry, it is time to introduce one new solid food every week or so. The tongue thrust reflex and production of saliva may cause a lot of drooling at this age. Early teethers may also be irritable, though most babies do not get their first teeth until after six months, and some may not do so until after one year.

As key social and motor abilities become apparent at four months, a child who appears delayed may need a formal developmental assessment. The baby who lacks a social smile may suffer from emotional or sensory deprivation. Are the parents interested in and appropriately interactive with their infant? If developmental delays are found, health professionals should determine their etiology and make referrals for early intervention.

Most employed mothers will have returned to work by the time their infant is four months old, and it is important that child care arrangements work for the baby and the parents. Family problems such as inadequate finances, few social supports, or low parental self-esteem may impair parents' ability to nurture. An irritable child who cries frequently or does not sleep through the night will clash temperamentally with the family who values regularity and tranquillity. It is important that parents seek help when feeling sad, discouraged, depressed, overwhelmed, or inadequate. Parents who have the support they need can be warmly rewarded by their interactions with their four-month-old infant.

# HEALTH SUPERVISION INTERVIEW

## TRIGGER QUESTIONS

To be used selectively by the health professional. Discuss any issues or concerns of the family.

How are you?

How are you feeling?

How is your family getting along?

What do you enjoy most about Jackie?

What questions or concerns do you have about Douglas?

What new things is he doing?

Have there been any major stresses or changes in your family since your last visit?

Who helps you out with Eiko?

Is it easy or difficult to tell what Kevin wants or needs?

What have you found to be the best way to comfort Raisha?

How is feeding going? What are you feeding Bobby at this time?

Does Mariah sleep through the night?

Do you think Charles hears all right? Sees all right? Does he turn his head when you walk into the room?

Have you returned to work or school, or do you plan to do so? What are your child care arrangements?

Have you and your partner been getting out without the baby?

# Developmental Surveillance and Milestones

## TRIGGER QUESTIONS AND POSSIBLE RESPONSES

**Do you have any specific concerns about Jerome's development or behavior?**

**How does Jerome communicate what he wants?**

> Demonstrates range of affects (e.g., pleasure, displeasure, sadness)

> Vocalizes (babbles, "dada," "baba")

**What do you think Jerome understands?**

> Recognizes mother's voice

**How can Jerome move his body?**

> Controls head well

> In prone position, holds head erect and raises body on hands

> Sits with support

> Rolls over from prone to supine

> Opens hands and holds own hands

**How does Jerome act around family members?**

> Babbles and coos

> Smiles, laughs, and squeals

> Recognizes parent's voice and touch

> Has spontaneous social smile

**Tell me about Jerome's typical play.**

> Mouths

> Blows bubbles

> Imitates a cough or razzing noises

> Reaches for and bats at objects

> Grasps rattle

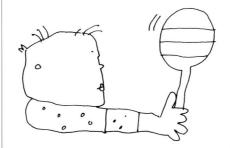

Babbles and coos

Smiles, laughs, and squeals

In prone position, holds head erect and raises body on hands

Rolls over from prone to supine

Opens hands, holds own hands, grasps rattle

Controls head well

Reaches for and bats at objects

Looks at and may become excited by mobile

Recognizes parent's voice and touch

Has spontaneous social smile

May sleep for at least six hours

Able to comfort himself (e.g., fall asleep by himself without breast or bottle)

## Observation of Parent-Infant Interaction

Are the parent and infant interested in and responsive to each other (e.g., gazing, talking, holding, cuddling, and smiling)? How does the parent attend to the baby when he is being examined? How does the parent comfort the baby when he cries?

## Physical Examination

Measure and plot on a standard chart the head circumference, length, weight, and weight for length. Share the information with the parent.

As part of the complete physical examination, the following should be noted:

Red reflex

Developmental hip dysplasia

Cardiac murmurs

Neurologic problems

Evidence of neglect or abuse

**IMMUNIZATIONS**

| | |
|---|---|
| Hemophilus Influenza Type b (Hib) Vaccine[3] | #2 |
| Diphtheria, Tetanus, Pertussis (DTP) Vaccine (Hib and DTP can be combined.[3]) | #2 |
| Oral Poliovirus (OPV) Vaccine | #2 |
| Hepatitis B Virus (HBV) Vaccine (If not administered at age 1–2 months) | #2 |

Describe side effects of immunizations and when to call about them.

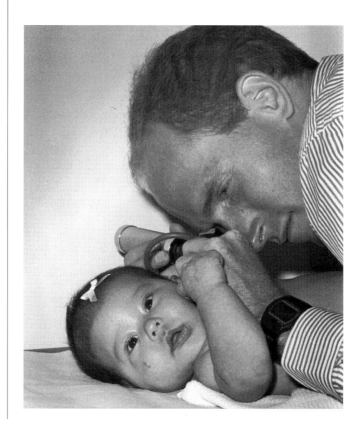

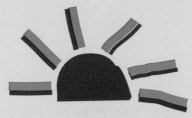

# How Can I Help My Baby?

Dennis Booker was born with Vaeter syndrome, imperforate anus, spina bifida, and esophageal atresia. While his twin brother is normal, Dennis's lower extremities are partially missing and his remaining appendages are dysfunctional. Dennis's family lives in a rural county that has 29,000 residents but no obstetricians, pediatricians, or public health clinics to provide care for mothers and children. Mrs. Booker received her prenatal care through a local family physician.

At birth, Dennis was transferred to a children's hospital 130 miles from his family's home. He had numerous surgeries for his various anomalies, as well as a gastrointestinal tube for feeding. His parents spent most of their time at the hospital being taught how to care for Dennis. Dennis was alert, followed objects, and showed the responses of normally developing infants.

Dennis was discharged from the hospital at about three months of age. Church members, friends, and grandparents help his parents by taking care of the Booker's two year old and Dennis's twin so that Mrs. Booker can focus her attention on Dennis and Mr. Booker can return to work. Because there is no local specialist to provide care for Dennis, repeated trips to the children's hospital are necessary for his medical care and case management. Staff at the children's hospital try to offer basic immunizations, screenings, and other preventive services, but Dennis's other needs take priority.

The county board of mental retardation and developmental disabilities provides Dennis and his family with early intervention services in their home. A local public health nurse, Carla Gomez, visits the home as well. After several visits Mrs. Booker begins to trust Carla. During one home visit, Mrs. Booker says that she is concerned that she is not doing enough to get Dennis to develop as normally as possible. Carla helps her look at the developmental tasks Dennis needs to accomplish and the environmental changes his family should make in order for him to succeed at those tasks.

Carla refers Dennis's family to local agencies for early intervention services, including physical therapy and occupational therapy. In order for the physician at the children's hospital to assess the range of Dennis's skills and determine additional referrals needed, Carla helps the family make videotapes of Dennis mouthing, reaching, getting his hand to his mouth, and attempting to sit. Dennis's parents are shown how to help Dennis meet his oral gratification needs so that he will be able to eat following removal of the gastrointestinal tube. They learn to encourage his vocalizations.

Carla also refers Dennis to the Bureau for Children with Medical Handicaps and assists the family in locating good "technical" child care for Dennis to relieve his parents. Carla helps the family find financial assistance. Through her relationship with the Bookers she is able to provide health supervision.

# ANTICIPATORY GUIDANCE FOR THE FAMILY

In addition to providing anticipatory guidance, many health professionals give families handouts
at an appropriate reading level or a videotape that they can review or study at home.[1]

## Promotion of healthy habits

### Injury and illness prevention

Continue to use an infant car seat that is properly secured at all times.

Continue to test the water temperature with your wrist to make sure it is not hot before bathing the baby.

Never leave the baby alone or with a young sibling or pet.

Do not leave him alone in a tub of water or on high places such as changing tables, beds, sofas, or chairs. Always keep one hand on the baby.

Continue to keep the baby's environment free of smoke. Keep the home and car nonsmoking zones.

Do not drink hot liquids or smoke while holding the baby.

Avoid overexposure to the sun.

Keep toys with small parts or other small or sharp objects out of reach.

Keep all poisonous substances, medicines, cleaning agents, health and beauty aids, and paints and paint solvents locked in a safe place out of the baby's sight and reach.

Keep sharp objects (e.g., scissors, knives) out of reach.

Do not give the infant plastic bags, latex balloons, or small objects such as marbles.

Use safety locks on cabinets.

Do not use an infant walker at any age.

Recognize early signs of illness:

- Fever
- Failure to eat
- Vomiting
- Diarrhea/dehydration
- Unusual irritability, lethargy
- Skin rash
- Reaction to immunization

## Nutrition

Continue to breastfeed or to use iron-fortified formula for the first year of the infant's life. This milk will continue to be his major source of nutrition.

Begin introducing solid foods with a spoon when the infant is four to six months of age. Use a spoon to give him an iron-fortified, single-grain cereal such as rice. If there are no adverse reactions, add a new pureed food to the infant's diet each week, beginning with fruits and vegetables.

Always supervise the infant while he is eating.

Give exclusively breastfeeding infants iron supplements.

Continue to give the breastfeeding infant 400 I.U.'s of vitamin D daily if he is deeply pigmented or does not receive enough sunlight.

Do not give the infant honey until after his first birthday to prevent infant botulism.

Ensure that your caregiver is feeding the infant appropriately.

## Oral health

To protect the infant's teeth, do not put him to bed with a bottle or prop it in his mouth.

## Promotion of parent-infant interaction that is mutually enjoyable and satisfying

Nurture the baby by holding, cuddling, and rocking him, and by talking and singing to him.

Encourage the baby's vocalizations. Talk to him during dressing, bathing, feeding, playing, walking, and driving.

Read to the baby. Play music.

Play social games such as pat-a-cake, peek-a-boo, so-big.

Establish a bedtime routine and other habits to discourage night awakening.

Encourage the baby to learn to console himself by putting him to bed awake.

Begin to help the baby learn self-consoling techniques by providing him with the same transitional object—such as a stuffed animal, blanket, or favorite toy—at bedtime or in new situations.

Encourage play with age-appropriate toys.

Discuss baby sitters and child care arrangements with the health professional.

## Promotion of constructive family relationships and parental health

If mother has returned to work: Discuss child care arrangements and role tensions with the health professional.

Take some time for yourself and spend some individual time with your partner.

Keep in contact with friends and family members. Avoid social isolation.

Encourage your partner to participate in caring for the infant.

Continue to meet the needs of other children in the family, appropriately engaging them in the care of the baby.

## Promotion of community Interactions

If you need financial assistance to help pay for health care expenses, ask about resources or for referrals to the state Medicaid programs or other state medical assistance programs.

Ask about resources or referrals for food (e.g., WIC), housing, or transportation if needed.

Learn about and consider attending parent-child play groups.

Maintain or expand ties to your community through social, religious, cultural, volunteer, and recreational organizations or resources.

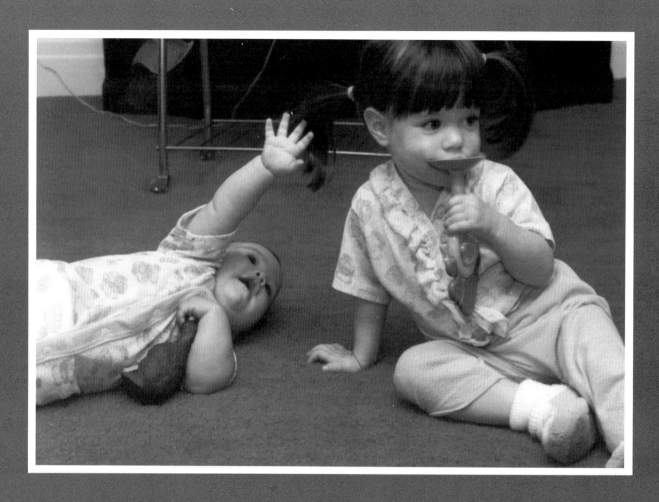

*The major developmental markers of a six month old
are social and emotional. A six-month-old baby
likes to interact with people.*

# Six Month Visit

Parents cherish their interactions with their social six-month-old infant, who smiles and babbles back at them but is still immobile. The feelings of attachment between the parents and their child create a secure emotional bond that will help provide stability to the changing family. The major developmental markers of a six month old are social and emotional.

A six-month-old baby likes to interact with people. She increasingly engages in reciprocal and face-to-face play and often initiates these games. From these reciprocal interactions, she develops a sense of trust and self-efficacy. Her distress is less frequent.

The infant is also starting to discriminate with whom she wants to be sociable. She usually prefers interacting with her parents or other regular caregivers and may be afraid of new people.

The six month old can sit with support and smiles or babbles with a loving adult. She may have a block or toy in hand. As she watches her hands, she can reach for objects such as cubes and grasp them with her fingers and thumbs. She can transfer objects between her hands and obtain small objects by raking with all fingers. She may also mouth, shake, bang, and drop the toy. Language has moved beyond making a razzing noise to single-consonant babbling. The baby often produces long strings of vocalizations in play, usually during interactions with adults. She can recognize her own name. The baby stands with help and enjoys bouncing up and down in the standing position. She likes rocking back and forth on her hands and knees, in preparation for crawling forward or backward.

An infant who tends to lie on her back, show little interest in social interaction, avoid eye contact, smile and vocalize infrequently, and keep her hands in her mouth or held together in a prayerful position is indicating either constitutional problems or a lack of appropriate attention from her parents. She may need more nurturance, increased health supervision, formal developmental assessment, or other interventions.

Over the next few months, as the infant develops an increasing repertoire of motor skills such as rolling and crawling, parents must be vigilant for falls. The expanding world of the infant must be looked at through her eyes to make exploration as safe as possible. The baby will do more sooner than the parents anticipate. Toys must be sturdy and have no small parts that could be aspirated. Baby walkers should never be used at any age. The hazards presented by steps should be countered with safety gates.

# HEALTH SUPERVISION INTERVIEW

## TRIGGER QUESTIONS

To be used selectively by the health professional. Discuss any issues or concerns of the family.

**How are you?**

**How are things going in your family?**

**How is Maria doing?**

**What do you and your partner enjoy most about Ali?**

**What questions or concerns do you have about Alonzo?**

**Have there been any major changes or stresses in your family since your last visit?**

**What are some of Aaron's new achievements?**

**How does Madeline spend her day?**

**Is it easy to tell what Daniel wants?**

**Are you breastfeeding Emma?**
**If not, what type of formula do you use? How often do you feed her?**
**What is the total amount of formula consumed per day?**

**Have you introduced solids? What is Florene eating?**
**Has she had any reactions?**

**Do you think that Consuela hears all right?**
**Does she turn her head when you walk into the room?**

**How are you balancing your roles of partner and parent?**

**Do you have a reliable person to care for your baby when you need to go out?**
**How are your child care arrangements going? Are you satisfied with them?**

**Do you have a gun at home? Do you keep it locked up?**
**Where do you keep the ammunition?**

# Developmental Surveillance and Milestones

## TRIGGER QUESTIONS AND POSSIBLE RESPONSES

**Do you have any specific concerns about Katherine's development or behavior?**

**How does Katherine communicate what she wants?**

> Demonstrates range of affects (e.g., pleasure, displeasure, sadness)
>
> Vocalizes (babbles, "dada," "baba")
>
> Gestures (points, shakes head)

**What do you think Katherine understands?**

> Own name
>
> Names of family members
>
> Simple phrases ("no-no," "bye-bye")

**How does Katherine move?**

> Sits with support
>
> Rolls over
>
> Creeps, scoots on bottom

**How does Katherine act around other people?**

> Smiles, laughs, squeals
>
> Responsive or withdrawn with family members
>
> Outgoing or wary with strangers

**Tell me about Katherine's typical play.**

> Mouths
>
> Blows bubbles
>
> Imitates a cough or razzing noises
>
> Rakes small objects
>
> Shows interest in toys
>
> Shakes, bangs, throws, and drops objects

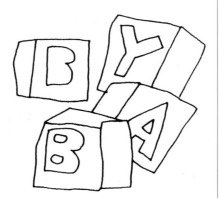

Vocalizes single consonants ("dada," "baba")

Babbles reciprocally

Rolls over

Has no head lag when pulled to sit

Sits with support

Stands when placed and bears weight

Grasps and mouths objects

Shows differential recognition of parents

Starts to self-feed

Transfers cubes or other small objects from hand to hand

Rakes in small objects

Is interested in toys

Self-comforts

Smiles, laughs, squeals, imitates razzing noise

Turns to sounds

May begin to show signs of stranger anxiety

Usually has first tooth erupt around six months of age

**INFANCY • 6 MONTHS**

## Observation of Parent-Infant Interaction

Are the parent and infant interested in and responsive to each other (i.e., displaying mutual gazing, vocal interaction, and interactive playing)? How does the parent attend to the baby when she is being examined? How does the parent comfort the baby when she cries?

## Physical Examination

Measure and plot on a standard chart the head circumference, length, weight, and weight for length. Share the information with the parent.

As part of the complete physical examination, the following should be noted:

Red reflex

Strabismus

Tooth eruption

Developmental hip dysplasia

Problems with tendon reflexes, muscle tone, or use of extremities

Evidence of neglect or abuse

Flat feet, explain the condition to the parent

### ADDITIONAL SCREENING PROCEDURES

Anemia screening
(If certification is needed for WIC)

Assessment of risk of high-dose lead exposure[2]

Lead screening
(At 6 months if infant is high risk or
12 months if low risk)[4]

### IMMUNIZATIONS

| | |
|---|---|
| Hemophilus Influenza Type b (Hib) Vaccine[3] | #3 |
| Diphtheria, Tetanus, Pertussis (DTP) Vaccine (Hib and DTP can be combined)[3] | #3 |
| Oral Poliovirus (OPV) Vaccine[3] | #3 |
| Hepatitis B Virus (HBV) Vaccine (To be administered once at age 6–18 months) | #3 |

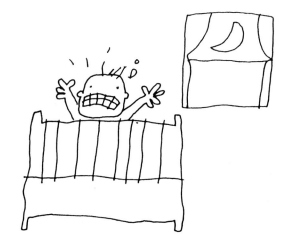

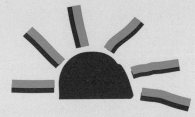

# We Are Exhausted!

*When children reach a period of light sleep and wake up, they may not be able to return to sleep until the same conditions that existed when they fell asleep are present.*

At the six month health supervision visit, Mrs. Leon reports that she and her husband are both exhausted because their daughter Maria awakens four times a night. Mrs. Leon stresses that her marriage is solid and that her husband frequently helps out with household tasks, including taking care of the baby. The parents' sleeplessness, however, has made them short-tempered with each other. Mr. Leon, who is having difficulty doing his job, has begun sleeping in the living room so that he will not be disturbed when Maria awakens during the night.

Dr. Ramirez finds no feeding problems or other behavioral difficulties, and the child's development is normal. Maria is sitting, crawling, and saying consonant sounds. Dr. Ramirez asks about Maria's bedtime ritual. When putting Maria to bed, Mrs. Leon feeds her until she falls asleep and then puts her in the crib.

Dr. Ramirez says to Mrs. Leon, "When children reach a period of light sleep and wake up, they may not be able to return to sleep until the same conditions that existed when they fell asleep are present. So when Maria wakes up, she needs you to hold her until she falls asleep again." Dr. Ramirez tells Mrs. Leon that she should continue to rock, hold, and feed Maria before bed. However, she should put Maria to bed before she falls completely asleep. That way, when Maria reaches a light period of sleep, she will be in the same place where she fell asleep. This association will help her return to sleep. Dr. Ramirez asks that Mrs. Leon call her in a week to let her know how the new strategy worked.

Early the next week Mrs. Leon reports to Dr. Ramirez, "During the first four days there was no change. Then Maria started to sleep longer hours. My husband is no longer sleeping in the living room and we both feel a lot more relaxed." She thanks the doctor for her help and says she will call if Maria has any other sleeping problems before the nine month visit.

# ANTICIPATORY GUIDANCE FOR THE FAMILY

In addition to providing anticipatory guidance, many health professionals give families handouts
at an appropriate reading level or a videotape that they can review or study at home.[1]

## Promotion of healthy habits

### Injury and illness prevention

Get down on the floor and check for hazards at baby's eye level.

Continue to use an infant car seat that is properly secured at all times.

Continue to test the water temperature with your wrist to make sure it is not hot before bathing the baby.

Never leave the baby alone or with a young sibling or pet.

Do not leave her alone in a tub of water or on high places such as changing tables, beds, sofas, or chairs. Always keep one hand on the baby.

Empty buckets, tubs, or small pools immediately after use. Ensure that swimming pools have a four-sided fence with a self-closing, self-latching gate.

Continue to keep the baby's environment free of smoke. Keep the home and car nonsmoking zones.

Do not drink hot liquids or smoke while holding the baby.

Avoid overexposure to the sun.

Do not leave heavy objects or containers of hot liquids on tables with tablecloths that the baby may pull down.

Place plastic plugs in electrical sockets.

Keep toys with small parts or other small or sharp objects out of reach.

Keep sharp objects (e.g., scissors, knives) out of reach.

Keep all poisonous substances, medicines, cleaning agents, health and beauty aids, and paints and paint solvents locked in a safe place out of the baby's sight and reach. Never store poisonous substances in empty jars or soda bottles.

Obtain a one-ounce bottle of Syrup of Ipecac to be kept in the home and used as directed by the poison control center or the health professional. Keep the number of the poison control center near the telephone.

Do not give the infant plastic bags, latex balloons, or small objects such as marbles.

Install safety devices on drawers and cabinets where the infant may play.

Install gates at the top and bottom of stairs, and place safety devices on windows.

Lower the crib mattress.

Avoid dangling electrical and drapery cords.

Keep pet food and dishes out of reach. Do not permit the baby to approach the dog while the dog is eating.

Do not use an infant walker at any age.

Learn first aid and infant cardiopulmonary resuscitation (CPR).

Recognize early signs of illness:

> Fever
>
> Failure to eat
>
> Vomiting
>
> Diarrhea
>
> Dehydration

Unusual irritability, lethargy

Petechiae

Cough

Seizure

Reaction to immunization

## Nutrition

Continue to breastfeed or use iron-fortified formula for the first year of the infant's life. This milk will continue to be her major source of nutrition.

Introduce solid foods. Use a spoon to give the infant an iron-fortified, single-grain cereal such as rice. If there is no adverse reaction, add a new pureed food to the diet each week, starting with fruits and vegetables and then meats. Let the infant indicate when and how much she wants to eat.

Avoid giving the infant foods that may be aspirated or cause choking (e.g., peanuts, popcorn, hot dogs or sausages, carrot sticks, celery sticks, whole grapes, raisins, corn, whole beans, hard candy, large pieces of raw vegetables or fruit, tough meat).

Always supervise the infant while she is eating. Learn emergency procedures for choking.

Serve solid food two or three times per day.

Begin to offer a cup for water or juice.

Limit juice to four to six ounces per day.

Give iron supplements to infants who are exclusively breastfeeding.

Continue to give the breastfeeding infant 400 I.U.'s of vitamin D daily if she is deeply pigmented or does not receive enough sunlight.

Do not give the infant honey until after her first birthday to prevent infant botulism.

Ensure that your caregiver is feeding the infant appropriately.

## Oral health

To protect the infant's teeth, do not put her to bed with a bottle or prop it in her mouth.

Clean the infant's teeth with a soft brush, beginning with the eruption of her first tooth.

Give the infant fluoride supplements as recommended by the health professional based on the level of fluoride in the infant's drinking water.

## Promotion of parent-infant interaction that is mutually enjoyable and satisfying

Encourage the baby's vocalizations. Talk to her during dressing, bathing, feeding, playing, walking, and driving.

Read to the baby. Play music.

Play social games such as pat-a-cake, peek-a-boo, so-big.

Provide opportunities for exploration.

To set limits and discipline the infant at this age, use distraction, stimulus control, proximal physical presence, structure, and routines. Limit the number of rules and consistently enforce them.

Establish a bedtime routine and other habits to discourage night awakening.

Encourage the baby to learn to console herself by putting her to bed awake.

Consistently provide the baby with the same transitional object—such as a stuffed animal, blanket, or favorite toy—so that she can console herself at bedtime or in new situations.

Encourage play with age-appropriate toys.

Discuss with the health professional any problems your child is having with separation anxiety.

## Promotion of constructive family relationships and parental health

Take some time for yourself and spend some individual time with your partner.

Keep in contact with friends and family members. Avoid social isolation.

Continue to meet the needs of other children in the family, appropriately engaging them in the care of the baby.

Discuss with the health professional your child care arrangements and working hours. Also talk about availability of time for close interaction with the infant and about fatigue.

## Promotion of community interactions

If you need financial assistance to help pay for health care expenses, ask about resources or for referrals to the state Medicaid programs or other state medical assistance programs.

Ask about resources or referrals for food (e.g., WIC), housing, or transportation if needed.

Learn about and consider attending parent-child play groups.

Maintain or expand ties to your community through social, religious, cultural, volunteer, and recreational organizations or resources.

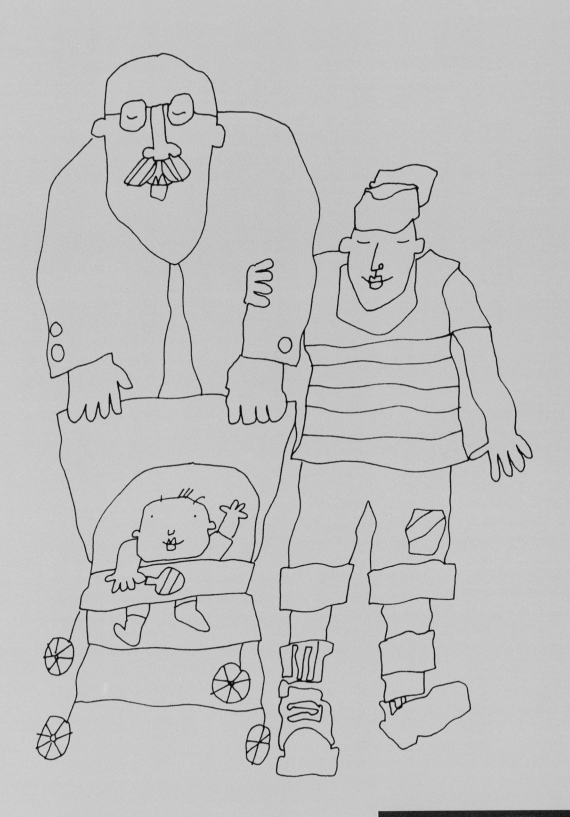

65

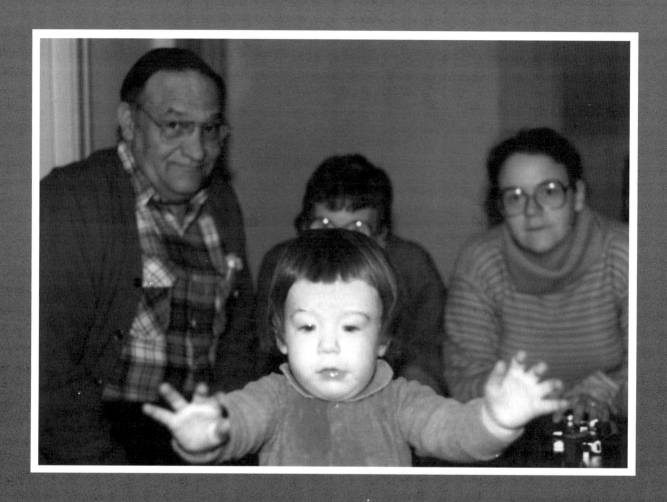

*At the nine month visit,*
*it is important for the health professional to assess*
*the parents' attitudes and ability to cope with*
*the child's separation and protest.*

# Nine Month Visit

The nine month old has made some striking developmental gains, displaying ever-increasing independence. He is more mobile and will express explicit opinions about everything, from the foods he eats to his bedtime. These opinions will often take the form of protests. Also, the baby has gained object permanence. He understands that an object or person—such as a parent—exists in spite of not being visible at the moment. He is not yet confident, however, that the object will reappear.

The nine month old will exhibit many behaviors indicating his insecurity with the world in general. His protests when a parent leaves signal his attachment and his fears. This same insecurity may lead to night awakening. Up until this period, the baby was waking during his normal sleep cycle but usually fell back to sleep. Now when the baby wakens, he realizes that he is in a dark room, without his parents. This realization generally leads to distressed crying, a behavior difficult for parents.

The parents' world has also changed dramatically. The child's increased mobility and protests require the beginnings of limit-setting. The parents must decide when it is important to say no. This requires that they have high self-esteem, responsibility in their role as parents, and a great deal of energy. They may also view the child's growing independence with a sense of loss. No longer content just to be held, cuddled, and coddled, the baby will now wiggle, want to be put down, and crawl away. He will say no in his own way, from closing his mouth and shaking his head when a parent wants to feed him to screaming when he finds himself alone.

Good parenting—which previously meant meeting the basic requirements associated with nurturing, eating, sleeping, and dressing—requires increasingly complex skills. As the baby approaches his first birthday, the parents' own agendas, based in part on the way in which they were reared, will become a significant factor. At the nine month visit, it is important for the health professional to assess the parents' attitudes and ability to cope with the child's separation and protest. The health professional should also provide the parents with some basic skills and resources for making decisions about methods of managing their child's behavior.

# HEALTH SUPERVISION INTERVIEW

## TRIGGER QUESTIONS

To be used selectively by the health professional. Discuss any issues or concerns of the family.

**How are you?**

**How are things going in your family?**

**What questions or concerns do you have today?**

**Tell me about Bradley. What do you find most rewarding about him?**

**What are some of his new achievements?**

**Have there been any major changes or stresses in your family since your last visit?**

**What is Whitney eating?**
**Does she eat anything** (e.g., clay, dirt, paint chips) **that is not food?**

**Does Tomás awaken at night?**

**Do you think that Michael hears all right?**

**Now that Yolanda can move on her own more,**
**what changes have you made in your home to ensure her safety?**

**How does it feel to have Lisa becoming more independent?**

**What are your thoughts about discipline?**

**Do you have some time for yourself?**

**Who do you turn to when you need some help?**

**Do you have child care? How is it going?**

**Does Sara play in a house with peeling or chipping paint?**
**Do you know if the house was built before 1960? Has the house been remodeled recently?**

**Have you heard of lead poisoning? Are any of Sara's siblings or playmates being treated for lead poisoning?**
**Does she have any other exposure to lead?**

**Do you feel safe in your neighborhood?**

# Developmental Surveillance and Milestones

## TRIGGER QUESTIONS AND POSSIBLE RESPONSES

**Do you have any specific concerns about Alan's development or behavior?**

**How does Alan communicate what he wants?**

Vocalizes (babbles, "dada," "mama")

Gestures (points, shakes head)

**What do you think Alan understands?**

Own name

Names of family members

Simple phrases ("no-no," "bye-bye")

**How does Alan move?**

Creeps, scoots on bottom

Crawls

Pulls to stand

Cruises

Walks

**How does Alan act around other people?**

Responsive or withdrawn with family members

Anxious about separation or not

Outgoing or wary with strangers

Plays social games such as peek-a-boo and pat-a-cake

**Tell me about Alan's typical play.**

Mouths

Pokes with index finger

Shakes, bangs, throws, and drops objects

Imitates

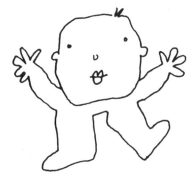

## MILESTONES

Responds to own name

Understands a few words such as "no-no" and "bye-bye"

Babbles, imitates vocalizations

May say "dada" or "mama" nonspecifically

Crawls, creeps, moves forward by scooting on bottom

Sits independently

May pull to stand

Inferior pincer grasp

Pokes with index finger

Shakes, bangs, throws, and drops objects

Plays interactive games such as peek-a-boo and pat-a-cake

Feeds self with fingers

Starts to use cup

Sleeps through the night but may awaken and cry

May show anxiety with strangers

Usually has first tooth erupt around six months of age

# Observation of Parent-Infant Interaction

Are the parent and infant interested in and responsive to each other (i.e., sharing vocalizations, smiles, and facial expressions)? Does the parent respond supportively to the infant's autonomy or independent behavior as long as it is not dangerous?

# Physical Examination

Measure and plot on a standard chart the head circumference, length, weight, and weight for length. Share the information with the parent.

As part of the complete physical examination, the following should be noted:

Red reflex

Strabismus

Tooth eruption

Cardiac murmurs

Developmental hip dysplasia

Neurologic problems

Parachute reflex to check for hemiparesis

Descent of testes

Evidence of neglect or abuse

## ADDITIONAL SCREENING PROCEDURES

Assessment of risk of high-dose lead exposure[2]

Lead screening by 12 months of age[4]

Hematocrit or hemoglobin screening at 9–12 months if any of the following risk factors are present:

Low socioeconomic status

Birthweight under 1,500 grams

Whole milk given before six months of age (Not recommended)

Low-iron formula given (Not recommended)

Tuberculin test (PPD) if any of the following risk factors are present:

Low socioeconomic status

Residence in areas where tuberculosis is prevalent

Exposure to tuberculosis

Immigrant status

## IMMUNIZATIONS

Hepatitis B Virus (HBV) Vaccine     #3
(If not administered at age six months)

Ensure immunization status is up to date

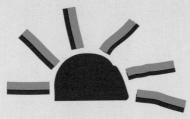

# My Baby Has Become a Handful

Nine-month-old Abby is brought in for health supervision. Her mother, Ms. Barton, has no specific complaints and Abby's past medical history is unremarkable. Abby has a normal physical examination, but her weight for age has dropped from the 40th percentile to the 25th. "I really try to feed Abby, but she can be pretty hardheaded," Ms. Barton admits. Dr. King notices that Ms. Barton seems tired and a little sad. When she questions her further, Ms. Barton replies, "Abby has started waking in the middle of the night. During the day she crawls around and gets into everything. She was so easy before but now I can't seem to keep up with her."

Dr. King discusses Abby's increasing mobility and emerging autonomy. "Try not to worry about it. Many babies her age are hard to feed," Dr. King reassures Ms. Barton.

"It's normal—even healthy—for Abby to get into everything." Dr. King also acknowledges that these behaviors can be difficult for a parent to handle and suggests strategies to manage them. A follow-up visit is scheduled for the next week.

Ms. Barton still seems depressed the next week. She tells Dr. King that her husband, Mr. Robinson, has been working very hard. He really only sees Abby on Sundays and "feels bad about it." His parents, on the other hand, are around constantly. "My husband's mother helps care for Abby, but she is always telling me how to handle her."

Dr. King empathizes with Ms. Barton about her difficult situation. She says, "I don't have a simple solution for you, but I think if we work together on finding you more support, we can make your situation a lot better." She suggests that Mr. Robinson come to as many visits

as possible, provides the family with a booklet on infant development, and refers them to a weekly parent support group that offers child care. Dr. King asks that Ms. Barton call in three weeks. During the call Dr. King asks, "So, are you feeling any better?" Ms. Barton still sounds depressed, so Dr. King refers her for counseling and further evaluation.

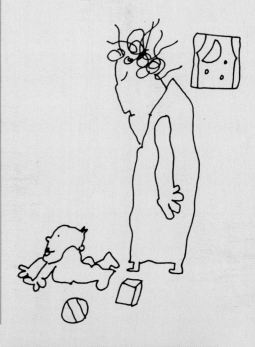

# ANTICIPATORY GUIDANCE FOR THE FAMILY

In addition to providing anticipatory guidance, many health professionals give families handouts
at an appropriate reading level or a videotape that they can review or study at home.[1]

## Promotion of healthy habits

### Injury and illness prevention

Get down on the floor and check for hazards at baby's eye level.

Continue to use an infant car seat until the child is one year of age.

Continue to test the water temperature with your wrist to make sure it is not hot before bathing the baby.

Never leave the baby alone or with a young sibling or pet.

Do not leave him alone in a tub of water or on high places such as changing tables, beds, sofas, or chairs. Always keep one hand on the baby.

Continue to empty buckets, tubs, or small pools immediately after use. Ensure that swimming pools have a four-sided fence with a self-closing, self-latching gate.

Continue to keep the baby's environment free of smoke. Keep the home and car nonsmoking zones.

Do not drink hot liquids or smoke while holding the baby.

Avoid overexposure to the sun.

Do not leave heavy objects or containers of hot liquids on tables with tablecloths that the baby may pull down.

Place plastic plugs in electrical sockets.

Keep toys with small parts or other small or sharp objects out of reach.

Keep sharp objects (e.g., scissors, knives) out of reach.

Keep all poisonous substances, medicines, cleaning agents, health and beauty aids, and paints and paint solvents locked in a safe place out of the baby's sight and reach. Never store poisonous substances in empty jars or soda bottles.

Keep Syrup of Ipecac in the home to be used as directed by the poison control center or the health professional. Keep the number of the poison control center near the telephone.

Do not give the infant plastic bags, latex balloons, or small objects such as marbles.

Install safety devices on drawers and cabinets where the infant may play.

Install gates at the top and bottom of stairs, and place safety devices on windows.

Lower the crib mattress.

Avoid dangling electrical and drapery cords. Ensure that appliances are inaccessible.

Keep pet food and dishes out of reach. Do not permit the baby to approach the dog while the dog is eating.

Do not use an infant walker at any age.

Learn child cardiopulmonary resuscitation (CPR).

Recognize early signs of illness:

> Fever
>
> Failure to eat
>
> Vomiting
>
> Diarrhea
>
> Dehydration
>
> Unusual irritability, lethargy
>
> Petechiae
>
> Cough
>
> Seizure

## Nutrition

Start giving the infant table foods in order to increase the texture and variety of foods in his diet.

Encourage finger foods and mashed foods as appropriate.

Avoid giving the infant foods that may be aspirated or cause choking (e.g., peanuts, popcorn, hot dogs or sausages, carrot or celery sticks, whole grapes, raisins, corn, whole beans, hard candy, large pieces of raw vegetables or fruit, or tough meat).

Closely supervise the infant while he is eating.

Continue teaching the infant how to drink from a cup.

Continue to breastfeed or use iron-fortified formula for the first year of the infant's life.

Continue to give the breastfeeding infant 400 I.U.'s of vitamin D daily if he is deeply pigmented or does not receive enough sunlight.

Continue to give iron supplements to infants who are exclusively breastfed.

Do not give the infant honey until after his first birthday to prevent infant botulism.

## Oral health

To protect the infant's teeth, do not put him to bed with a bottle or prop it in his mouth.

Clean the infant's teeth with a soft brush.

Give the infant fluoride supplements as recommended by the health professional based on the level of fluoride in the infant's drinking water.

## Promotion of parent-infant interaction that is mutually enjoyable and satisfying

Discuss with the health professional the baby's temperament and how the family is adapting to it.

Encourage the baby's vocalizations. Talk to him during dressing, bathing, feeding, playing, walking, and driving.

Play social games such as pat-a-cake, peek-a-boo, and so-big.

Provide opportunities for exploration.

To set limits and discipline the infant at this age, use distraction, stimulus control, proximal physical presence, structure, and routines. Limit the number of rules and consistently enforce them.

Establish a bedtime routine and other habits to discourage night awakening.

Encourage the baby to learn to console himself by putting him to bed awake.

Consistently provide the baby with the same transitional object—such as a stuffed animal, blanket, or favorite toy—so that he can console himself at bedtime or in new situations.

## Promotion of constructive family relationships and parental health

Take some time for yourself and spend some individual time with your partner.

Encourage your partner's involvement in health supervision visits and infant care.

Keep in contact with friends and family members. Avoid social isolation.

Continue to meet the developmental needs of other children in the family, appropriately engaging them in the care of the baby.

Discuss with the health professional child care arrangements and working hours. Also talk about availability of time for close interaction with the infant and about fatigue.

## Promotion of community interactions

If you need financial assistance to help pay for health care expenses, ask about resources or for referrals to the state Medicaid programs or other state medical assistance programs.

Ask about resources or referrals for food (e.g., WIC), housing, or transportation if needed.

Learn about and consider attending parent-child play groups.

Maintain or expand ties to your community through social, religious, cultural, volunteer, and recreational organizations or resources.

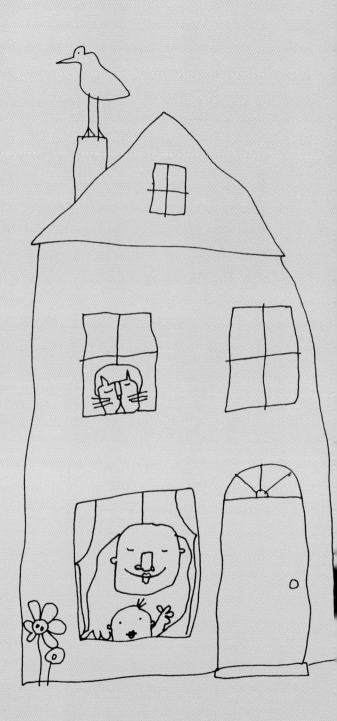

# INFANCY HEALTH SUPERVISION SUMMARY

## What else should we talk about?

### Summarize findings of the visit

Emphasize strengths. Underscore the infant's achievements and progress in development, the increasing competence of the parents, and how well they are all doing. Compliment the parents on their efforts to care for the baby and on their ability to recognize and respond to the baby's needs. Give them suggestions, reading materials, and resources to promote health and reinforce good health practices.

### Arrange continuing care

### Next visit

Give the parents materials to prepare them for the next health supervision visit.

Recommend that the parents make an appointment for the next regularly scheduled visit.

If indicated, ask the parents to make an appointment for a supplementary health supervision visit.

### Other care

Ensure that the parents make an appointment to return to the health facility for follow-up on problems identified during the health supervision visit, or refer the infant for secondary or tertiary medical care.

Refer the family to appropriate community resources for help with problems identified during the visit (e.g., parenting classes, parent-infant groups, marital or financial counseling, mental health services, early intervention programs, adult education programs). Make arrangements to follow up on referrals and coordinate care.

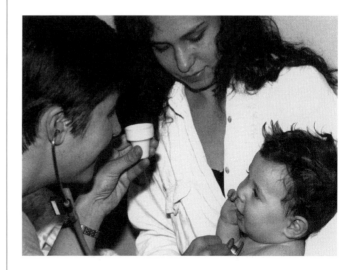

## Infancy Endnotes

1. The Injury Prevention Program (TIPP) of the American Academy of Pediatrics produces parent information sheets that highlight injury prevention priorities at each age, as well as parent information sheets on specific issues such as water safety. Community-based prevention groups, such as SAFE KIDS, also produce injury prevention materials.

2. To assess the risk of high-dose lead exposure, ask:

   Does your child live in or regularly visit a house (or a preschool or child care center) built before 1960? Does it have peeling or chipping paint? Has there been recent or planned renovation or remodeling?

   Does your home's plumbing have lead pipes or copper with lead solder joints?

   Does your child live near a heavily travelled major highway where soil and dust may be contaminated with lead?

   Does your child frequently come in contact with an adult who works with lead (e.g., in construction, welding, pottery, or other trades)?

   Does your child live near a lead smelter, battery recycling plant, or other industrial site likely to release lead?

   Do you give your child any home remedies that may contain lead?

   Have any of your children or any of their playmates had lead poisoning?

   If all answers are negative, screen the child for lead at one and two years of age.

   If any answer is positive, the child is considered at high risk for high-dose lead exposure. Administer a blood lead screening test immediately and at every health supervision visit through six years of age.

   If any blood test result is ≥10 µg/dL, the health professional should refer to the Centers for Disease Control and Prevention (CDC) guidelines and develop a management/treatment plan. (The CDC guidelines are subject to change, so consult the latest edition.) See appendix E, page 264 for lead toxicity screening for Medicaid-eligible children.

   US Department of Health and Human Services, Public Health Service, Centers for Disease Control. 1991. Preventing lead poisoning in young children: A statement by the Centers for Disease Control—October 1991. N.p.: Centers for Disease Control.

3. The American Academy of Pediatrics recommends the following schedule for Hemophilus influenza type b (Hib) vaccine and diphtheria, tetanus, pertussis (DTP) vaccine for children younger than 15 months of age:

   > HbOC (HIBTITER™) or PRP-T vaccine at 2, 4, 6, and 12–15 months; or

   > PRP-OMP (PedvaxHIB®) vaccine at 2, 4, 6, and 12–15 months; or

   > HbOC-DTP combination vaccine at 2, 4, 6, and 15 months. *As an option for the 15 month booster, acellular (DTap) vaccine may also be used in conjunction with any Hib conjugate.*

   The Advisory Committee on Immunization Practices (ACIP) recommends that the third dose of oral poliovirus vaccine be given at 6 months instead of 15–18 months.

   See the AAP Recommended Immunization Schedule and the Recommendations of the Advisory Committee on Immunization Practices in the appendix.

4. A blood lead test must be used to screen Medicaid-eligible children for lead poisoning. See appendix E, page 264.

# Bibliography

American Academy of Pediatrics, Committee on Genetics. 1992. Issues in newborn screening. *Pediatrics* 89(2):345–349.

American Academy of Pediatrics, Committee on Nutrition. 1992. The use of whole cow's milk in infancy. *Pediatrics* 89(6):1105–1109.

American Academy of Pediatrics, Task Force on Infant Positioning and SIDS. 1992. Positioning and SIDS. *Pediatrics* 89(6):1120–1126.

Bell TA, Grayston T, Krohn MA, Kronmal RA, The Eye Prophylaxis Study Group. 1993. Randomized trial of silver nitrate, erythromycin, and no eye prophylaxis for the prevention of conjunctivitis among newborns not at risk for gonoccal ophthalmitis. *Pediatrics* 92(6):755–760.

Brazelton TB. 1969. *Infants and Mothers: Differences in Development*. New York: Dell Publishing.

Brooks-Gunn J, Liaw F, Klebanov PK. 1992. Effects of early intervention on cognitive function of low birth weight preterm infants. *Journal of Pediatrics* 120(3):350–359.

Canadian Task Force on the Periodic Health Examination. 1990. Periodic health examination, 1990 update: 4. Well-baby care in the first 2 years of life. *Canadian Medical Association Journal* 143(9):18–23.

Casey PH, Whitt JK. 1980. Effect of the pediatrician on the mother-infant relationship. *Pediatrics* 65(4):815–820.

Chilmonczyk BA, Knight GJ, Palomaki GE, Pulkkinen AJ, Williams J, Haddow JE. 1990. Environmental tobacco smoke exposure during infancy. *American Journal of Public Health* 80(10):1205–1208.

Clayton EW. 1992. Issues in state newborn screening programs. *Pediatrics* 90(4): 641–645.

Eisenberg A, Murkoff HE, Hathaway SE. 1989. *What to Expect the First Year*. New York: Workman Publishing.

Fomon SJ, ed. 1993. *Nutrition of Normal Infants*. St. Louis, MO: Mosby-Year Book.

Frankowski BL, Weaver SO, Secker-Walker RH. 1993. Advising parents to stop smoking: Pediatricians' and parents' attitudes. *Pediatrics* 91(2):296–300.

Freed GL. 1993. Breast-feeding: Time to teach what we preach. *Journal of the American Medical Association* 269(2):243–245.

Green M. 1993. Maternal depression: Bad for children's health. *Contemporary Pediatrics* 10:28–36.

Hamburg DA. 1990. *A Decent Start: Promoting Healthy Child Development in the First Three Years of Life*. New York: Carnegie Corporation of New York.

Kemper KJ, Avner ED. 1992. The case against screening urinalyses for asymptomatic bacteriuria in children. *American Journal of Diseases in Children* 146:343–346.

Kirby RS, Swanson ME, Kelleher KJ, Bradley RH, Casey PH. 1993. Identifying at-risk children for early intervention services: Lessons from the infant health and development program. *Journal of Pediatrics* 122(5):680–686.

Leventhal JM, Garber RB, Brady CA. 1989. Identification during the postpartum period of infants who are at high risk of child maltreatment. *Journal of Pediatrics* 114(3):481–487.

Meyer EC, Garcia Coll CT, Lester BM, Zachariah Boukydis CF, McDonough SM, Oh W. 1994. Family-based intervention improves maternal psychological well-being and feeding interaction of preterm infants. *Pediatrics* 93(2):241–246.

Miller AR, Barr RG, Eaton WO. 1993. Crying and motor behavior of six-week-old infants and postpartum maternal mood. *Pediatrics* 92(4):551–558.

Nowak A. 1993. What pediatricians can do to promote oral health. *Contemporary Pediatrics* 10: 90–106.

Olds DL, Kitzman H. 1990. Can home visitation improve the health of women and children at environmental risk? *Pediatrics* 86(1):108–116.

Olds DL, Henderson CR, Chamberlin R, Tatelbaum R. 1986. Preventing child abuse and neglect: A randomized trial of nurse home visitation. *Pediatrics* 78(1):65–77.

Orr ST, James SA, Burns BJ, Thompson B. 1989. Chronic stressors and maternal depression: Implications for prevention. *American Journal of Public Health* 79(9):1295–1296.

Ramey CT, Bryant DM, Wasik BH, Sparling JJ, Fendt KH, LaVange LM. 1992. Infant health and development program for low birth weight, premature infants: Program elements, family participation, and child intelligence. *Pediatrics* 89(3):454–465.

Serwint JR, Wilson MH, Duggan AK, Mellits ED, Baumgardner RA, DeAngelis C. 1991. Do postpartum nursery visits by the primary care provider make a difference? *Pediatrics* 88(3):444–449.

Shonkoff JP, Houser-Cram P, Krauss MW, Upshur CC. 1992. Development of infants with disabilities and their families: Implications for theory and service delivery. *Monographs of the Society for Research in Child Development* 57(6, Serial No. 230). Chicago, IL: University of Chicago Press.

Sullivan SA, Birch LL. 1994. Infant dietary experience and acceptance of solid foods. *Pediatrics* 93(2):271–277.

UNICEF. 1990. *Innocenti Declaration on the Protection, Promotion and Support of Breastfeeding.* New York: UNICEF.

Walker D, Gugenheim S, Down MP, Northern JL. 1989. Early language milestone scale and language screening of young children. *Pediatrics* 83(2):284–288.

Zero to Three/National Center for Clinical Infant Programs. 1992. *Heart Start: The Emotional Foundations of School Readiness.* Arlington, VA: Zero to Three/National Center for Clinical Infant Programs.

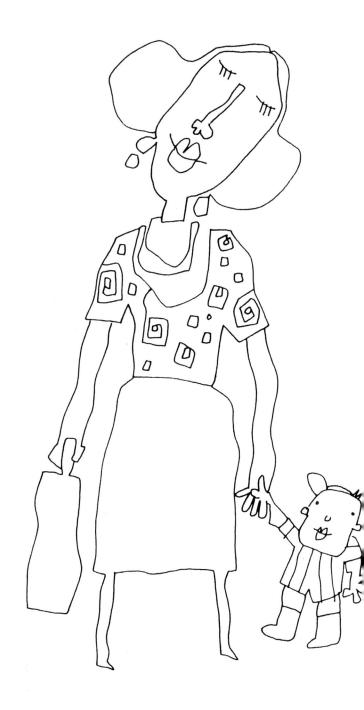

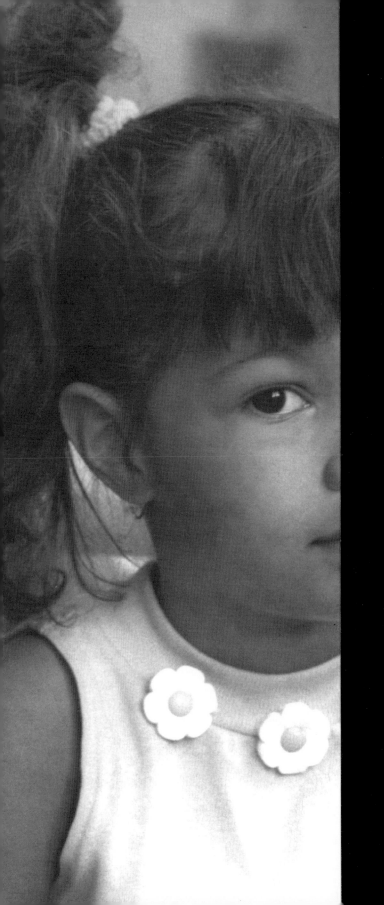

1–5 Years

Early Childhood

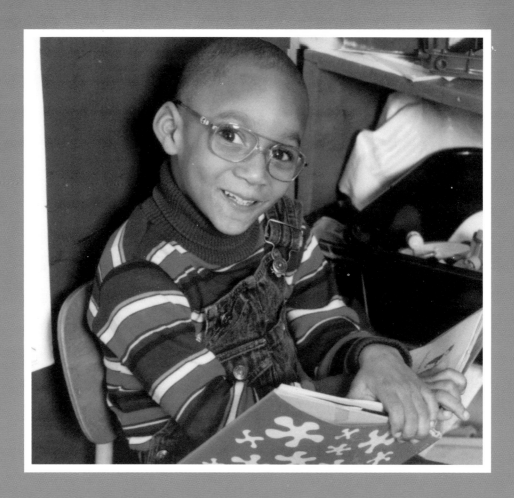

*You can't educate a child who isn't healthy and you can't keep a child healthy who isn't educated.*

—M. Joycelyn Elders, M.D.
Surgeon General
United States Public Health Service

# Early Childhood

The one year old who is well cared for has a secure sense of attachment to his important caregivers, is developing an expanded capacity to communicate through sounds and gestures, and can navigate by cruising, perhaps by taking a few steps alone or, if necessary, by dropping to all fours and crawling with great speed.

At the beginning of this developmental period, a child's understanding of the world of people and objects is bound by what he can see, hear, feel, and manipulate physically. By the end of early childhood, the process of thinking moves beyond "the here and now" to incorporate the use of mental symbols and the development of fantasy. For the infant, mobility is a goal to be mastered. For the healthy young child, it is a mechanism for exploration and increasing independence. The one year old is beginning to use the art of imitation in his repetition of familiar sounds and physical gestures. The five year old has mastered most of the complex rules of his native language, and can communicate thoughts and ideas effectively.

The toddler stands on the threshold of the process of separation and individuation from his primary caregivers, who nurtured and protected him during his early months. By the end of early childhood, the well-adjusted child, having internalized the security of early bonds, pursues new relationships outside of the family as an individual in his own right. Understanding and respecting this evolving independence is an important parental challenge.

The healthy toddler has been immunized against diphtheria, tetanus, pertussis, polio, measles, mumps, rubella, Hemophilus influenza type B, and hepatitis B.

His growth and development have been monitored, and adequate nutrition has been ensured through dietary supervision and supplemental vitamins, fluoride, and iron when necessary. By the end of early childhood, some children have had to contend with significant disease or disability, and virtually all have experienced the common nonpreventable early childhood illnesses. As a consequence, each child learns the difference between health/well-being and illness/discomfort.

## Physical

The chubby, pot-bellied infant who tripled his birthweight in the first year of life slows his rate of gain significantly. The active toddler sheds his baby fat and straightens his posture. His physical strength, coordination, and dexterity all improve dramatically. The cautious and tentative walker becomes the reckless runner, climber, and jumper. As a fearless and tireless explorer and experimenter, the toddler is vulnerable to injury, but appropriate adult supervision can ensure an environment that balances safety with the freedom to take controlled risks.

The range of physical abilities among young children during this age period is considerable. Some are endowed with natural grace and agility; others demonstrate less "fine tuning" in their physical prowess, yet they "get the job done."

Parents and other caregivers can encourage young children's independence in eating by serving a nutritionally well-balanced selection of foods and allowing children to choose what and how much to eat. Good oral health is a part of the child's well-being. Early counseling on feeding practice is the essential first step. Regular dental visits, access to fluoride, and healthy

81

nutrition and snacking practices can lead to the prevention of dental decay.

Although parents and other primary caregivers, including providers of child care services, have considerable control over the environment in which a young child is raised, the community also plays an important role. Children with access to safe play areas in a neighborhood free of violence have opportunities for the protected risk taking that is important during this developmental period. For those who grow up in the presence of physical and emotional dangers, the risk for harm is high.

## Cognitive/linguistic

Young children learn through play. If the toddler experienced the security of a nurturing and reliable source of protection and attachment during infancy, he now has a strong base from which to explore the world. The egocentricity of the young child is related less to a sense of selfishness than to a cognitive inability to see things from the perspective of others.

Young children live largely in a world of magic in which they often have difficulty differentiating what is real from what is make-believe. Some have imaginary friends. Many engage in elaborate fantasy play. Learning to identify the boundaries between fantasy and reality, and developing an elementary ability to think logically, are among the more important developmental tasks of this age period.

Caregivers need to provide a safe "laboratory" for these "young scientists" to conduct their "research." Children need access to a variety of tools and experiences. They need opportunities to learn through trial and error, as well as through planned effort. Their seemingly endless string of repetitive questions can test the limits of the most patient parent. These queries, however, must be acknowledged and responded to in a manner that not only provides answers but also validates and reinforces the child's burgeoning curiosity.

## Social/emotional/behavioral

During the dynamic years from age one to five, children develop an emerging sense of themselves as individuals who live in families, as well as within larger social systems. Building on the secure and trusting relationships established in the first year of life, and venturing beyond the parallel play of toddlers, the maturing young child establishes an expanding network of friends and acquaintances.

The culture of the family and that of the community provide a framework within which the socialization process unfolds. The increasingly self-conscious young child grapples with such complex issues as gender roles, peer and/or sibling competition, and the difference between right and wrong. The temperamental differences that were manifested in the feeding, sleeping, and self-regulatory behaviors of the infant are transformed into the varied styles of coping and adaptation demonstrated by the young child. Some young children appear to think before they act; others are impetuous. Some children are slow to warm up while others operate on a very short fuse. Some accept limits and rules with more equanimity than others. The range of "normal" behavior is broad and highly dependent upon the match between the child's and the caregiver's styles. Aggression, acting out, excessive risk taking, and antisocial behaviors are common. Caregivers need to respond with a variety of interventions that set constructive limits and help children achieve self-discipline. Ultimately, healthy social and emotional development depend on how children view themselves and the extent to which they feel valued by others.

## Health behavior

As young children identify with their parents, caregivers, and other important role models, they internalize a wide range of lifestyle attributes. They can benefit from the exhilaration of regular physical exercise and the joy of laughter shared with family and friends. Meals may be a pleasurable opportunity for nutrition and social interaction, or the focus of family conflict amidst the hurried ingestion of high-fat snacks. Well-monitored, selective television viewing may be an appropriate form of education and entertainment; conversely, television can be a constant source of passive diversion, background noise, and exposure to violence.

When faced with adversity or stress, young children may be taught both healthy and unhealthy coping strategies, ranging from denial or retreat to active mastery. During a period when the power of role models and the process of identification are strong, young children incorporate salient features of the lifestyles of those who are most important in their lives. Good health supervision, a collaborative process that involves parents and professionals, can serve as a significant protective factor. In addition, health supervision can contribute to individual autonomy and a growing sense of personal competence and mastery, while enhancing positive interpersonal interactions and the development of rich human relationships.

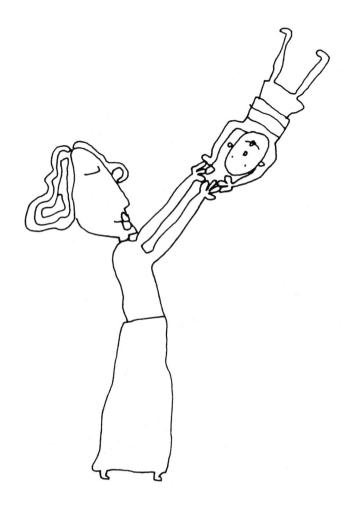

83

# EARLY CHILDHOOD DEVELOPMENTAL CHART

Health professionals should assess the achievements of the child and provide guidance to the family on anticipated tasks.
The effects are demonstrated by health supervision outcomes.

## ACHIEVEMENTS DURING EARLY CHILDHOOD

Regular sleeping habits

Independence in eating

Completion of toilet training

Ability to dress and undress

Ability to separate from parents

Progression from parallel to interactive play and sharing

Warm relationship and good communication with parents and siblings

Clear communication of needs and wishes

Expression of feelings such as joy, anger, sadness, and frustration

Self-comforting behavior

Self-discipline

Intelligible speech

Positive self-image

Demonstrates curiosity and initiative

Asks frequent questions

Demonstrates imaginative, make-believe, and dress-up play

## TASKS FOR THE CHILD

Learn good eating habits

Practice good dental hygiene

Participate in physical games and play

Develop autonomy, independence, and assertiveness

Respond to limit-setting and discipline

Learn self-quieting behaviors and self-discipline

Learn appropriate self-care

Make friends and meet new people

Play with and relate well to siblings and peers

Learn to understand and use language to meet needs

Listen to stories

Limit television viewing

## HEALTH SUPERVISION OUTCOMES

Early autonomy

Optimal nutrition

Satisfactory growth and development

Establishment of good health habits

Injury prevention

Immunizations

School readiness

Promotion of developmental potential

Prevention of behavioral problems

Promotion of family strengths

Enhancement of parental effectiveness

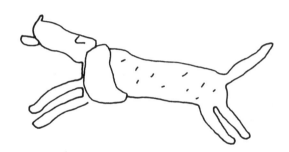

# FAMILY PREPARATION FOR EARLY CHILDHOOD HEALTH SUPERVISION

Instructions to be provided to the family by the health professional.

Be prepared to give updates on the following at your next visit:

> Illnesses and infectious diseases
> Injuries
> Visits to other health facilities or providers
> Use of the emergency department
> Hospitalizations or surgeries
> Immunizations
> Food and drug allergies
> Eating habits
> Medications
> Supplementary fluoride and vitamins
> Dental care
> Vision and hearing
> Chronic health conditions

Update your child's personal health record.

Be prepared to provide the following information on your family:

> Health of and location of each significant family member
>
> Genetic disorders
>
> Depression or other mental health problems in the immediate or extended family
>
> Alcoholism or other substance abuse (including use of tobacco) in the immediate or extended family
>
> Family transitions (e.g., birth, death, marriage, divorce, loss of income, move, frequently absent parent, incarceration, change in child care arrangements)

> Home environment/pets/neighborhood
>
> Hazardous exposures (e.g., violence, lead, asbestos, tuberculosis)

Prepare and bring in questions, concerns, and observations about issues such as:

> Child care arrangements
>
> Chronic health problems (ear infections, frequent colds)
>
> Developmental concerns (delayed language acquisition, poor physical skills)
>
> Discipline issues (limit-setting, tantrums)
>
> Achievements

Talk to the child's other caregivers and family members about any issues they might want you to raise with the health professional.

Bring in reports from preschool or child care. Bring the Individualized Family Service Plan (IFSP) or the Individualized Education Program (IEP) if the child has special needs.

Complete and bring in psychosocial or developmental questionnaires such as the Home Observation Measurement of the Environment (HOME).

Fill out and bring in preschool health forms for completion by the health professional.

Talk to your child about the visit with the health professional, including the physical exam, immunizations, and other procedures.

# STRENGTHS DURING EARLY CHILDHOOD

Health professionals should remind families of their strengths during the health supervision visit.
Strengths and issues for child, family, and community are interrelated and interdependent.

## CHILD

Has good physical health and nutritional status

Has good appetite

Has good sleeping habits

Has regular dental care

Engages in physical activities with vigor

Has positive, cheerful, friendly temperament

Feels parents' unconditional love

Trusts parents

Relates warmly to and communicates well with parents

Is developing social competence

Has had some joyful experiences

Accepts limits

Has good attention span

Has normal cognitive ability

Asks questions

Demonstrates curiosity and initiative

Plays with toys

Achieves developmental milestones

## FAMILY

Meets basic needs (food, shelter, clothing, health care)

Provides a safe, childproof environment (e.g., smoke detectors, car seats)

Enjoys child

Responds to child's developmental needs

Encourages speech and reacts to child

Spends individual time with child

Praises and takes pride in child's achievements

Is consistent in relationship with and expectations from child

Offers emotional support and comfort

Possesses working knowledge of child health and development

Encourages exploration and emerging independence

Uses appropriate disciplinary measures

Offers child choices when appropriate

Provides good role model

Siblings get along well

Has support of extended family and others

Parents pursue additional education or career advancement

## COMMUNITY

Provides preschools and public libraries

Provides quality schools and educational opportunities for all families

Provides parent education classes

Provides support for families with special needs (e.g., WIC, early intervention programs, Head Start, community outreach)

Provides affordable, high-quality child care

Provides an environment free of hazards (violence, pollution, lead, asbestos, radiation)

Ensures that neighborhoods are safe

Provides affordable housing and public transportation

Develops integrated systems of health care

Fluoridates drinking water

Promotes community interactions (neighborhood watch programs, support groups, community centers)

Promotes positive ethnic/cultural milieu

# ISSUES DURING EARLY CHILDHOOD

Health professionals should address issues—problems, stressors, and concerns—that families raise during health supervision. Strengths and issues for child, family, and community are interrelated and interdependent.

## CHILD

Sleeping concerns (resistance to going to bed, night awakening, sleeping with bottle, nightmares, and night terrors)

Eating concerns (decreased appetite, "picky" eating, food jags, pica)

Behavioral concerns (distractibility, lack of control, demanding or aggressive behavior, biting, hitting, temper tantrums, breath-holding spells, impulsiveness)

Emotional concerns (shyness, fears, separation problems and anxiety)

Speech or language concerns (speech delay, unintelligibility, dysfluency)

Autism

Undersocialization; few or poor peer relationships

Infections, illnesses

Baby bottle tooth decay

Lead poisoning

Iron deficiency anemia

Chronic illness

Developmental delay

## FAMILY

Dysfunctional parents or other family members (depressed, mentally ill, abusive, disinterested, overly critical, overprotective, incarcerated)

Marital problems

Domestic violence (verbal, physical, or sexual abuse)

Frequently absent parent

Rotating "parents" (parents' girlfriends or boyfriends)

Inadequate child care arrangements

Family health problems (illness, chronic illness, or disability)

Substance use (alcohol, drugs, tobacco)

Financial insecurity/homelessness

Family transitions (move, births, divorce, remarriage, incarceration, death)

Lack of knowledge about child development

Lack of parenting skills, parental self-esteem, or self-efficacy

Intrusive family members

Social isolation and lack of support

Neglect or rejection of child

## COMMUNITY

Poverty

Inadequate housing

Environmental hazards (e.g., lead)

Unsafe neighborhood

Community violence

Poor opportunities for employment

Lack of affordable, high-quality child care and preschool programs

Lack of programs for families with special needs (early intervention, Head Start)

Lack of social support

Isolation in a rural community

Lack of educational programs and social services for adolescent parents

Lack of social, educational, cultural, and recreational opportunities

Discrimination and prejudice

Lack of access to medical/dental services

Inadequate public services (transportation, garbage removal, lighting, repair of public facilities, police and fire protection)

Inadequate fluoride levels in community drinking water

**EARLY CHILDHOOD • 1–5 YEARS**

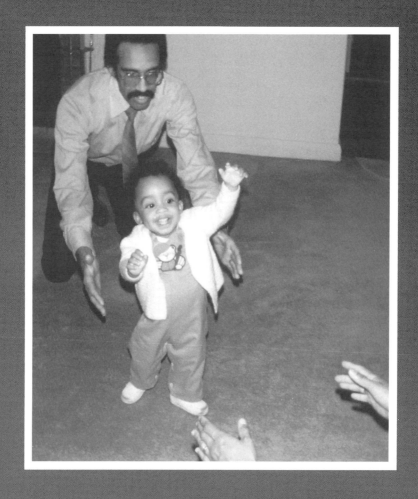

*Walking, one of the most exciting developmental milestones,
occurs near the toddler's first birthday, bringing with it
autonomy and independence.*

# One Year Visit

The one year old stands proudly, feet a bit apart, somewhat bowlegged, her belly protruding. Walking, one of the most exciting developmental milestones, occurs near the toddler's first birthday, bringing with it autonomy and independence. During her first year of life, she was rarely in conflict with her environment. She might have been demanding when she cried, and she required considerable care to be kept comfortable, safe, well-fed, and clean. At times, she might have upset the balance in the family and required parental adaptation. However, she spent most of her first year getting to know and trust her parents and her environment. Now, as a toddler, she is becoming increasingly competent in all areas of development. Her world is broadening, bringing both excitement and challenges.

Autonomy and independent locomotion are developmental achievements of which the parents and toddler are justifiably proud, but the toddler constantly encounters barriers posed by reality. She cannot go as fast as she would like without tripping; she cannot always reach desired objects; and she falls and hurts herself. While charmed by her exploits, her parents must watch her constantly to keep her safe.

As the toddler's autonomy, independence, and cognitive abilities grow, she begins to exert her own will. In response, her parents' perceptions of her demands change dramatically, influenced by their own upbringing and childhood experiences. Do the parents understand the toddler's needs and attempt to meet them? Do the parents perceive their child's attempts to manipulate her environment as a threat to their authority? The one year old's dramatic struggle for autonomy will test her parents' ability to let go, permit independence, and enjoy aspects of her behavior that are out of their direct control. The toddler's messy attempts to self-feed may be difficult for her parents as they sort out their own need to control or their desire for order and neatness. The fact that the toddler may develop a resistance to going to bed or staying there adds to the challenge.

Responding sensitively to the one year old's behavior is a complex challenge. Some parents who did well with the more passive younger infant may be less sure of their role now. Parents who exhibit a "parenting presence" accommodate the demands of the child while maintaining their own authority. They must have a full measure of patience, enough self-confidence to set limits, the judgment to know which needs are most imperative, and an ability not to interpret the child's negative behavior as being directed against them. They need to act as positive role models—for example, by consistently wearing seat belts. Parents who try to enjoy the toddler's independence can best provide a stable home base as her curiosity and mobility carry her into an expanding world.

# HEALTH SUPERVISION INTERVIEW

## TRIGGER QUESTIONS

To be used selectively by the health professional. Discuss any issues or concerns of the family.

How are you?

How are things going in your family?

What questions or concerns do you have about Darren today?

What are some of the things you enjoy most about Tom?

What new things is Jung doing?

Have there been any major changes or stresses in your family since your last visit?

What is Paula eating now?

Does Fei sleep through the night?

How does Rebecca's father help take care of her?

Who else can you turn to when you need help caring for Rosa?

What are your child care arrangements? How do you feel about them?

What are your thoughts about discipline? Do you and your partner tend to agree?

What do you do when David wants something you think he shouldn't have?

Does Kossi have an object or favorite toy he uses to comfort himself?

What are some of the main hassles in your life right now? Transportation? Money?
Family problems? Housing? Personal safety?

How many times have you moved in the past year?

Have you ever been in a relationship where you have been hurt, threatened, or treated badly?

Have you ever been worried that someone was going to hurt your child? Has your child ever been abused?

How have you childproofed your home? Are household cleaners and poisonous items locked up
or stored out of Mary's sight and reach?

Do you have smoke alarms in your home? Have you checked the batteries recently?

Do you have a gun in the house? Where is it kept? Is it locked up? Where is the ammunition stored?

# Developmental Surveillance and Milestones

**Do you have any specific concerns about Tashi's development or behavior?**

**How does Tashi communicate what she wants?**

Vocalizes (e.g., screeches, babbles)

Gestures (points, shakes head)

Speaks words ("mama," "dada")

**What do you think Tashi understands?**

Names of family members

Names of familiar objects

Simple phrases (e.g., "all gone," "bye-bye," "peek-a-boo")

Simple requests ("give me the ball")

**How does Tashi get from one place to another?**

Crawls

Cruises

Walks

**How does Tashi act around family members?**

Responsive or withdrawn

Affectionate or hostile/aggressive

Happy or sad

Anxious about separation or not

**How does Tashi react to strangers?**

Outgoing or slow to warm up

Wary/resistant

**To what extent does Tashi eat independently?**

Finger-feeds

Uses cup

Uses spoon

**Tell me about Tashi's typical play.**

Mouths

Shakes, bangs, throws, and drops objects

Imitates

Plays with containers

Uses objects appropriately on own body (e.g., brushes own hair)

Has manual dexterity

## MILESTONES

Pulls to stand, cruises, and may take a few steps alone

Plays social games such as pat-a-cake, peek-a-boo, and so-big

Has precise pincer grasp

Points with index finger

Bangs two blocks together

Has vocabulary of one to three words in addition to "mama" and "dada"

Imitates vocalizations

Drinks from a cup

Looks for dropped or hidden objects

Waves "bye-bye"

Feeds self

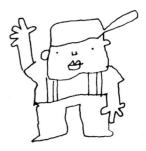

91

## Observation of Parent-Child Interaction

Are the parent and toddler interested in and responsive to each other (i.e., sharing vocalizations, smiles, and facial expressions)? Does the parent respond to the toddler's distress? What is the toddler's activity level, and how does the parent respond to it? Does the parent respond supportively to the toddler's autonomy or independent behavior as long as it is not dangerous? Does the parent speak to the toddler in positive terms?

## Physical Examination

Measure and plot on a standard chart the head circumference, length, weight, and weight for length. Share the information with the parent.

Examine the toddler's feet and observe her walking and gait. Reassure the parents about normal variations.

As part of the complete physical examination, the following should be noted:

Red reflex

Cardiac murmurs

Developmental hip dysplasia

Tooth eruption

Caries, baby bottle tooth decay, or dental injuries

Evidence of neglect or abuse

**ADDITIONAL SCREENING PROCEDURES**

Assessment of risk of high-dose lead exposure[1]

Lead screening by 12 months of age[2]

Hematocrit or hemoglobin screening at 9–12 months if certification is needed for WIC, or if any of the following risk factors are present:

Low socioeconomic status

Birthweight under 1,500 grams

Whole milk given before six months of age (Not recommended)

Low-iron formula given (Not recommended)

Low intake of iron-rich foods (Not recommended)

Tuberculin test (PPD) (At either 12 or 15 months, before or at the time of administering the Measles, Mumps, and Rubella Vaccine)

**IMMUNIZATIONS**

Hemophilus Influenza Type b (Hib) Vaccine                         #3 or #4 (If administering certain combined vaccines)[3]

Hepatitis B Virus (HBV) Vaccine                         #3 (If it was not administered previously)

Measles, Mumps, and Rubella (MMR) Vaccine     #1 (Can be administered at age 12 or 15 months)

Ensure that immunization status is up to date

# ANTICIPATORY GUIDANCE FOR THE FAMILY

In addition to providing anticipatory guidance, many health professionals give families handouts
at an appropriate reading level or a videotape that they can review or study at home.[4]

## Promotion of healthy habits

### Injury prevention

Get down on the floor and check for new hazards now that the toddler is walking.

Switch to a toddler car seat and make sure it is properly secured each time it is used.

Reexamine the hot water heater thermostat to ensure that it is set at less than 120 °F. Continue to test the water temperature with your wrist to make sure it is not hot before bathing your toddler.

Supervise the toddler constantly whenever she is in or around water, buckets, the toilet, or the bathtub. Young siblings should not be left alone to supervise a toddler (e.g., in the bathtub or in the house).

Continue to empty buckets, tubs, or small pools immediately after use. Ensure that swimming pools have a four-sided fence with a self-closing, self-latching gate.

Put sunscreen on the toddler before she goes outside to play.

Continue to keep the toddler's environment free of smoke. Keep the home and car nonsmoking zones.

Test smoke detectors to ensure that they work properly. Change batteries yearly.

Do not leave heavy objects or containers of hot liquids on tables with tablecloths that the toddler may pull down.

Turn pan handles toward the back of the stove. Keep the toddler away from hot stoves, fireplaces, irons, curling irons, and space heaters.

Ensure that electric wires, outlets, and appliances are inaccessible or protected.

Keep all poisonous substances, medicines, cleaning agents, health and beauty aids, and paints and paint solvents locked in a safe place out of the toddler's sight and reach. Never store poisonous substances in empty jars or soda bottles.

Keep cigarettes, lighters, matches, and alcohol out of the toddler's sight and reach.

Keep Syrup of Ipecac in the home to be used as directed by the poison control center or the health professional. Keep the number of the poison control center near the telephone.

Do not give the toddler plastic bags, latex balloons, or small objects such as marbles.

Continue to use gates at the top and bottom of stairs and safety devices on windows. Supervise the toddler closely when she is on stairs.

Confine the toddler's outside play to areas within fences and gates, especially at a child care facility, unless she is under close supervision.

Keep the toddler away from moving machinery, lawn mowers, overhead garage doors, driveways, and streets.

Ensure that a toddler riding in a seat on an adult's bicycle is wearing a helmet. Wear a helmet yourself.

Teach the child to use caution when approaching dogs, especially if the dogs are unknown or eating.

Choose caregivers carefully. Discuss with them their attitudes about and behavior in relation to discipline. Prohibit corporal punishment.

Enroll in a child cardiopulmonary resuscitation (CPR) course.

## Nutrition

Feed the toddler at family mealtimes and give her two to three nutritious snacks per day.

As much as possible, let the toddler feed herself. Toddlers learn to like foods by touching and mouthing them repeatedly.

Offer the toddler nutritious foods and let her decide how much to eat. Toddlers will eat a lot one time, not much the next.

Anticipate that the toddler's rate of weight gain will be slower than in her first year.

If you are breastfeeding: Discuss with the health professional weaning from the breast when desired.

If you are bottlefeeding: Change from formula to whole milk. Milk requirements decrease to 16–24 ounces per day. Wean the toddler from the bottle.

Continue teaching the toddler how to drink from a cup.

Avoid giving the toddler foods and drinks that are high in sugar.

Ensure that the toddler's caregiver feeds her nutritious foods.

Avoid giving the toddler foods or small toys that may be aspirated or cause choking (e.g., peanuts, popcorn, hot dogs or sausages, carrot sticks, celery sticks, whole grapes, raisins, corn, whole beans, hard candy, large pieces of raw vegetables or fruit, or tough meat).

## Oral health

Begin brushing the toddler's teeth with a tiny, pea-size amount of fluoridated toothpaste.

To protect the toddler's teeth, do not put her to bed with a bottle or prop it in her mouth.

Give the toddler fluoride supplements as recommended by the health professional based on the level of fluoride in the toddler's drinking water.

Make an appointment for the toddler's first dental examination and risk assessment.

## Promotion of social competence

Praise the toddler for good behavior.

Encourage language development by reading books to the toddler, singing her songs, and talking about what you and she are seeing and doing together.

Encourage exploration and initiative.

Encourage the toddler to play alone as well as with playmates, siblings, and parents.

To set limits and discipline a toddler of this age, use distraction, gentle restraint of the toddler, removal of the object from the toddler or the toddler from the stimulus, "time out," proximal parental presence, structure, and routines. Use discipline as a means of teaching and protecting, not punishing.

Limit the number of rules and consistently enforce them. Develop rules for all family members.

Anticipate and avoid unnecessary conflict situations.

Although hitting, biting, and other aggressive behaviors are common, discipline the toddler so that she learns not to do them.

Expect the toddler to sleep through the night in her own bed. Reinforce good sleeping habits. Maintain a regular bedtime ritual.

Promote learning of self-quieting behaviors. Consistently provide the toddler with the same transitional object—such as a stuffed animal, blanket, or favorite toy—so that she can console herself at bedtime or in new situations.

Do not begin toilet training for many months. Discuss details of toilet training with the health professional at the next visit.

Limit television watching to less than one hour per day of appropriate programs. Watch programs with your child.

Anticipate that the toddler may touch her genitalia.

## Promotion of constructive family relationships and parental health

Take some time for yourself and spend some individual time with your partner.

Pick the toddler up. Cuddle her, hold her, and talk with her.

Show affection in the family.

Spend some individual time with each child.

Create opportunities for each family member to interact with and play with the toddler every day.

Promote family communication. Play games with the toddler.

Share meals as a family whenever possible.

Reach agreement with all family members on how to support the toddler's emerging independence while maintaining consistent limits.

Limit the number of people who provide care for your child while you and your partner are working.

Discuss with the health professional your own preventive and health-promoting practices (e.g., using seat belts, avoiding tobacco, eating properly, exercising and doing breast self-exams or testicular self-exams).

## Promotion of community interactions

If you need financial assistance to help pay for health care expenses, ask about resources or for referrals to the state Medicaid programs or other state medical assistance programs.

Ask about resources or referrals for food (e.g., WIC), housing, or transportation if needed.

Learn about and consider attending parent-toddler play groups.

Learn about and consider attending parent education classes or parent support groups.

Maintain or expand ties to your community through social, religious, cultural, volunteer, and recreational organizations.

Discuss with the health professional choosing and evaluating child care programs. Discuss the child care arrangements you have made.

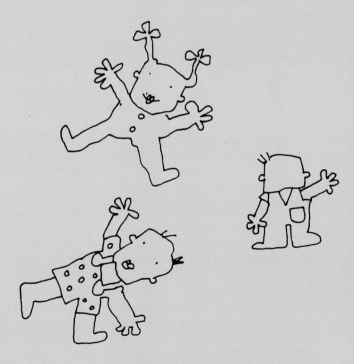

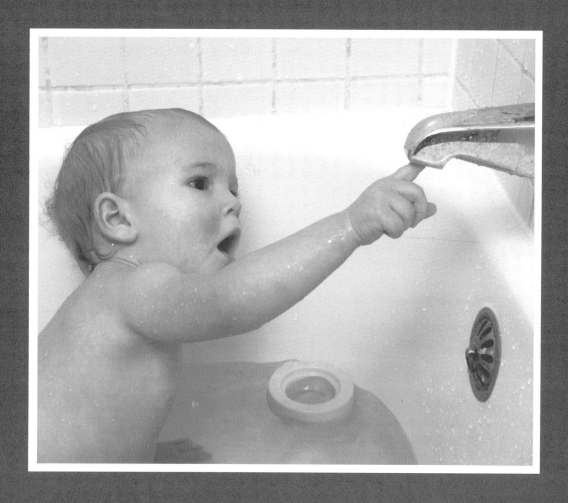

*Lacking a sense of danger or a fear of falling,*
*he will try to scale playground equipment or poke his finger*
*into an electrical socket.*

# Fifteen Month Visit

The 15 month old is a whirlwind of activity and curiosity, with no apparent sense of internal limits. His first tentative steps have become headlong dashes to explore new places. Children of this age require constant parental attention and guidance. Selma Fraiberg aptly stated: "The discovery of independent locomotion and the discovery of a new self usher in a new phase in personality development. The toddler is quite giddy with [his] new achievements. [He] behaves as if [he] had invented this new mode of locomotion, and [he] is quite in love with [himself] for being so clever. From dawn to dusk [he] marches around in an ecstatic, drunken dance, which ends only when [he] collapses with fatigue."[5]

The full impact of such dramatic developmental changes as independent locomotion and growing autonomy will not be felt until the child has his first temper tantrum in the supermarket, ruins the carpet, or shows his first real resistance to being fed, diapered, or put to bed. Now the toddler begins to display a new emotion: frustration. He will become angry when he is unable to accomplish a task, when he cannot make someone understand his rudimentary communication, and when he is not allowed to do precisely as he wishes. If crying and even screaming fail to elicit the desired response, the toddler may escalate his protests to full-blown temper tantrums or episodes of breath-holding.

At the same time, the toddler's new mobility makes it much more likely that he will injure himself. He will run into the street or climb a flight of stairs without a moment's hesitation. Lacking a sense of danger or a fear of falling, he will try to scale playground equipment or poke his finger into an electrical socket. Minor injuries may surprise him, but they rarely deter him for long.

Parents, on the other hand, must walk a fine line: They must allow their child the freedom to explore yet keep him safe; they must respond to his needs while limiting his undifferentiated demands; they must cope with their own anger and frustration as they help the child master his. At the 15 month visit, the health professional can help parents learn how to structure their child's environment and gain the parenting skills they need for their balancing act.

# HEALTH SUPERVISION INTERVIEW

## TRIGGER QUESTIONS

To be used selectively by the health professional. Discuss any issues or concerns of the family.

How are you?

How are things going in your family?

What questions or concerns do you have about Shanessa?

How would you describe Joshua's personality these days?

What are some of the things about Chris that you are most proud of?

Have there been any major changes or stresses in your family since your last visit?

Does Roger have special activities he likes to do with you, such as read a book or play a game?

Does Cindy still take a bottle?

Does Juanita have a will of her own? How and when does she show that?

What kinds of things do you find yourself saying no about?

How are you and your partner managing Clifford's behavior? What do you do when you disagree?
Do you talk with each other about your child rearing ideas?
Are your approaches basically similar and consistent?

Have you been able to get out of the house without Amy?

What do you do when you become angry or frustrated with Simone?

Who else can you turn to when you need help caring for Paul?

Do you feel pressure to toilet train Fatima?

How is child care going?

Have you ever been in a relationship where you have been hurt, threatened, or treated badly?

Have you ever been worried that someone was going to hurt your child?
Has your child ever been abused?

Does anyone in your home have a gun? Does a neighbor or family friend?
If so, is the gun locked up? Where is the ammunition stored?

# Developmental Surveillance and Milestones

## TRIGGER QUESTIONS AND POSSIBLE RESPONSES

**Do you have any specific concerns about Kenji's development or behavior?**

**How does Kenji communicate what he wants?**

Vocalizes

Gestures

Speaks words (other than "mama" or "dada")

**What do you think Kenji understands?**

Names of family members

Names of familiar objects

Names of body parts

Simple phrases (e.g., "no more")

Simple instructions without gestured cues ("go get your shoes")

**How does Kenji get from one place to another?**

Crawls, cruises

Walks

Runs, climbs

**How does Kenji act around family members?**

Responsive or withdrawn

Affectionate or hostile/aggressive

Compliant or defiant

Anxious about separation or not

**How does Kenji react to strangers?**

Outgoing or slow to warm up

Wary/resistant

**To what extent does Kenji eat independently?**

Finger-feeds

Uses cup

Uses spoon

**Tell me about Kenji's typical play.**

Shakes, bangs, throws, and drops objects

Imitates

Plays with containers

Uses objects appropriately on own body (e.g., brushes own hair)

## MILESTONES

Has vocabulary of three to six words

Can point to one or more body parts

Understands simple commands

Walks well, stoops, climbs stairs

Stacks two blocks

Feeds self with fingers

Drinks from a cup

Listens to a story

Indicates what he wants by pulling, pointing, or grunting

Engages in simple representational play with doll (e.g., pretends to feed)

Has manual dexterity

Participates in social play

# Observation of Parent-Child Interaction

When the toddler moves around the room, how does the parent react? Does the parent watch the child, follow him closely, or ignore him? How do the parent and toddler play with toys? Does the parent hold the toy, give the toy to the toddler, or wait for him to take it? Does the parent react positively when the health professional praises the child? If there are siblings in the room, how do they react to the toddler?

# Physical Examination

Measure and plot on a standard chart the head circumference, length, weight, and weight for length. Share the information with the parent.

Examine the toddler's feet and observe his walking and gait. Reassure the parent about normal variations.

As part of the complete physical examination, the following should be noted:

Nevi, cafe au lait spots, or birthmarks

Tooth eruption

Caries, baby bottle tooth decay, or dental injuries

Excessive injuries or bruising that may indicate inadequate supervision or abuse

Other evidence of neglect or abuse

## ADDITIONAL SCREENING PROCEDURES

Assessment of risk of high-dose lead exposure[1]

Tuberculin test (PPD)
(If not performed at 12 months)

## IMMUNIZATIONS

Hemophilus Influenza Type b
(Hib) Vaccine                                          #3 or #4
(If administering certain combination
vaccines and not administered at age
12 months)[3]

Diphtheria, Tetanus, Pertussis (DTP) Vaccine          #4
(Hib and DTP can be combined)[3]

Hepatitis B Virus (HBV) Vaccine                       #3
(If not administered previously)

Measles, Mumps, and Rubella (MMR) Vaccine             #1
(If not administered previously)

Ensure that immunization status is up to date

# ANTICIPATORY GUIDANCE FOR THE FAMILY

In addition to providing anticipatory guidance, many health professionals give families handouts
at an appropriate reading level or a videotape that they can review or study at home.[4]

## Promotion of healthy habits

### Injury prevention

Continue to use a toddler car seat and make sure it is properly secured each time it is used.

Continue to test the water temperature with your wrist to make sure it is not hot before bathing the toddler.

Supervise the toddler constantly whenever he is in or around water, buckets, the toilet, or the bathtub. Young siblings should not be left alone to supervise a toddler (e.g., in the bathtub or in the house).

Continue to empty buckets, tubs, or small pools immediately after use. Ensure that swimming pools have a four-sided fence with a self-closing, self-latching gate.

Continue to put sunscreen on the toddler before he goes outside to play.

Continue to keep the toddler's environment free of smoke. Keep the home and car nonsmoking zones.

Do not leave heavy objects or containers of hot liquids on tables with tablecloths that the toddler may pull down.

Turn pan handles toward the back of the stove. Keep the toddler away from hot stoves, fireplaces, irons, curling irons, and space heaters.

Ensure that electric wires, outlets, and appliances are inaccessible or protected.

Exclude poisons, medications, and toxic household products from the home or keep them in locked cabinets. Have safety caps on all medications.

Keep cigarettes, lighters, matches, and alcohol out of the toddler's sight and reach.

Keep Syrup of Ipecac in the home to be used as directed by the poison control center or the health professional. Keep the number of the poison control center near the telephone.

Do not give the toddler plastic bags, latex balloons, or small objects such as marbles.

Never underestimate the ability of a 15 month old to climb. Some children may climb out of the crib at this age. Ensure that the crib mattress is on the lowest rung.

Continue to use gates at the top and bottom of stairs and safety devices on windows. Supervise the toddler closely when he is on stairs.

Confine the toddler's outside play to areas within fences and gates, especially at a child care facility, unless he is under close supervision.

Keep the toddler away from moving machinery, lawn mowers, overhead garage doors, driveways, and streets.

Ensure that a toddler riding in a seat on an adult's bicycle is wearing a helmet. Wear a helmet yourself.

Teach the child to use caution when approaching dogs, especially if the dogs are unknown or eating.

Choose caregivers carefully. Discuss with them their attitudes about and behavior in relation to discipline. Prohibit corporal punishment.

### Nutrition

Encourage the toddler to eat at family mealtimes and give him two to three nutritious snacks per day.

Make mealtimes pleasant and companionable. Encourage conversation.

Encourage the toddler to feed himself.

Let the toddler experiment with a variety of foods from each food group by touching and mouthing them repeatedly. He may become more aware of and suspicious of new or strange foods, but do not limit the menu to only foods the toddler likes.

Offer the toddler nutritious foods and let him decide what and how much to eat. Toddlers will eat a lot one time, not much the next. "Food jags" are common.

Anticipate that the toddler's rate of weight gain will be slower than in his first year.

Give the toddler drinks in a cup.

Ensure that the toddler's caregiver feeds him nutritious foods.

Avoid giving the toddler foods or small toys that may be aspirated or cause choking (e.g., peanuts, popcorn, hot dogs or sausages, carrot sticks, celery sticks, whole grapes, raisins, corn, whole beans, hard candy, large pieces of raw vegetables or fruit, or tough meat).

## Oral health

Continue to brush the toddler's teeth with a tiny, pea-size amount of fluoridated toothpaste. Children under the age of four or five years do not have the manual dexterity to clean their own teeth adequately.

To protect the toddler's teeth, do not put him to bed with a bottle or prop it in his mouth.

Give the toddler fluoride supplements as recommended by the health professional based on the level of fluoride in the toddler's drinking water.

Schedule the toddler's first dental visit if it has not already occurred.

## Promotion of social competence

Praise the toddler for good behavior and accomplishments.

Encourage language development by reading books to the toddler, singing him songs, and talking about what you and he are seeing and doing together.

Encourage play, which is a way of learning social behaviors.

Encourage the toddler's autonomous behavior, curiosity, sense of emerging independence, and feeling of competence.

Develop strategies to manage the power struggles that result from the toddler's need to control his environment.

To set limits and discipline a toddler of this age, use distraction, gentle restraint of the toddler, removal of the object from the toddler or the toddler from the stimulus, and "time outs." Use discipline as a means of teaching and protecting, not punishing.

Although hitting, biting, and other aggressive behaviors are common, discipline the toddler so that he learns not to do them.

Continue to reinforce good sleeping habits. Maintain a regular bedtime ritual.

Encourage the toddler to use a transitional object, such as a stuffed animal or favorite blanket, to learn self-quieting behaviors.

Recognize that toilet training is part of developmentally appropriate learning. Delay toilet training until the toddler is dry for periods of about two hours, knows the difference between wet and dry, can pull his pants up and down, wants to learn, and can give a signal when he is about to have a bowel movement.

Limit television watching to less than one hour per day of appropriate programs. Watch programs with your child.

Anticipate that the toddler may touch his genitalia.

## Promotion of constructive family relationships and parental health

Take some time for yourself and spend some individual time with your partner.

Pick the toddler up. Cuddle him, hold him, and talk with him.

Spend some time playing with the toddler each day. Focus on activities that he expresses interest in and enjoys.

Listen to and show respect for the toddler.

Show affection in the family.

Spend some individual time with each child.

Help the toddler express such feelings as joy, anger, sadness, fear, and frustration.

Create opportunities for each family member to interact with and play with the toddler every day.

Promote family communication. Play games with the toddler.

Share meals as a family whenever possible.

Reach agreement with all family members on how to support the toddler's emerging independence while maintaining consistent limits.

Discuss with the health professional your own preventive and health-promoting practices (e.g., using seat belts, avoiding tobacco, eating properly, exercising and doing breast self-exams or testicular self-exams).

## Promotion of community interactions

If you need financial assistance to help pay for health care expenses, ask about resources or for referrals to the state Medicaid programs or other state medical assistance programs.

Ask about resources or referrals for food (e.g., WIC), housing, or transportation if needed.

Learn about and consider attending parent-toddler play groups.

Learn about and consider attending parent education classes or parent support groups.

Maintain or expand ties to your community through social, religious, cultural, volunteer, and recreational organizations.

Discuss with the health professional choosing and evaluating child care programs. Discuss the child care arrangements you have made.

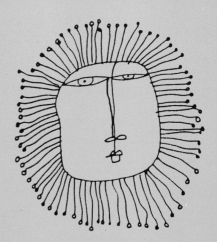

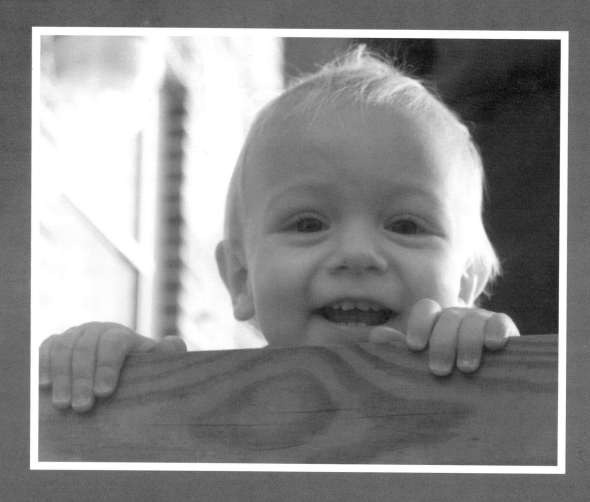

*The behavior of an 18 month old*
*can be frustrating at times, but her delight in her own emerging*
*competence and achievements can bring a sense of joy*
*and accomplishment to all around her . . . .*

# Eighteen Month Visit

The 18 month old requires gentle transitions, patience, consistent limits, and respect. One minute she insists on independence; the next she is clinging fearfully to her parent. If the toddler is challenged by a playmate or a sibling, her cheerful playing can quickly turn into a screaming tantrum. Much of the energy and drive that was channeled into physical activity is now directed toward more complex tasks and social interactions. Having learned the concept of choice, the toddler becomes assertive about her own wishes. Because her repertoire of language and behavior is rather limited, her method of expressing herself generally consists of saying "No!" She can also be noncompliant, collapsing her legs rather than walking where adults want her to go.

The defiance and negativism of an 18 month old are not truly aggressive, but rather assertions of her emerging sense of her own identity. When the toddler bounces a ball 20 times in the kitchen, she is not trying to drive her parents crazy. Rather, she is trying to learn about bouncing balls, and repetition is the best teacher. The toddler resists change and will often experience frustration as she attempts to learn new skills. However, she responds positively and happily to a stable environment.

The 18 month old needs to have strong emotional ties to her parents. In order to venture out into the world and test her newfound assertiveness, she must know that she has a safe, emotionally secure place at home. Parents can assist their child by not taking her assertiveness personally. As she tries out new skills, they can modify her environment to avoid as many problem situations as possible. They must carefully choose which issues are worth a battle. Extra patience and a sense of humor can help parents with the tough task of continually reinforcing the limits they have set.

Parents who can view the toddler's negativism as budding independence and who provide a physically and emotionally stable environment will support her through this sometimes stormy period and be richly rewarded. The behavior of an 18 month old can be frustrating at times, but her delight in her own emerging competence and achievements can bring a sense of joy and accomplishment to all around her, as she applauds herself and looks around for parental acclaim and reinforcement. The 18 month old can light up a room.

# HEALTH SUPERVISION INTERVIEW

## TRIGGER QUESTIONS

To be used selectively by the health professional. Discuss any issues or concerns of the family.

**How are you?**

**How are things going in your family?**

**What questions or concerns do you have about Nina?**

**What kinds of things do you find yourself saying no about?**

**What are some of the things that you most enjoy about Carlton?**
**What seems most difficult?**

**Have there been any major changes or stresses in your family since your last visit?**

**Does Hiroshi have any playmates?**

**What are some of Tianna's favorite activities?**

**What do you do when you become angry or frustrated with Rachel?**

**How does Steve assert himself?**
**Does he hit, bite, or kick? How are you managing his behavior?**

**Do you and your partner agree on your household rules?**

**How does Sharon get along at child care?**

**Do you feel pressure to toilet train Kate?**

**Have you ever been in a relationship where you have been hurt, threatened, or treated badly?**

**Have you ever been worried that someone was going to hurt your child?**
**Has your child ever been abused?**

**Do you feel safe in your neighborhood?**

**Does anyone in your home have a gun? Does a neighbor or a family friend?**
**If so, is the gun locked up? Where is the ammunition stored?**

# Developmental Surveillance and Milestones

## TRIGGER QUESTIONS AND POSSIBLE RESPONSES

**Do you have any specific concerns about Elena's development or behavior?**

**How does Elena communicate what she wants?**

> Vocalizes and gestures
>
> Speaks words (15 to 20)
>
> Uses phrases of two or three words
>
> Speaks intelligibly to family

**What do you think Elena understands?**

> Names of family members
>
> Names of familiar objects, including those in pictures
>
> Names of body parts
>
> Simple instructions without gestured cues (e.g., "sit down")

**How does Elena get from one place to another?**

> Crawls, walks
>
> Runs, climbs
>
> Goes up and down stairs (one step at a time)

**How does Elena act around family members?**

> Responsive or withdrawn
>
> Affectionate or hostile/aggressive
>
> Compliant or defiant
>
> Dependent or self-reliant
>
> Anxious about separation or not

**How does Elena react to strangers?**

> Outgoing or slow to warm up
>
> Wary/resistant

**How does Elena act around other children?**

> Interactive or withdrawn/resistant
>
> Friendly or hostile/aggressive (e.g., hitting, biting)

**Tell me about Elena's typical play.**

> Plays with favorite toys (describe how used)
>
> Listens to stories
>
> Engages in simple representational play with doll
>
> Has manual dexterity

## MILESTONES

Walks quickly or runs stiffly

Walks backwards

Throws a ball

Has a vocabulary of 15–20 words

Imitates words

Uses two-word phrases

Pulls a toy along the ground

Stacks three or four blocks

Uses a spoon and cup

Listens to a story, looking at pictures and naming objects

Shows affection, kisses

Follows simple directions

Points to some body parts

Imitates a crayon stroke and scribbles

Dumps an object from bottle without demonstration

## Observation of Parent-Child Interaction

How do the parent and child communicate? (Parents vary in their awareness of language milestones and the ability to report this information.) What words do they use? What is the tone of the interaction and the feeling conveyed? When the health professional speaks and interacts with the child directly, does the parent intervene? How does the parent discipline or restrain the child? Does the parent seem positive when speaking about the child?

## Physical Examination

Measure and plot on a standard chart the head circumference, length, weight, and weight for length. Share the information with the parent.

Examine the toddler's feet and observe her walking and gait. Reassure the parent about normal variations.

As part of the complete physical examination, the following should be noted:

Caries, baby bottle tooth decay, or dental injuries

Excessive injuries or bruising that may indicate inadequate supervision or abuse

Other evidence of neglect or abuse

### ADDITIONAL SCREENING PROCEDURES

Assessment of risk of high-dose lead exposure[1]

### IMMUNIZATIONS

Hepatitis B Virus (HBV) Vaccine          #3
(If not administered previously)

Ensure that immunization status is up to date

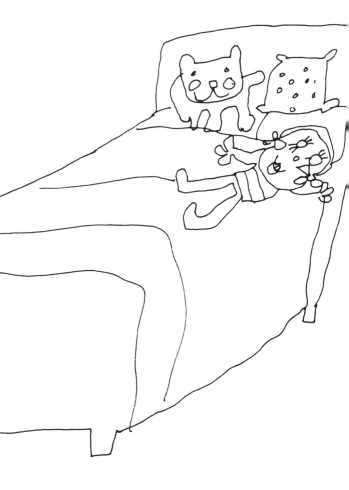

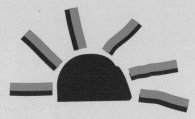

# No Bottle at Bedtime

After standing behind a counter all day, Eva St. Pierre is exhausted when she picks up her 18-month-old daughter, Debbie, from her child care provider's house. She takes Debbie home, feeds her, plays with her for a while, then puts her to bed with a juice-filled bottle. Eva feels relieved when Debbie settles down to sleep—she has many household chores to complete before she can go to bed herself. Eva worries about putting Debbie to bed with a bottle, though. Her coworker's son has bad teeth, and his doctor said that he developed this condition by falling asleep while drinking from a nursing bottle.

At the next health supervision visit, Debbie's doctor, Dr. Mikkelsen, talks with Eva about the nursing bottle and tooth decay. "I understand how important it is to get Debbie to sleep," she says, "so we should spend a good part of this visit talking about ways to comfort Debbie to help her sleep. First, I should emphasize that letting Debbie go to sleep with a nursing bottle at bedtime is not good for her. Let me show you some pictures of children who have developed severe tooth decay after falling asleep with a nursing bottle." Dr. Mikkelson shows Eva the pictures and points out that her daughter may be at risk for severe cavities, pain, and more tooth decay. "Extensive treatment, possibly under general anesthesia, could cost you $3,000."

Dr. Mikkelsen explains to Eva that she can prevent Debbie from developing dental disease and get her to sleep at the same time. Dr. Mikkelsen suggests that Eva consider comfort measures such as holding Debbie, rubbing her back, and giving her a pacifier. Eva says that Debbie is used to having the bottle in bed with her and that it might be hard for her to suddenly break this habit. Dr. Mikkelsen advises Eva that if Debbie insists on having the bottle, it can be filled with water or gradually changed to water by offering increasingly diluted juice. "I'm going to refer you to a pediatric dentist for Debbie's first dental checkup," Dr. Mikkelsen says. "Why don't you call me in a month so we can talk about how the new sleep routine is working out?"

# ANTICIPATORY GUIDANCE FOR THE FAMILY

In addition to providing anticipatory guidance, many health professionals give families handouts
at an appropriate reading level or a videotape that they can review or study at home.[4]

## Promotion of healthy habits

### Injury prevention

Continue to use a toddler car seat and make sure it is properly secured each time it is used.

Continue to test the water temperature with your wrist to make sure it is not hot before bathing the toddler.

Supervise the toddler constantly whenever she is in or around water, buckets, the toilet, or the bathtub.

Continue to empty buckets, tubs, or small pools immediately after use. Ensure that swimming pools have a four-sided fence with a self-closing, self-latching gate.

Ensure that the toddler wears a life vest if boating. Inflatable flotation devices or "knowing how to swim" do not make a toddler safe in the water.

Put sunscreen on the toddler before she goes outside to play or swim.

Continue to keep the toddler's environment free of smoke. Keep the home and car nonsmoking zones.

Ensure that electric wires, outlets, and appliances are inaccessible or protected.

Keep cigarettes, lighters, matches, alcohol, firearms, and electrical tools locked up and/or out of the toddler's sight and reach.

Exclude poisons, medications, and toxic household products from the home or keep them in locked cabinets. Have safety caps on all medications.

Keep Syrup of Ipecac in the home to be used as directed by the poison control center or the health professional. Keep the number of the poison control center near the telephone.

Continue to use gates at the top and bottom of stairs and safety devices on windows. Supervise the toddler closely when she is on stairs.

Never leave the toddler alone in the car or in the house.

Do not expect young children to supervise the toddler (e.g., in the house, apartment, playground, or yard).

Keep the toddler away from moving machinery, lawn mowers, overhead garage doors, driveways, and streets.

Ensure that a toddler riding in a seat on an adult's bicycle is wearing a helmet. Wear a helmet yourself.

Teach the child to use caution when approaching dogs, especially if the dogs are unknown or eating.

Discuss with the health professional what to do for falls, cuts, puncture wounds, bites, bumps on the head, bleeding, and broken bones.

Choose caregivers carefully. Discuss with them their attitudes about and behavior in relation to discipline. Prohibit corporal punishment.

### Nutrition

Encourage the toddler to eat with the family by serving her in a highchair or booster seat at table height. A toddler will often eat better with a trusted adult nearby.

Make mealtimes pleasant and companionable. Encourage conversation.

Give her two to three nutritious snacks per day. Provide snacks rich in complex carbohydrates, and limit sweets and high-fat snacks. Avoid using snacks as a reward or giving the toddler cookies or sweets because she "hasn't eaten all day."

Continue encouraging the toddler to feed herself with her hands and drink from a cup. She may also be using utensils.

Encourage the toddler to experiment with food, deciding what and how much to eat from the nutritious foods that you offer. Toddlers will eat a lot one time, not much the next. Food jags are common. A toddler's intake will vary considerably over any 24-hour period, but it should be balanced over several days.

Let the toddler develop clear likes and dislikes.

Do not allow feeding to serve as the focus of a power struggle.

Ensure that the toddler's caregiver feeds her nutritious foods.

Avoid giving the toddler foods that are easily aspirated.

## Oral health

Continue to brush the toddler's teeth with a small, pea-size amount of fluoridated toothpaste.

Give the toddler fluoride supplements as recommended by the health professional based on the level of fluoride in the toddler's drinking water.

Schedule the toddler's first dental visit if it has not already occurred.

## Promotion of social competence

Praise the toddler for good behavior and accomplishments.

Model appropriate language. Encourage language development by reading books to the toddler, singing her songs, and talking about what you and she are seeing and doing together.

Reinforce self-care and self-expression.

To promote a sense of competence and control, invite the toddler to make choices whenever possible. (The choices should be ones you can live with—e.g., "Red pants or blue ones?")

Encourage the toddler to be assertive in appropriate situations, yet provide limits when they are needed.

Decide what limits are important to you and your toddler. Be specific when setting these limits. Briefly tell your toddler why she is being disciplined. Attempt to be as consistent as possible when enforcing limits.

Keep time out or other disciplinary measures brief. Do not hesitate to pick the toddler up, hold her, or remove her from dangerous or conflictual situations. Reassure the toddler once the negative behavior has stopped.

When disciplining the toddler, make a verbal separation between her and her behavior: "I love you, but I don't like it when you do _____."

When possible, give the toddler a "yes" as well as a "no." For example: "No, you can't play with the remote control, but you can play with the blocks."

Do not get into a power struggle with your child. Prepare strategies for sidestepping conflicts and appropriately asserting your power. You can control only your own responses to the toddler's behavior. For example, you cannot make a toddler sleep, but you can insist that she stay in her room.

Teach the toddler about disciplinary measures such as time out when she is most capable of learning (i.e., when she is rested, fed, and not angry).

Prepare strategies to deal with night awakening, night fears, nightmares, and night terrors.

Encourage self-quieting behaviors, such as quiet play or the use of a transitional object.

Recognize that toilet training is part of developmentally appropriate learning. Delay toilet training until the toddler is dry for periods of about two hours, knows the difference between wet and dry, can pull her pants up and down, wants to learn, and can give a signal when she is about to have a bowel movement.

Limit television watching to less than one hour per day of appropriate programs. Watch programs with your child.

Anticipate that the toddler may touch her genitalia.

### Promotion of constructive family relationships and parental health

Take some time for yourself and spend some individual time with your partner.

Spend some time playing with the toddler each day. Focus on activities that she expresses interest in and enjoys.

Listen to and show respect for the toddler.

Show interest in child care activities.

Show affection in the family.

Spend some individual time with each child.

Help the toddler express such feelings as joy, anger, sadness, fear, and frustration.

Create opportunities for each family member to interact with and play with the toddler every day.

Keep family outings relatively short and simple. Lengthy activities tire the toddler and may lead to irritability or a temper tantrum.

Do not expect the toddler to share her toys.

Acknowledge conflicts between siblings. Whenever possible, attempt to resolve conflicts without taking sides. For example, if a conflict arises about a toy, the toy can be put away. Do not allow hitting, biting, or other violent behavior.

Allow older children to have objects that they do not have to share with the toddler. Give them a storage space that the toddler cannot get into.

Share meals as a family whenever possible.

Reach agreement with all family members on how to support the toddler's emerging independence while maintaining consistent limits.

Discuss with the health professional your own preventive and health-promoting practices (e.g., using seat belts, avoiding tobacco, eating properly, exercising and doing breast self-exams or testicular self-exams).

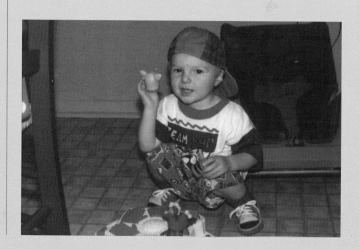

## Promotion of community interactions

If you need financial assistance to help pay for health care expenses, ask about resources or for referrals to the state Medicaid programs or other state medical assistance programs.

Ask about resources or referrals for food (e.g., WIC), housing, or transportation if needed.

Learn about and consider attending parent-toddler play groups. Discuss with the health professional possible programs for your child: preschools, early intervention programs, or other community programs.

Learn about and consider attending parent education classes or parent support groups.

Maintain or expand ties to your community through social, religious, cultural, volunteer, and recreational organizations.

Discuss with the health professional choosing and evaluating child care programs. Discuss the child care arrangements you have made.

Find out what you can do to make your community safer. Advocate for and participate in a neighborhood watch program.

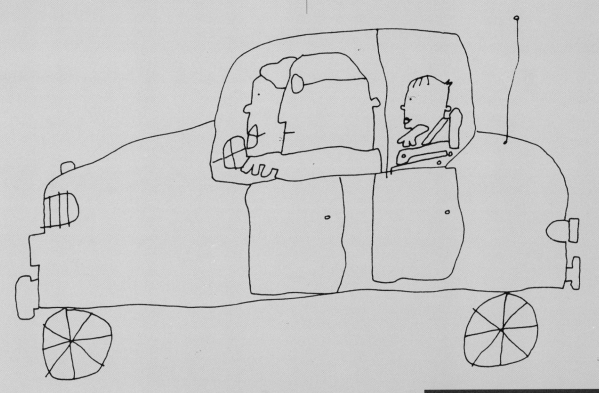

113

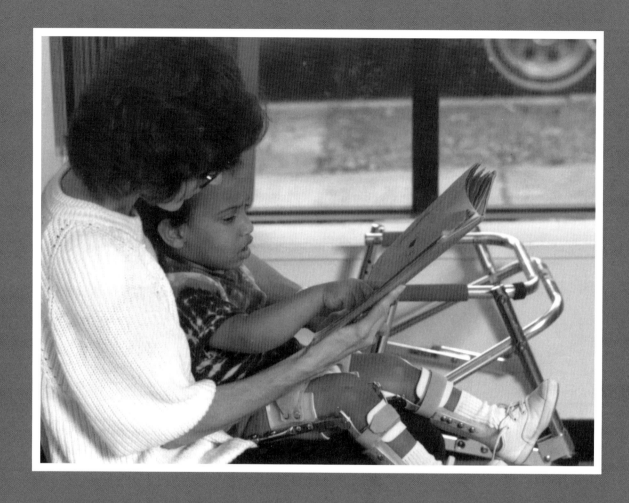

*He enjoys brushing his teeth, reading a book, and
imitating his parents doing household chores.*

# Two Year Visit

The two year old is spirited, delightful, joyful, carefree, challenging, and trying. Though the family may be frustrated when the child is unsuccessful at communicating his needs, helping the two year old master the use of language can be rewarding for both parent and child. The two year old is learning to be sociable but is not yet skilled at interacting with other children. Rather than sharing, he engages in parallel play alongside his peers. The two year old cannot be expected to sit in a circle with other children or listen to a long story. These abilities will develop between the ages of two and three.

Watching the two year old go through his daily routine may be amusing. He enjoys brushing his teeth, reading a book, and imitating his parents doing household chores. To fully understand new activities, he tries them repeatedly. What happens when one splashes water from the tub? How does one knock over the garbage can? How far will the teddy bear fall down the stairs? What does mud feel like? However, when presented with a choice—between orange juice and apple juice, for example—the child ceases his activity and has a difficult time making a decision. After he finally makes a choice, he often wants to change it.

In spite of what appears to be a yearning for independence, the two year old frequently hides behind his parent's legs when approached by other adults. He may develop fears at this age. He may be afraid of being drained out of the tub with the water or being eaten by monsters underneath the bed. The two year old is often reluctant to share his parents and will play one against the other. With parental reassurance, the child gains more confidence and overcomes his fears.

It can be difficult for parents to realize that a child's repetitious exploratory behavior is compelled by curiosity and not a rejection of their standards. The child is ready to be taught simple rules about safety and behavior in the family, but he is only beginning to be able to internalize them. Many of his actions are still governed by his parents' reactions. A two year old has learned what to do to get his parents to respond, either negatively or positively. He will throw tantrums to get his way if he knows that his parents will react strongly. Similarly, if parents overreact to dysfluency or other language attempts, it can prolong this normal phase of speech development. Parents' positive support of good behavior sends a constructive message to the child.

# HEALTH SUPERVISION INTERVIEW

## TRIGGER QUESTIONS

To be used selectively by the health professional. Discuss any issues or concerns of the family.

**How are you?**

**How are things going in your family?**

**Do you have any questions or concerns about Li Wong?**

**What do you and your partner enjoy most about Tanya?**
**What seems to be most difficult?**

**Have there been any major changes or stresses in your family since your last visit?**

**How is Roxanne's toilet training going?**

**What are Leah's sleeping habits? Eating habits?**

**Does Jack eat nonfood substances such as clay, dirt, or paint chips?**

**What language(s) does your family speak at home?**

**How is child care going?**

**How are you dealing with setting limits for Orlando and disciplining him?**

**Do both parents and all caregivers agree on disciplinary style and setting limits?**

**How do you deal with tantrums?**

**Do you ever get so angry with Adam that you are worried about what you might do next?**

**Have you ever been in a relationship where you have been hurt, threatened, or treated badly?**

**Have you ever been worried that someone was going to hurt your child?**
**Has your child ever been abused?**

**Do you feel safe in your neighborhood?**

**Does anyone in your home have a gun? Does a neighbor or a family friend?**
**If so, is the gun locked up? Where is the ammunition stored?**

# Developmental Surveillance and Milestones

## TRIGGER QUESTIONS AND POSSIBLE RESPONSES

**Do you have any specific concerns about Lincoln's development or behavior?**

**How does Lincoln communicate what he wants?**

    Vocalizes and gestures

    Speaks words (rapidly expanding vocabulary)

    Uses phrases of two or three words

    Speaks intelligibly to strangers (25 percent of the time)

**What do you think Lincoln understands?**

    Names of family members

    Names of familiar objects, including those in pictures

    Names of seven body parts

    Simple instructions without gestured cues (e.g., "sit down")

**How does Lincoln get from one place to another?**

    Walks, climbs, runs

    Goes up and down stairs (one step at a time)

**How does Lincoln act around family members?**

    Responsive or withdrawn

    Affectionate or hostile/aggressive

    Compliant or defiant

    Dependent or self-reliant

    Anxious about separation or not

**How does Lincoln react to strangers?**

    Outgoing or slow to warm up

    Wary/resistant

**How does Lincoln act around other children?**

    Interactive or withdrawn/resistant

    Friendly or hostile/aggressive (e.g., hitting, biting)

**To what extent has Lincoln developed independence in eating and dressing?**

    Uses cup, spoon, and fork

    Assists in putting on clothing

## MILESTONES

Can go up and down stairs one step at a time

Can kick a ball

Can stack five or six blocks

Has vocabulary of at least 20 words

Uses two-word phrases

Makes or imitates horizontal and circular strokes with crayon

Can follow two-step commands

Imitates adults

**Tell me about Lincoln's typical play.**

    Plays with favorite toys (describe how used)

    Listens to stories

    Engages in simple fantasy play

    Engages in parallel play with peers

    Has manual dexterity

## Observation of Parent-Child Interaction

How do the parent and child communicate? (Parents vary in their awareness of language milestones and the ability to report this information.) What words do they use? What is the tone of the interaction and the feeling conveyed? Does the parent teach the child the name of a person or object during the visit? How does the parent discipline or restrain the child? Does the parent seem positive when speaking about the child?

## Physical Examination

Measure and plot on a standard chart the head circumference, height, weight, and weight for height. Share the information with the parent.

As part of the complete physical examination, the following should be noted:

Strabismus

Caries, baby bottle tooth decay, developmental anomalies, malocclusion, pathologic conditions, or dental injuries

Excessive injuries or bruising that may indicate inadequate supervision or possible abuse

Other evidence of neglect or abuse

**ADDITIONAL SCREENING PROCEDURES**

Assessment of risk of high-dose lead exposure[1]

Lead screening[2]

Assessment of risk for hyperlipidemia[6]

Annual tuberculin test (PPD) if any of the following risk factors are present:

Low socioeconomic status
Residence in areas where tuberculosis is prevalent
Exposure to tuberculosis
Immigrant status

**IMMUNIZATIONS**

Ensure that immunization status is up to date

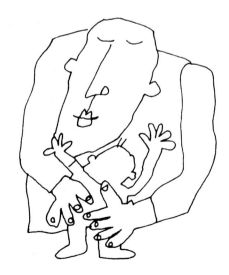

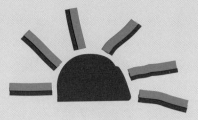

# Home Hazards

*Gita has had many opportunities in the home to teach about health and safety.*

As a public health nurse working with families with young children, Gita Bakshi finds that home visits are invaluable for building relationships and providing appropriate and meaningful anticipatory guidance. Gita has had many opportunities in the home to teach about health and safety. She could not have offered the same type of instruction in a clinic, office, or classroom setting.

Before a visit to the Carey family, a single mother with two preschool children and a 35-week-old, premature infant, Gita plans to show the mother how to keep her home safe as her infant grows and becomes more mobile. Once in the home, however, she realizes that there are some pressing safety issues that she did not consider in the clinic.

When Gita arrives, she sees that the extremely cramped house is heated by two old portable electric units. There are no smoke detectors, and there is only one door for an exit. The baby's crib is newly painted, but it is also old, and its slats are more than 2 3/8" apart. An attractive, hand-made mobile that hangs above the bed could pose a strangulation risk. Gita also notices the Carey's cat asleep in the crib. Ms. Carey remarks that her baby and the cat share the crib at naptime and every night. Gita intended to offer tips on making a house safe for an active infant, and suddenly she finds that she needs to remove the infant from immediate danger.

Through making several visits to the home and building a trusting relationship with Ms. Carey, Gita is able to talk to her about injury prevention. Gita helps her remove the mobile to prevent injury to the baby. She works with Ms. Carey and her landlord to install smoke detectors. Some of the more difficult changes, such as getting a safer crib and keeping the cat out of the crib, will take time. But Gita, as a home visitor, will be able to work closely with this family to minimize some of the hazards in their home.

**EARLY CHILDHOOD • 2 YEARS**

# ANTICIPATORY GUIDANCE FOR THE FAMILY

In addition to providing anticipatory guidance, many health professionals give families handouts
at an appropriate reading level or a videotape that they can review or study at home.[4]

## Promotion of healthy habits

### Injury prevention

Continue to use an age-appropriate car seat that is properly secured at all times.

Ensure that the child wears a life vest if boating. Inflatable flotation devices or "knowing how to swim" do not make a child safe in the water.

Ensure that swimming pools in the child's community, in his apartment complex, or at his home have a four-sided fence with a self-closing, self-latching gate. Children should be supervised by an adult whenever they are in or near water.

Continue to put sunscreen on the child before he goes outside to play or swim.

Continue to keep the child's environment free of smoke. Keep the home and car nonsmoking zones.

Test smoke detectors to ensure that they work properly. Change batteries yearly.

Keep cooking utensils, hot liquids, knives, and hot pots on the stove out of reach.

Ensure that electric wires, outlets, and appliances are inaccessible or protected.

Keep cigarettes, lighters, matches, alcohol, and electrical tools locked up and/or out of the child's sight and reach.

Exclude poisons, medications, and toxic household products from the home or keep them in locked cabinets. Have safety caps on all medications.

Keep Syrup of Ipecac in the home to be used as directed by the poison control center or the health professional. Keep the number of the poison control center near the telephone.

Guard against falls. Use locked doors or gates at the top and bottom of stairs and safety devices on windows. Supervise the child when he is on stairs.

Ensure that guns, if in the home, are locked up and that ammunition is stored separately. A trigger lock is an additional important precaution.

Teach the child to use caution when approaching dogs, especially if the dogs are unknown or eating.

Never leave the child alone in the car or the house or while taking a bath.

Do not expect young children to supervise the two year old.

Supervise all play near streets or driveways.

Ensure that a child riding in a seat on a parent's bicycle is wearing a helmet.

Ensure that playgrounds are safe. Check for impact- or energy-absorbing surfaces under playground equipment. Make sure that playground equipment is not over three feet tall and not made of pressure-treated wood.

Choose caregivers carefully. Discuss with them their attitudes about and behavior in relation to discipline. Prohibit corporal punishment.

## Nutrition

Serve the child meals with the family and give him two to three nutritious snacks per day.

Make mealtimes pleasant and companionable. Encourage conversation.

Provide nutritious snacks rich in complex carbohydrates, and limit sweets and high-fat snacks.

Offer the child nutritious foods and let him decide what and how much to eat. Children will eat a lot one time, not much the next.

Choose the menu. Do not let the child dictate it. Most children will eat a considerable number of foods.

Serve a variety of foods, particularly those containing iron.

Enforce reasonable mealtime behavior, but do not force eating.

Let the child experiment with food.

Avoid engaging in struggles about eating.

Ensure that the child's caregiver feeds him nutritious foods.

## Oral health

Continue to brush the child's teeth with a tiny, pea-size amount of fluoridated toothpaste.

Give the child fluoride supplements as recommended by the health professional based on the level of fluoride in the child's drinking water.

Schedule a dental appointment for the child every six months, unless his dentist determines otherwise based on his individual needs/susceptibility to disease.

## Sexuality education

Anticipate the child's normal curiosity about his body parts, including genitalia.

Use correct terms for genitalia.

## Promotion of social competence

Praise the child for good behavior and accomplishments.

Model appropriate language. Encourage language development by reading books to the child, singing him songs, and talking about what you and he are seeing and doing together.

Spend individual time with the child, playing with him, hugging or holding him, taking walks, painting, and doing puzzles together.

Appreciate the child's investigative nature, and do not excessively limit his explorations. Guide him through fun learning experiences.

Promote physical activity in a safe environment.

Encourage parallel play with other children, but do not expect shared play yet. Give the child opportunities to assert himself.

Reinforce self-care and self-expression.

To promote a sense of competence and control, invite the child to make choices whenever possible. (The choices should be ones you can live with—e.g., "Red pants or blue ones?")

Reinforce limits and appropriate behavior. Try to be consistent in expectations and discipline.

Use time out or remove source of conflict for unacceptable behavior.

Learn how to respond to the child's needs without giving in to every wish or becoming upset and reacting negatively to his constant questions and physical activity.

Prepare strategies to deal with night awakening, night fears, nightmares, and night terrors.

Encourage self-quieting behaviors, such as quiet play or the use of a transitional object.

Recognize that toilet training is part of developmentally appropriate learning.

Promote toilet training when the child is dry for periods of about two hours, knows the difference between wet and dry, can pull his pants up and down, wants to learn, and can give a signal when he is about to have a bowel movement.

Limit television watching to less than one hour per day of appropriate programs. Watch programs with your child.

## Promotion of constructive family relationships and parental health

Take some time for yourself and spend some individual time with your partner.

If another baby is expected, discuss with the health professional how to prepare the two-year-old child for the new baby.

Spend some time playing with the child each day. Focus on activities that he expresses interest in and enjoys.

Listen to and show respect for the child.

Show interest in child care activities.

Show affection in the family.

Spend some individual time with each child.

Help the child express such feelings as joy, anger, sadness, fear, and frustration.

Create opportunities for each family member to interact with and play with the child every day.

Keep family outings relatively short and simple. Lengthy activities tire the child and may lead to irritability or a temper tantrum.

Do not expect a child to share his toys.

Acknowledge conflicts between siblings. Whenever possible, attempt to resolve conflicts without taking sides. For example, if a conflict arises about a toy, the toy can be put in time out. Do not allow hitting, biting, or other violent behavior.

Allow older children to have objects that they do not have to share with the child. Give them a storage space that the child cannot get into.

Share meals as a family whenever possible. Spend time talking to each other.

Reach agreement with all family members on how to support the child's emerging independence while maintaining consistent limits.

Discuss with the health professional your own preventive and health-promoting practices (e.g., using seat belts, avoiding tobacco, eating properly, exercising and doing breast self-exams or testicular self-exams).

## Promotion of community interactions

If you need financial assistance to help pay for health care expenses, ask about resources or for referrals to the state Medicaid programs or other state medical assistance programs.

Ask about resources or referrals for food (e.g., WIC), housing, or transportation if needed.

Learn about and consider attending parent-child play groups. Discuss with the health professional possible programs for your child: preschools, early intervention programs, or other community programs.

Learn about and consider attending parent education classes or parent support groups.

Maintain or expand ties to your community through social, religious, cultural, volunteer, and recreational organizations.

Discuss with the health professional choosing and evaluating child care programs. Discuss the child care arrangements you have made.

Find out what you can do to make your community safer. Advocate for and participate in a neighborhood watch program.

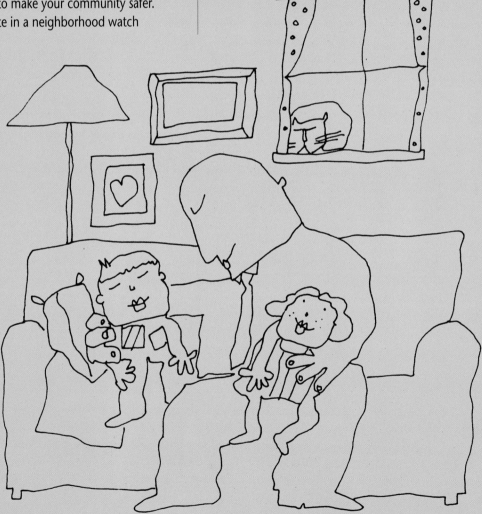

123

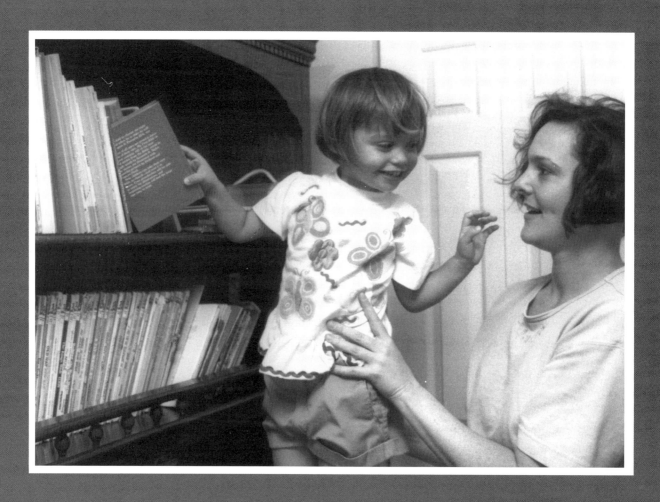

The three year old has developed understandable speech,
a major achievement, and she can now negotiate with her parents:
"Story first, then nap." She can also make choices,
deciding between green socks and blue or between
an orange and an apple.

# Three Year Visit

Around her third birthday, a real egocentric individualist makes her presence known. Her successes or failures at controlling the world around her will influence her behavior. As she makes her own simple choices, she is able to learn from trial and error and has a new feel for right and wrong. She can look forward to something pleasant or perceive an encounter as disagreeable. Unpredictability still reigns, however, as she decides whether to fight or to talk her way out of threatening situations.

The three year old has developed understandable speech, a major achievement, and she can now negotiate with her parents: "Story first, then nap." She can also make choices, deciding between green socks and blue or between a tea party and playing outside.

Awareness of gender differences has begun to emerge, in terms of both physical differences and society's expectations. Most three year olds can easily state "I am a girl" or "I am a boy." Body shape has altered from the baby mold to a more grown-up image. The three year old's physical abilities have developed, giving her real control over what her hands are touching or where her feet take her. Speech and motor activity are now focused on investigating or modifying the environment.

Around age three, the child can participate easily in the mainstream of family activities. She can come along to the store or a friend's house without the elaborate arrangements that babies require. She may need a transitional object that helps her move from one activity to another and feel safe in a variety of situations, but she is apt to wait quietly before sounding the cry of panic in uncertain situations. Many three year olds begin attending preschool, and health professionals can remind parents of children with special health needs of their children's right to appropriate education in the public school system.

The three year old is eager to explore her world and responds well to encouragement. She will say "okay" when given a choice, having learned that most of the choices her parents provide are good. Parents who have stifled their child's desire to explore with too many "no's" or "don't's" may have produced either frustration or withdrawal in response. The world can be truly a wonderful place for a three year old if she has the support, affection, and protection of the adults around her.

# HEALTH SUPERVISION INTERVIEW

## TRIGGER QUESTIONS

To be used selectively by the health professional. Discuss any issues or concerns of the family.

**How are you?**

**How are things going in your family?**

**Do you have any questions or concerns about Antonio?**

**What do you and your partner enjoy most about Mohammed these days?**

**What seems most difficult?**

**Have there been any major changes or stresses in your family since your last visit?**

**What are some of the new things that Anna is doing?**

**How is toilet training going?**

**What are Terry's eating habits?**

**How is child care** (e.g., preschool, early intervention) **going?**
**What does Samantha's teacher say about her?**

**What language(s) does your family speak at home?**

**Do family members understand Rafael's speech?**

**How do you deal with Alberto's greater independence?**
**What do you do when he has ideas that are different from yours?**

**Are you able to set clear and specific limits for Anita?**

**Have you ever been in a relationship where you have been hurt, threatened, or treated badly?**

**Have you ever been worried that someone was going to hurt your child?**
**Has your child ever been abused?**

**Do you feel safe in your neighborhood?**

**Does anyone in your home have a gun? Does a neighbor or a family friend?**
**If so, is the gun locked up? Where is the ammunition stored?**

# Developmental Surveillance and Milestones

## TRIGGER QUESTIONS AND POSSIBLE RESPONSES

**Do you have any specific concerns about Patty's development or behavior?**

**How does Patty communicate what she wants?**

Uses plurals, pronouns

Uses sentences of three or four words, short paragraphs

Speaks intelligibly to strangers (75 percent of the time)

**What do you think Patty understands?**

Names of most common objects

Physical relationships (e.g., "on," "in," "under")

Concept of "two"

Gender differences

Two-step instructions ("pick up your doll and put it on the chair")

**How does Patty get from one place to another?**

Walks, climbs, runs

Goes up and down stairs (alternating feet)

**How does Patty act around family members?**

Responsive or withdrawn

Affectionate or hostile/aggressive

Compliant or defiant

Dependent or self-reliant

Anxious about separation or not

**How does Patty react to strangers?**

Outgoing or slow to warm up

Wary/resistant

**How does Patty act around other children?**

Interactive or withdrawn/resistant

Friendly or hostile/aggressive

**To what extent has Patty developed independence in eating, dressing, and toileting?**

Uses cup, spoon, and fork

Puts on coat or jacket without assistance

Has bladder control

Has bowel control

## MILESTONES

Jumps in place, kicks a ball, balances on one foot

Rides a tricycle

Knows own name, age, and sex

Copies a circle and a cross

Has self-care skills (e.g., feeding, dressing)

Shows early imaginative behavior

**Tell me about Patty's typical play**

Plays with favorite toys (describe how used)

Listens to stories

Engages in elaborate fantasy play (with dolls, animals, people)

Plays interactive games with peers (able to take turns)

Has manual dexterity

## Observation of Parent-Child Interaction

How do the parent and the child communicate? How much of the communication is verbal? How much is nonverbal? Does the parent use baby talk? Does the parent give the child choices? (For example, "Do you want to sit on the table or on my lap?") Does the parent give commands to the child or ask the child what she wants to do? How does the child react?

## Physical Examination

Measure and plot on a standard chart the height, weight, and weight for height. Share the information with the parent.

As part of the complete physical examination, the following should be noted:

Caries, developmental dental anomalies, malocclusion, pathologic conditions, or dental injuries

Excessive injuries or bruising that may indicate inadequate supervision or possible abuse

Other evidence of neglect or abuse

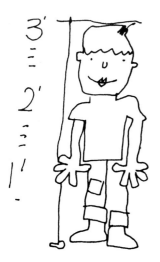

128

**ADDITIONAL SCREENING PROCEDURES**

Assessment of risk of high-dose lead exposure[1]

Vision screening
(Vision screening guidelines appear in appendix F, page 265)

Rescreen vision in six months if child is uncooperative

Hearing screening

Assessment of risk for hyperlipidemia[6]

Annual tuberculin test (PPD) if any of the following risk factors are present:

Low socioeconomic status
Residence in areas where tuberculosis is prevalent
Exposure to tuberculosis
Immigrant status

Blood pressure screening

**IMMUNIZATIONS**

Ensure that immunization status is up to date

# ANTICIPATORY GUIDANCE FOR THE FAMILY

In addition to providing anticipatory guidance, many health professionals give families handouts
at an appropriate reading level or a videotape that they can review or study at home.[4]

## Promotion of healthy habits

### Injury prevention

Continue to use an age-appropriate car seat that is properly secured at all times.

Ensure that the child wears a life vest if boating. Inflatable flotation devices or "knowing how to swim" do not make a child safe in the water.

Ensure that swimming pools in the child's community, in her apartment complex, or at her home have a four-sided fence with a self-closing, self-latching gate. Children should be supervised by an adult whenever they are in or near water.

Continue to put sunscreen on the child before she goes outside to play or swim.

Continue to keep the child's environment free of smoke. Keep the home and car nonsmoking zones.

Test smoke detectors to ensure that they work properly. Change batteries yearly.

Keep cooking utensils, hot liquids, knives, and hot pots on the stove out of reach.

Ensure that electric wires, outlets, and appliances are inaccessible or protected.

Keep cigarettes, lighters, matches, alcohol, and electrical tools locked up and/or out of the child's sight and reach.

Exclude poisons, medications, and toxic household products from the home or keep them in locked cabinets. Have safety caps on all medications.

Keep Syrup of Ipecac in the home to be used as directed by the poison control center or the health professional. Keep the number of the poison control center near the telephone.

Ensure that guns, if in the home, are locked up and that ammunition is stored separately. A trigger lock is an additional important precaution.

Never leave the child alone in the car or the house or while taking a bath.

Do not expect young children to supervise the three year old.

Supervise all play near streets or driveways.

Know where your child is at all times. She is too young to be roaming the neighborhood alone.

Teach your child pedestrian safety skills.

Ensure that a child riding in a seat on an adult's bicycle is wearing a helmet.

Ensure that playgrounds are safe. Check for impact- or energy-absorbing surfaces under playground equipment. Make sure that playground equipment is not over three feet tall and not made of pressure-treated wood.

Choose caregivers carefully. Discuss with them their attitudes about and behavior in relation to discipline. Prohibit corporal punishment.

Teach the child not to talk to strangers.

## Nutrition

Serve the child meals with the family and give her two to three nutritious snacks per day.

Make mealtimes pleasant and companionable. Encourage conversation.

Provide nutritious snacks rich in complex carbohydrates, and limit sweets and high-fat snacks.

Offer the child nutritious foods and let her decide what and how much to eat. Children will have an increasing list of accepted foods.

Serve a variety of healthy foods and model for the child how to eat them.

Ensure that the child's caregiver feeds her nutritious foods.

## Oral health

Teach the child to brush her teeth with a pea-size amount of fluoridated toothpaste.

Give the child fluoride supplements as recommended by the health professional based on the level of fluoride in the child's drinking water.

Schedule a dental appointment for the child every six months, unless her dentist determines otherwise based on her individual needs/susceptibility to disease.

## Sexuality education

Anticipate the child's normal curiosity about genital differences between boys and girls and about masturbation.

Use correct terms for genitalia.

Answer questions about "where babies come from."

Introduce the notion that some areas of the body are private.

## Promotion of social competence

Praise the child for good behavior and accomplishments.

Encourage the child to talk with you about her preschool, friends, or observations. Answer her questions.

Encourage interactive reading with the child.

Spend individual time with the child, doing something you both enjoy.

Provide opportunities for exploration.

Provide opportunities for the three year old to socialize with other children in play groups, preschool, or other community activities.

Promote physical activity in a safe environment.

Give the child opportunities to make choices (e.g., which clothes to wear, books to read, places to go).

Reinforce limits and appropriate behavior. Try to be consistent in expectations and discipline.

Use time out or remove source of conflict for unacceptable behavior.

Encourage self-discipline.

Anticipate that your child may have many fears, including night terrors.

Limit television watching to an average of one hour per day of appropriate programs. Watch the programs together and discuss them.

## Promotion of constructive family relationships and parental health

If another baby is expected, discuss with the health professional how to prepare the three-year-old child for the new baby.

Spend some time playing with the child each day. Focus on activities that she expresses interest in and enjoys.

Listen to and show respect for the child.

Show interest in preschool and/or child care activities.

Show affection in the family.

Spend some individual time with each child.

Participate in games and other activities with the child.

Encourage the development of good sibling relationships. Acknowledge conflicts between siblings. Whenever possible, attempt to resolve conflicts without taking sides. Do not allow hitting, biting, or other violent behavior.

Share meals as a family whenever possible. Spend time talking to each other.

Handle anger constructively in the family.

Discuss with the health professional your own preventive and health-promoting practices (e.g., using seat belts, avoiding tobacco, eating properly, exercising and doing breast self-exams or testicular self-exams).

## Promotion of community interactions

If you need financial assistance to help pay for health care expenses, ask about resources or for referrals to the state Medicaid programs or other state medical assistance programs.

Ask about resources or referrals for food (e.g., WIC), housing, or transportation if needed.

Discuss with the health professional possible programs for the child: preschools, early intervention programs, Head Start (most programs start at age four), swimming and other exercise programs, or other community programs.

Learn about and consider attending parent education classes or parent support groups.

Maintain or expand ties to your community through social, religious, cultural, volunteer, and recreational organizations.

Discuss with the health professional choosing and evaluating child care programs. Discuss the child care arrangements you have made.

Find out what you can do to make your community safer. Advocate for and participate in a neighborhood watch program.

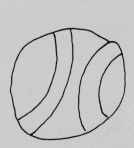

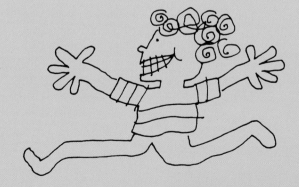

131

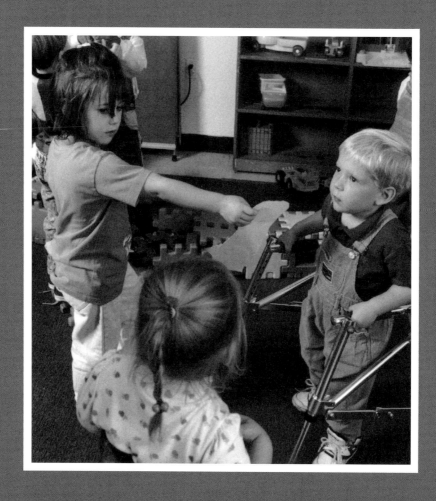

*Although scrappy behavior with peers*
*may present a problem at preschool or during play,*
*the four year old can be assertive*
*without being aggressive.*

# Four Year Visit

Language skills, combined with an insatiable curiosity, enlarge the world of the four year old and give him a sense of independence. Able to dress and undress himself and having achieved bowel and bladder control—although he may not be dry at night—he feels grown-up beyond his years. While his thinking remains egocentric, he is sensitive to the feelings of others. He can identify such emotions as sadness, anger, anxiety, fear, and guilt in others as well as himself. Now that he can play collaboratively, he has formed budding friendships with his peers.

Talkative and animated, the four year old is a delightful conversationalist, able to tell an involved story or relate a recent experience. He frequently demands to know why, what, when, and how.

His seemingly boundless energy and increased motor skills are channeled into group games and such physical activities as running, climbing, swinging, sliding, and jumping. At the same time, he needs opportunities to rest and play quietly by himself. Fantasy and "magical thinking" are reflected in imaginative play, including "make-believe" and "dress-up." Because four year olds are curious about their own bodies and those of the opposite sex, sexual exploration is normal and common at this age. Modesty and a desire for privacy begin to emerge.

The child enjoys and looks forward to the social and learning opportunities at preschool. Although scrappy behavior with peers may present a problem at preschool or during play, the four year old can be assertive without being aggressive.

The four year old's family can find him tedious at times. While the child is still trying to understand why the ball can bounce so high, he is also interested in seeing the consequences of his actions on family members. How many times will his parents say "No" before they get angry? How far off the sidewalk can he stray before they chase after him? How many toys can he take before his sister protests? In his efforts to learn about appropriate social interaction and expected behavior in the family, he tests the limits of his parents and siblings. On the other hand, the four year old responds well to praise and clearly stated rules.

# HEALTH SUPERVISION INTERVIEW

## TRIGGER QUESTIONS

To be used selectively by the health professional. Discuss any issues or concerns of the family.

**How are you?**

**How are things going in your family?**

**Do you have any questions or concerns about Carmen?**

**What do you and your partner enjoy most about Yukari?**

**Have there been any major changes or stresses in your family since your last visit?**

**What are some of Craig's new skills?**

**Is Todd interested in other children? Does he have playmates?**

**How is Meredith doing in preschool? What does her teacher say about her?**

**How do you deal with Abu's greater independence?**
**What do you do when he has ideas that are different from yours?**

**Are you able to set clear and specific limits for Susie?**

**Do you have a pool? Is it attached to the house? Is it fenced?**
**Does it have a self-latching gate? Is the gate locked?**

**Have you ever been in a relationship where you have been hurt, threatened, or treated badly?**

**Have you ever been worried that someone was going to hurt your child?**
**Has your child ever been abused?**

**Do you feel safe in your neighborhood?**

**Does Marcos feel safe in your neighborhood?**

**Does anyone in your home own a gun? Does a neighbor or a family friend?**
**If so, is the gun locked up? Where is the ammunition stored?**

# Developmental Surveillance and Milestones

## TRIGGER QUESTIONS AND POSSIBLE RESPONSES

**Do you have any specific concerns about Lamont's development or behavior?**

**How does Lamont communicate what he wants?**

Uses past tense

Uses sentences of four to five words, short paragraphs

Describes a recent experience

May show some dysfluency (e.g., stuttering)

Speaks intelligibly to strangers (almost 100 percent of the time)

**What do you think Lamont understands?**

Concepts of "same" and "different"

Two- or three-step instructions

The difference between fantasy and reality

**How does Lamont get from one place to another?**

Walks, climbs, runs

Goes up and down stairs (alternating feet without support)

**How does Lamont act around others?**

Responsive or withdrawn

Friendly or hostile/aggressive

Compliant or defiant

Dependent or self-reliant

Anxious about separation or not

**To what extent has Lamont developed independence in eating, dressing, and toileting?**

Uses utensils

Puts on and removes clothing

Has bladder and bowel control

**Tell me about Lamont's typical play.**

Plays with favorite toys (describe how used)

Listens to stories

Engages in elaborate fantasy play

Plays interactive games with peers

Has manual dexterity

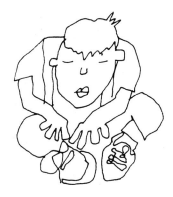

135

## Observation of Parent-Child Interaction

How do the parent and the child communicate? Does the parent allow the child to answer the health professional's questions directly, or does the parent intervene? Does the parent pay attention to the child's behavior, matching unacceptable behavior with consequences? How do the parent, the four year old, and any siblings interact? Who sits where? Does the parent pay attention to all the children?

## Physical Examination

Measure and plot on a standard chart the height, weight, and weight for height. Share the information with the parent.

Observe the child's gait.

As part of the complete physical examination, the following should be noted:

Caries, developmental dental anomalies, malocclusion, pathologic conditions, or dental injuries

Evidence of neglect or abuse

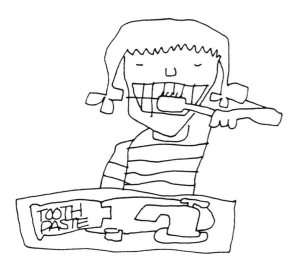

# ANTICIPATORY GUIDANCE FOR THE FAMILY

In addition to providing anticipatory guidance, many health professionals give families handouts
at an appropriate reading level or a videotape that they can review or study at home.[4]

## Promotion of healthy habits

### Injury prevention

Establish and enforce consistent, explicit, and firm rules for safe behavior.

Continue to use a car seat or a properly secured booster until the child weighs 60 pounds or his head is higher than the back of the seat.

Ensure that swimming pools in the child's community, in his apartment complex, or at his home have a four-sided fence with a self-closing, self-latching gate. Children should be supervised by an adult whenever they are in or around water.

Teach the child how to swim.

Continue to put sunscreen on the child before he goes outside to play or swim.

Continue to keep the child's environment free of smoke. Keep the home and car nonsmoking zones.

Test smoke detectors to ensure that they work properly. Change batteries yearly.

Keep cigarettes, lighters, matches, alcohol, and electrical tools locked up and/or out of the child's sight and reach.

Exclude poisons, medications, and toxic household products from home or keep them in locked cabinets. Have safety caps on all medications.

Keep Syrup of Ipecac in the home to be used as directed by the poison control center or the health professional. Keep the number of the poison control center near the telephone.

Ensure that guns, if in the home, are locked up and that ammunition is stored separately. A trigger lock is an additional important precaution.

Never leave the child alone in the car or the house or while taking a bath.

Supervise all play near streets or driveways.

Know where your child is at all times. He is too young to be roaming the neighborhood alone.

Teach your child pedestrian and neighborhood safety skills.

Teach the child about playground safety.

Ensure that the child wears a bicycle helmet when riding a tricycle or a bicycle with training wheels.

Choose caregivers carefully. Discuss with them their attitudes about and behavior in relation to discipline. Prohibit corporal punishment.

Teach the child safety rules regarding strangers.

### Nutrition

Serve the child three regular meals and two nutritious snacks per day. Make mealtimes pleasant and companionable. Encourage conversation.

Provide nutritious snacks rich in complex carbohydrates. Limit high-fat or low-nutrient foods and beverages such as candy, chips, or soft drinks.

Offer the child nutritious foods and let him decide what and how much to eat. Anticipate that the child will imitate peers in food likes and dislikes. He will have an increasing list of accepted foods.

**EARLY CHILDHOOD • 4 YEARS**

Model and encourage good eating habits. Serve a variety of healthy foods.

Ensure that the child's caregiver feeds him nutritious foods.

## Oral health

Ensure that the child brushes his teeth twice a day with a pea-size amount of fluoridated toothpaste. Regularly supervise tooth brushing.

Give the child fluoride supplements as recommended by the health professional based on the level of fluoride in the child's drinking water.

Learn how to prevent dental injuries and handle dental emergencies, especially the loss or fracture of a tooth.

If the child regularly sucks his fingers or thumb begin to intervene to get him to discontinue.

Schedule a dental appointment for the child every six months, unless his dentist determines otherwise based on his individual needs/susceptibility to disease.

## Sexuality education

Anticipate the child's normal curiosity about his body and the differences between boys and girls.

Use correct terms for all body parts, including genitalia.

Answer questions about "where babies come from."

Explain to the child that no one should touch his "private parts" without his permission.

## Promotion of social competence

Praise the child for cooperation and accomplishments.

Encourage the child to talk with you about his preschool, friends, or observations. Answer his questions.

Encourage interactive reading with the child.

Spend individual time with the child, doing something you both enjoy.

Enlarge the child's experiences through trips and visits to parks and other places of interest.

Provide opportunities for the four year old to socialize with other children in play groups, preschool, or other community activities.

Promote physical activity in a safe environment.

Encourage assertiveness without excessive aggression.

Set developmentally appropriate limits.

Use time out, removal of source of conflict, and other options for unacceptable behavior.

Encourage self-discipline.

Limit television viewing to an average of one hour per day of appropriate programs. Watch the programs together and discuss them.

Provide some type of structured learning environment for the child, whether in Head Start, preschool, Sunday school, or a community program or child care center.

Discuss with the health professional how to tell when the child is ready for school.

## Promotion of constructive family relationships and parental health

Listen to and show respect for the child.

Show interest in preschool and/or child care activities.

Show affection in the family.

Spend some individual time with each child.

Participate in games and other physical activities with the child.

Encourage the development of good sibling relationships. Acknowledge conflicts between siblings. Whenever possible, attempt to resolve conflicts without taking sides. Do not allow hitting, biting, or other violent behavior.

Share meals as a family whenever possible. Spend time talking to each other.

Handle anger constructively in the family.

Discuss with the health professional your own preventive and health-promoting practices (e.g., using seat belts, avoiding tobacco, eating properly, exercising and doing breast self-exams or testicular self-exams).

## Promotion of community interactions

If you need financial assistance to help pay for health care expenses, ask about resources or for referrals to the state Medicaid programs or other state medical assistance programs.

Ask about resources or referrals for food (e.g., WIC), housing, or transportation if needed.

Discuss with the health professional possible programs for the child: preschools, early intervention programs, prekindergarten programs, kindergarten, Head Start, swimming and other exercise programs, or other community programs.

Visit the child's preschool or other child care program unannounced. Ask if all children are immunized.

Learn about and consider attending parent education classes or parent support groups.

Maintain or expand ties to your community through social, religious, cultural, volunteer, and recreational organizations.

Discuss with the health professional choosing and evaluating child care programs. Discuss the arrangements you have made.

Find out what you can do to make your community safer. Advocate for and participate in a neighborhood watch program.

Advocate for adequate housing and play spaces/playgrounds.

Recommend that schools provide early and regular comprehensive health education that encourages healthy lifestyles.

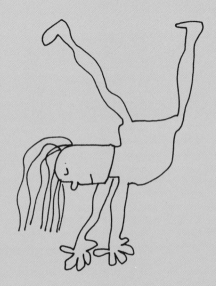

**EARLY CHILDHOOD • 4 YEARS**

# EARLY CHILDHOOD HEALTH SUPERVISION SUMMARY

**What else should we talk about?**

## Summarize findings of the visit

Emphasize strengths. Underscore the child's achievements and progress in development and the increasing competence of the parents. Compliment the parents on their efforts to care for the child. Give them suggestions, reading materials, and resources to promote health and reinforce good health practices.

## Arrange continuing care

### Next visit

Give the parents materials to prepare them for the next health supervision visit.

Recommend that the parents make an appointment for the next regularly scheduled visit.

If indicated, ask the parents to make an appointment for a supplementary health supervision visit.

## Other care

Ensure that the parents make an appointment to return to the health facility for follow-up on problems identified during the health supervision visit, or refer the child for secondary or tertiary medical care.

Consult with the school as necessary, especially if preschool progress is unsatisfactory or teacher evaluations are needed. (Obtain the parents' permission.)

Refer the family to appropriate community resources for help with problems identified during the visit (e.g., WIC, parenting classes, parent-toddler groups, marital counseling, mental health services, early intervention programs, Head Start, adult education programs). Make arrangements to follow up on referrals and coordinate care.

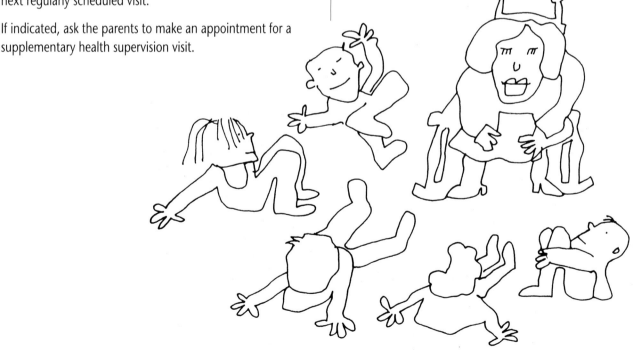

## Early Childhood Endnotes

1. To assess the risk of high-dose lead exposure, ask:

   Does your child live in or regularly visit a house (or a preschool or child care center) built before 1960? Does it have peeling or chipping paint? Has there been recent renovation or remodeling? Is any planned?

   Does your home's plumbing have lead pipes or copper with lead solder joints?

   Does your child live near a heavily travelled major highway where soil and dust may be contaminated with lead?

   Does your child frequently come in contact with an adult who works with lead (e.g., in construction, welding, pottery, or other trades)?

   Does your child live near a lead smelter, battery recycling plant, or other industrial site likely to release lead?

   Do you give your child any home remedies that may contain lead?

   Have any of your children or any of their playmates had lead poisoning?

   If all answers are negative, screen the child for lead at one and two years of age.

   If any answer is positive, the child is considered at high risk for high-dose lead exposure. Administer a blood lead screening test immediately and at every health supervision visit through six years of age.

   If any blood test result is ≥10 µg/dL, the health professional should refer to the Centers for Disease Control and Prevention (CDC) guidelines and develop a management/treatment plan. (The CDC guidelines are subject to change, so consult the latest edition.) See appendix for Medicaid-eligible children.

   US Department of Health and Human Services, Public Health Service, Centers for Disease Control. 1991. Preventing lead poisoning in young children: A statement by the Centers for Disease Control—October 1991. N.p.: Centers for Disease Control.

2. A blood lead test must be used to screen Medicaid-eligible children. See appendix E, page 264.

3. The American Academy of Pediatrics recommends the following schedule for Hemophilus influenza type b (Hib) vaccine and diphtheria, tetanus, pertussis (DTP) vaccine for children younger than 15 months of age:

   > HbOC (HIBTITER™) or PRP-T vaccine at 2, 4, 6, and 12–15 months; or
   >
   > PRP-OMP (PedvaxHIB®) vaccine at 2, 4, 6, and 12–15 months; or
   >
   > HbOC-DTP combination vaccine at 2, 4, 6, and 15 months. *As an option for the 15 month booster, acellular (DTap) vaccine may also be used in conjunction with any Hib conjugate.*

   The Advisory Committee on Immunization Practices (ACIP) recommends that the third dose of oral poliovirus vaccine be given at 6 months instead of 15–18 months.

   See the AAP Recommended Immunization Schedule and the Recommendations of the Advisory Committee on Immunization Practices in the appendix.

4. The Injury Prevention Program (TIPP) of the American Academy of Pediatrics produces parent information sheets that highlight injury prevention priorities at each age, as well as parent information sheets on specific issues such as water safety. Community-based prevention groups, such as SAFE KIDS, also produce injury prevention materials.

5. Fraiberg SH. 1959. *The Magic Years*. New York: Charles Scribner's Sons.

6. Hyperlipidemia screening if any of the following risk factors are present:

Parents or grandparents with a history of coronary or peripheral vascular disease before 55 years of age (Obtain a fasting serum lipid profile that includes determination of the low-density lipoprotein [LDL] cholesterol value.)

Parents with a blood cholesterol level ≥240 mg/dL (Obtain a nonfasting total blood cholesterol level; perform at least once.)

Hyperlipidemia screening at the discretion of the health professional if family history cannot be ascertained and any of the following risk factors are present in the family:

Smoking
Hypertension
Physical inactivity
Obesity
Diabetes mellitus
(Obtain a nonfasting total blood cholesterol.)

American Academy of Pediatrics. 1989. Indications for cholesterol testing in children. *Pediatrics* 83(1):141–142.

American Academy of Pediatrics, Committee on Nutrition. 1992. Statement on cholesterol. *Pediatrics* 90(3):469–473.

National Cholesterol Education Program (NCEP) Expert Panel on Blood Cholesterol Levels in Children and Adolescents. 1992. NCEP: Highlights of the report of the Expert Panel on Blood Cholesterol Levels in Children and Adolescents. *Pediatrics* 89(3):495–500.

## Bibliography

Brazelton TB. 1992. *Touchpoints*. New York: Addison-Wesley.

Brooks-Gunn J, Liaw F, Klebanov PK. 1992. Effects of early intervention on cognitive function of low birth weight preterm infants. *Journal of Pediatrics* 120(3):350–359.

Canadian Task Force on the Periodic Health Examination. 1990. Periodic health examination, 1990 update: 4. Well-baby care in the first 2 years of life. *Canadian Medical Association Journal* 143(9):18–23.

Capute AJ, Shapiro BK, Palmer FB. 1987. Marking the milestones of language development. *Contemporary Pediatrics* 4:24–41.

Casey PH, Evans LD. 1993. School readiness: An overview for pediatricians. *Pediatrics in Review* 14(1):4–10.

Coplan J, Gleason JR. 1988. Unclear speech: Recognition and significance of unintelligible speech in preschool children. *Pediatrics* 82(3, Pt. 2): 447–452.

Dixon SD, Stein MT. 1987. *Encounters with Children: Pediatric Behavior and Development* (2nd ed.). St. Louis, MO: Mosby Year Book.

Dodds M, Nicholson L, Muse B, Osborn LM. 1993. Group health supervision visits more effective than individual visits in delivering health care information. *Pediatrics* 91(3):668–670.

Fraiberg S. 1959. *The Magic Years*. New York: Charles Scribner's Sons.

Hamburg DA. 1990. *A Decent Start: Promoting Healthy Child Development in the First Three Years of Life*. New York: Carnegie Corporation of New York.

Kemper KJ, Avner ED. 1992. The case against screening urinalyses for asymptomatic bacteriuria in children. *American Journal of Diseases in Children* 146:343–346.

Kirby RS, Swanson ME, Kelleher KJ, Bradley RH, Casey PH. 1993. Identifying at-risk children for early intervention services: Lessons from the infant health and development program. *Journal of Pediatrics* 122(5):680–686.

Lauer RM, Clarke WR. 1990. Use of cholesterol measurements in childhood for the prediction of adult hypercholesterolemia: The Muscatine study. *Journal of the American Medical Association* 264(23):3034–3038.

Olds DL, Henderson CR, Chamberlin R, Tatelbaum R. 1986. Preventing child abuse and neglect: A randomized trial of nurse home visitation. *Pediatrics* 78(1):65–77.

Walker D, Gugenheim S, Down MP, Northern JL. 1989. Early language milestone scale and language screening of young children. *Pediatrics* 83(2):284–288.

Wasserman RC. 1992. Screening for vision problems in pediatric practice. *Pediatrics in Review* 13(1):4–5.

Zero to Three/National Center for Clinical Infant Programs. 1992. *Heart Start: The Emotional Foundations of School Readiness*. Arlington, VA: Zero to Three/National Center for Clinical Infant Programs.

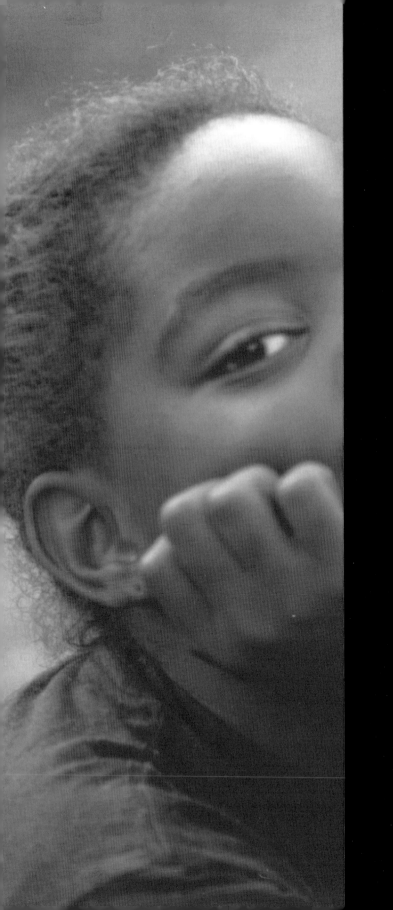

5–11 Years

Middle Childhood

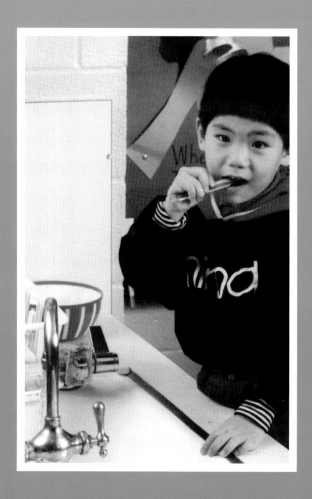

*We need to do a better job of weaving a safety net of*
*understanding, appreciation and guidance in the family,*
*in the community and school. We need to start thinking of*
*health and education as interlocking spheres.*

—C. Everett Koop, M.D.
Surgeon General,
United States Public Health Service
1981–1989

# Middle Childhood

What images do we have of the school-age child? One picture is of a youngster running through a playground, giggling as she happily pursues her friends in a game of tag. Safe, strong, resilient, well-nourished, and self-confident, she is able to interact with peers on an equal basis. This child is becoming aware of the outside world—its opportunities, its challenges, and its fun.

There may be a distinctly different picture for some children. Another child lets himself into an empty apartment at the end of a school day. He has rushed home, fearful of the people he meets in the street. Once in his sparsely furnished apartment, he occupies himself with television and snacks on soda and potato chips. From the TV, he learns he will be more socially valued and mature if he drinks beer, wears brand-name sneakers, and acts aggressively. For this child, there are few opportunities for quality peer interaction, cognitive enrichment, and the achievement of success.

These pictures contrast two disparate worlds of middle childhood and highlight the differential effect of social inequality on child health and well-being. To be successful, health supervision must be grounded in a solid base of knowledge about the physical, cognitive, emotional, social, and moral development of children. In each of these areas, there is a known progression during the middle childhood years. There also needs to be an appreciation of the family, the school, and the community as the context within which children grow and develop.

Children of school age should be active participants in health supervision. Whether this happens depends, in part, on the structure of the child's family, on his culture, and on the extent to which he is encouraged to form a health-promoting alliance with a health professional.

## Physical

During the middle years, the child's growth rate is somewhat slower than in previous years, and certainly less rapid than the growth the child will experience during adolescence. Nonetheless, major increases in strength and improvements in motor coordination do occur. These changes contribute to the child's growing sense of competence in relation to his physical abilities, and enhance his potential for participating in sports, dance, gymnastics, and other physical pursuits. Growth monitoring and periodic physical examinations to detect aberrant growth patterns are important components of health supervision.

Families can provide enormous support for healthy physical development. They can also work with communities to ensure that children have access to playgrounds, gymnasiums, and parks, in addition to well-supervised play activities. For children to flourish, communities must value the children's physical growth and provide play facilities to help their bodies develop in a healthy fashion. Health professionals can augment their personal office messages about physical fitness by advocating for such community facilities.

Middle childhood is a critical time for children with physical disabilities or chronic illness to adapt successfully to their disorder. They acquire a clearer sense of self and the ability to care for their health during this period. Children adapt best to chronic illnesses when health professionals, families, and communities work together to foster their emerging independence. Full

**MIDDLE CHILDHOOD • 5–11 YEARS**

inclusion in school and community life allows children with impairments to feel valued and to integrate their disabilities with other aspects of their lives.

## Cognitive

Children's readiness to take advantage of school depends upon their prior experiences. The synthesis of basic language, perception, and abstraction allows the child to read, write, and communicate thoughts of increasing complexity and creativity. Progress may appear subtle from month to month, but it is dramatic from one school year to the next. As the child's cognitive skills grow, he matures in his ability to understand the world and people around him and to function independently.

The major developmental achievement of this period is self-efficacy—i.e., the knowledge of what to do and the ability to do it. Success at school is most likely to occur when such achievement is valued by families. Parental encouragement of learning is essential. Families who reward children with enthusiasm and warmth for putting forth their best effort ensure their steady educational progress and prepare them to use their intelligence and knowledge productively. Moreover, by being aware of individual learning styles, parents and teachers can adapt materials and experiences to each child.

## Social/emotional

As children become more independent, they develop their own sense of personhood. They begin to discern where they "fit" in their family, school class, neighborhood, or community. When the "fit" is good and comfortable, children see themselves as effective and competent members of their family, group, class, team, school, or community. But when the "fit" is tenuous or poor, the dissonance may be a source of distress and may

predispose children to emotional disorders with long-term consequences. The promotion of good mental health requires active participation and support by families, health professionals, educators, and all who care for and teach children.

Children need both the freedom of personal expression and the structure of expectations and guidelines that they can understand and accept. Opportunities to interact with other children in play environments without excessive adult interference are important, although some neighborhoods or living arrangements restrict these chances. At the same time, children need to have positive interactions with adults, reinforcing their sense of self-esteem, self-worth, and belief in their capability of personal success.

The child's "self" evolves in a social context. Health professionals can help families understand this dynamic and encourage specific roles for their children within the family. Parents who consciously assess their child's emotional maturity and role in the family at each birthday will appreciate the changes that have occurred subtly over time. As a result, they will be able to celebrate the child's evolving autonomy by granting new privileges. Parents who match each new entitlement with a new responsibility signal their respect for the child's growing capability to contribute to the family and the community.

## Moral/spiritual

Part of the child's development as an individual includes a nascent understanding of the life cycle—of birth, growth, aging, and death. There is an increasing awareness that life fits into a larger scheme of relationships among individuals, groups of people, other living creatures, and the earth itself. School-age children become keenly interested in these topics, especially when confronted with personal experiences such as the birth of a sibling or the death of a grandparent.

As children experience these events and learn to view their personal encounters as part of a larger whole, families and communities provide important structure. They define value systems that provide children with basic principles and encourage them to examine their personal actions in light of their impact on those around them. Children's ability to understand their place in the larger world leads to greater self-esteem and competence. The close link between competence and self-esteem is strengthened when a child is recognized for achieving success in school, playing a leadership role among peers, participating in church activities, or otherwise helping to make a difference in the community. This understanding should be reinforced by those around the child. On the other hand, families need to ensure that children do not become over-extended by participating in too many extracurricular activities (e.g., soccer, ballet lessons, baseball).

## Health behaviors

As a child's sense of competence emerges in the middle childhood period, a shift in responsibility needs to occur in health supervision. At the beginning of the period, it is the parent who buys all the food, clothing, toys, and other materials. It is the parent who makes the rules about crossing the street, where a bike can be ridden, and what the child can eat. By the end of the period, the child is very much a consumer, handling a small or moderate allowance and deciding on snacks, games, TV programs, and other types of sports or entertainment. While the child is not making the safety rules, he is undoubtedly negotiating for more input into his bedtime, more independence regarding bike trips, more free time in the playground, and increased choice in

selecting friends and opportunities. As this shift occurs, children who are active and eager learners are ready to hear, consider, and respond to health promotion messages. The middle childhood period, therefore, offers an excellent opportunity to introduce information on health promotion and disease prevention, including discussion of smoking and use of alcohol and drugs. If the child feels that he has a real future, these interventions will make a difference in his life.

While most children do not have the emotional drive, cognitive understanding, or independence to experiment with lifestyles the way adolescents and young adults do, they are watching, listening, learning, and mapping their own view of the outside world. They are beginning to create their own scaffolding for life's experiments and experiences. It is the role of health supervision to help children build this structure solidly so that it can be expanded during adolescence. With the knowledge and understanding provided by health supervision, children can develop the responsibility necessary for good personal health practices and avoidance of unhealthy habits.

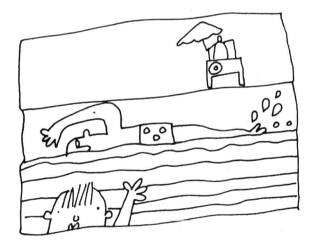

# MIDDLE CHILDHOOD DEVELOPMENTAL CHART

Health professionals should assess the achievements of the child and provide guidance to the family on anticipated tasks. The effects are demonstrated by health supervision outcomes.

## ACHIEVEMENTS DURING MIDDLE CHILDHOOD

Responsibility for good health habits

Ability to play in groups

One or more close friendships

Identification with peer groups

Competence as member of family, community, and other groups

Ability to express feelings

Belief in capacity for success

Understanding of right and wrong

Awareness of safety rules

Ability to read, write, and communicate increasingly complex and creative thoughts

Responsibility for homework

School achievement

## TASKS FOR THE CHILD

Maintain good eating habits

Practice good dental hygiene

Participate in athletic or exercise programs

Maintain appropriate weight

Wear bicycle helmet, seat belt, and contact sports mouth guard

Avoid alcohol, tobacco, and other drugs

Resist peer pressure to engage in risk-taking behaviors

Control impulses

Resolve conflict and manage anger constructively

Assume responsibility for belongings, chores, and good health habits

Play with and relate well to siblings and peers

Communicate well with parents, teachers, and other adults

Be industrious in school

## HEALTH SUPERVISION OUTCOMES

Sense of personal competence

Sense of self-efficacy and mastery

Active role in health supervision and promotion

Optimal nutrition

Satisfactory growth and development

Good health habits

Injury prevention

Personal safety

Social competence

Promotion of developmental potential

Prevention of behavioral problems

Promotion of family strengths

Enhancement of parental effectiveness

Success in school

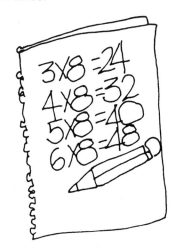

# FAMILY PREPARATION FOR MIDDLE CHILDHOOD HEALTH SUPERVISION

Instructions to be provided to the family by the health professional.

Be prepared to give updates on the following at your next visit:

> Illnesses and infectious diseases
> Injuries
> Visits to other health facilities or providers
> Use of the emergency department
> Hospitalizations or surgeries
> Immunizations
> Food and drug allergies
> Eating habits
> Medications
> Supplementary fluoride and vitamins
> Dental care
> Vision and hearing
> Chronic health conditions

Update your child's personal health record.

Be prepared to provide the following information on your family:

> Health of and location of each significant family member
>
> Genetic disorders
>
> Depression or other mental health problems in the immediate or extended family
>
> Alcoholism or other substance abuse (including use of tobacco) in the immediate or extended family
>
> Family transitions (e.g., birth, death, marriage, divorce, loss of income, move, frequently absent parent, incarceration, change in child care arrangements)

> Home environment/neighborhood
>
> Hazardous exposures (e.g., violence, asbestos, tuberculosis)

Prepare and bring in questions, concerns, and observations about issues such as:

> Stressors (school, friends, environment)
>
> School (learning style and peer interaction)
>
> Physical changes (sports readiness, aches and pains, injuries, dental status, eating patterns, approach of puberty)
>
> Achievements

Bring in reports from preschool/school, school attendance records, and results of parent-teacher conferences. Bring in the Individualized Education Program (IEP) if the child has special needs.

Bring in a schedule of the child's extracurricular activities.

Complete and bring in psychosocial or developmental questionnaires.

Fill out and bring in health forms (school entry, sports participation) for completion by the health professional.

Prepare your child to discuss issues, concerns, and achievements. Help your child learn about the health supervision process.

# STRENGTHS DURING MIDDLE CHILDHOOD

Health professionals should remind families of their strengths during the health supervision visit. Strengths and issues for child, family, and community are interrelated and interdependent.

## CHILD

Has good physical health and nutritional status

Has good eating habits

Is developing a sense of responsibility for own health

Has regular dental care

Engages in physical activities with vigor

Has positive, cheerful, friendly temperament

Feels loved and valued by parents and other adults

Has one or more close friends

Is developing social competence

Expresses feelings

Enjoys life and has joyful experiences

Has personal sense of competence

Has high self-esteem and expects personal success

Has opportunities for new challenges

Feels comfortable asking questions of parents and teachers

Is industrious in school

Has positive role models

## FAMILY

Meets basic needs (food, shelter, clothing, safety, health care)

Enjoys child

Responds to child's developmental needs

Encourages good communication

Spends individual time with child

Praises and takes pride in child's achievements

Reinforces child's feeling of being loved

Helps child develop social competence

Possesses working knowledge of child health and development

Serves nutritious family meals on a regular basis

Reinforces health as a family priority

Allows child age-appropriate autonomy

Protects child against excessive stress

Provides value system, good parental role models

Siblings get along well

Has support of extended family and others

Encourages ties to community

## COMMUNITY

Provides quality schools and educational opportunities for all families

Provides programs for children (recreational, sports, educational, social)

Provides activities for families

Encourages participation of children in organized groups

Provides support for families with special needs (school breakfast and lunch programs, appropriate educational programs, community outreach)

Provides neighborhood/school settings with supervised before- and after-school activities

Provides an environment free of hazards (violence, pollution, asbestos, radiation)

Ensures that neighborhoods are safe

Provides affordable housing and public transportation

Develops integrated systems of health care

Fluoridates drinking water

Promotes community interactions (neighborhood watch programs, support groups, community centers)

Promotes positive ethnic/cultural milieu

# ISSUES DURING MIDDLE CHILDHOOD

Health professionals should address issues—problems, stressors, and concerns—that families raise during health supervision.
Strengths and issues for child, family, and community are interrelated and interdependent.

## CHILD

School concerns (learning disabilities, underachievement, failure to do homework, frequent school absence or tardiness/school avoidance, lack of motivation)

Behavioral concerns (hyperactivity, distractibility, disobedience, temper outbursts, lying, aggression, fighting, stealing, vandalism, fire setting, violence)

Peer concerns (inability to get along with other children, shyness, lack of friends)

Emotional concerns (separation problems, depression, anxiety, low self-esteem, threat of suicide)

Risk-taking behavior (smoking, sexual activity, use of alcohol, drugs, or tobacco)

Weight and height concerns (short stature, obesity, eating disorders)

Failure to exercise

Chronic illness

Somatic complaints

Tics

Enuresis, encopresis

Developmental delay

## FAMILY

Dysfunctional parents or other family members (depressed, mentally ill, abusive, disinterested, overly critical, overprotective, incarcerated)

Marital problems

Domestic violence (verbal, physical, or sexual abuse)

Frequently absent parent

Rotating "parents" (parents' girlfriends or boyfriends)

Inadequate child care arrangements

Family health problems (illness, chronic illness, or disability)

Substance use (alcohol, drugs, tobacco)

Financial insecurity/homelessness

Family transitions (move, divorce, remarriage, incarceration, death)

Lack of knowledge about child development

Lack of parental self-esteem and self-efficacy

Poor family communication

Social isolation and lack of support

Rejection of child

## COMMUNITY

Poverty

Inadequate housing

Environmental hazards

Unsafe neighborhood

Community violence

Poor opportunities for employment

Low-quality or unsafe schools

Lack of supervised programs before and after school

Lack of programs for families with special needs (e.g., school breakfast and lunch)

Lack of social support

Isolation in a rural community

Lack of social, educational, cultural, and recreational opportunities

Discrimination and prejudice

Lack of access to medical/dental services

Inadequate public services (transportation, garbage removal, lighting, repair of public facilities, police and fire protection)

Inadequate fluoride levels in community drinking water

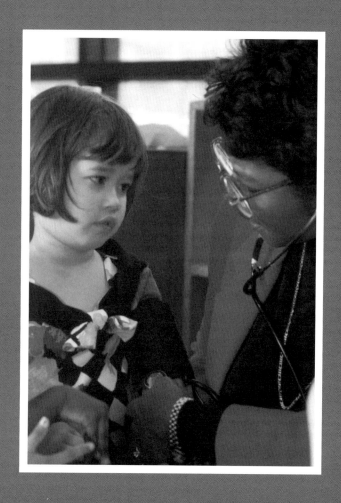

*The health professional should speak directly
with the child about her family, her friends,
and her excitement or fears about going to school.*

# Five Year Visit

As entry into elementary school approaches, the child's school readiness and her ability to separate from her parents gains importance. The five year old who has experienced preschool or child care may be able to separate more easily. How do the parents react to the approach of school entry? Should a child who will turn five in October start school? By considering how the child responds to new situations, the parents and the teacher can anticipate how the child's temperament will affect school entry and performance. If a child is "slow to warm up," it is crucial to give her time to adjust to a new school, new people, and new expectations.

Greater demands for impulse control are now being placed upon the child. She is expected to obey rules, get along with others, and not be disruptive. Paying attention to teachers, principals, and other adults may be difficult for her. Acquiring skills in listening, reading, and arithmetic challenges some children and excites others. The kindergartner will have many chances to make friends and come into contact with other families. There may be opportunities to go on school field trips or to participate in after-school activities. Some children manage these new challenges gracefully, while others struggle to learn appropriate behaviors. Parents should be encouraged to listen to their child's feelings and to praise her for her accomplishments.

As the child becomes more independent and interested in exploring the neighborhood, the health professional has new injury prevention issues to discuss with the parents. The health professional should impress upon parents the importance of teaching young children about playground safety, crossing streets safely, wearing bicycle helmets, and behaving safely around strangers. Since five year olds are frequently fascinated by matches and cigarette lighters, parents should be advised to keep these items out of reach, and children should be reminded that matches and lighters are not toys. The many dangers posed by guns and other weapons in the household should also be stressed to the parents.

With the child's gains in cognitive development, her ability to communicate becomes more sophisticated. The health professional should speak directly with the child about her family, her friends, and her excitement or fears about going to school.

# HEALTH SUPERVISION INTERVIEW

## TRIGGER QUESTIONS

To be used selectively by the health professional. Discuss any issues or concerns of the family.

### For the Parent(s)

How are you?

How are things going at home?

What questions or concerns do you have today?

What are you especially proud of about Damian?

Have there been any major changes or stresses in your family since your last visit?

How are you feeling about having Greta go to school?

How does Miyuki feel about going to school?

When you were Francesca's age, did you enjoy school?

How does James get along with others?

How did Scott do in preschool?

What have you done to prepare Carlos for crossing the street on the way to school
or for taking a school bus? Is his bus stop safe?
Will you visit the school with him before school starts?

Is there anything you would like to have checked out before Alexis goes to school?

Is there anything the school or teacher should know?

What are your plans for before- and after-school care?

Does Joyce usually eat what you fix for dinner?

How many hours a day does John sleep? Is it hard to get him out of bed in the morning?

What do you and your partner do when you disagree or argue about discipline?

Have you ever been in a relationship where you have been hurt, threatened, or treated badly?

Have you ever been worried that someone was going to hurt your child?
Has your child ever been abused?

**For the Child**

Are you and your friends excited about going to school?

Do you like going to child care (or preschool)?

Will you ride the bus to school?

Do you have a best friend?

What do you do for fun?

Tell me some of the things you are best at.

If you had three wishes, what would they be?

Do you have chores to help your parents around the house?

What is your address? Your phone number?

How do you get along with your brothers and sisters? With your parents?

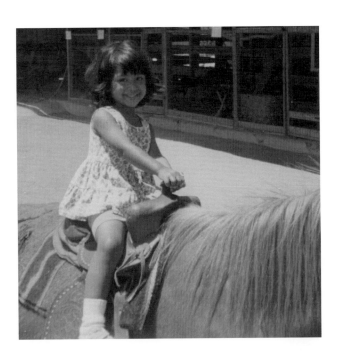

# Developmental Surveillance and Milestones

## TRIGGER QUESTIONS AND POSSIBLE RESPONSES

**Do you have any specific concerns about Robin's development or behavior?**

**How does Robin communicate what she wants?**

    Uses words (uses future tense)

    Uses complete sentences of five words

    Speaks short paragraphs

    Is able to recall parts of a story

    Shows fluency

    Speaks intelligibly to strangers (100 percent of the time)

**What do you think Robin understands?**

    Concept of numbers

    Two- or three-step instructions

    Own address and telephone number

**How does Robin get from one place to another?**

    Walks, climbs, runs

    Goes up and down stairs (alternating feet without support)

    Skips

**How does Robin act around others?**

    Responsive or withdrawn

    Friendly or hostile/aggressive

    Compliant or defiant

    Dependent or self-reliant

    Anxious about separation or not

**To what extent has Robin developed independence in eating, dressing, and toileting?**

    Uses utensils

    Dresses self (except for tying shoelaces)

    Has bladder and bowel control

**Does Robin show an ability to understand the feelings of others?**

## MILESTONES

Dresses self without help

Knows own address and telephone number

Can count on fingers

Copies a triangle or square

Draws a person with a head, a body, arms, and legs

Recognizes most letters of the alphabet

Prints some letters

Plays make-believe and dress-up

May be able to skip

**Tell me about Robin's typical play.**

    Plays with favorite toys (describe how used)

    Listens to stories

    Engages in elaborate fantasy play

    Plays interactive games with peers (follows rules of games)

    Has manual dexterity

## Observation of Parent-Child Interaction

Does the child sit with the parent or in her own chair? When the health professional asks the child a question, does the parent answer or does the child? Is the child active in the reception room or the examination room? How does the parent respond to this activity? How does the parent discipline the child? What is the child's reaction to the discipline?

## Physical Examination

Measure and plot on a standard chart the height, weight, and weight for height. Share the information with the parent.

As part of the complete physical examination, the following should be noted:

Caries, developmental dental anomalies, malocclusion, pathologic conditions, or dental injuries

Evidence of neglect or abuse

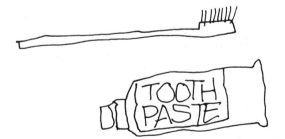

### ADDITIONAL SCREENING PROCEDURES

Assessment of risk of high-dose lead exposure[1]

Vision screening
(Vision screening guidelines appear in appendix F, page 265)

Hearing screening

Assessment of risk for hyperlipidemia[2]

Annual tuberculin test (PPD) if any of the following risk factors are present:

Low socioeconomic status
Residence in areas where tuberculosis is prevalent
Exposure to tuberculosis
Immigrant status

Blood pressure screening

Perform tuberculin test (PPD) once before school entry at four to six years of age

### IMMUNIZATIONS

Ensure that immunization status is up to date

Administer once before school entry at four to six years of age:

| | |
|---|---|
| Diphtheria, Tetanus, Pertussis (DTP) Vaccine (The acellular DTaP Vaccine may be substituted) | #5 |
| Oral Poliovirus (OPV) Vaccine | #4 |
| Measles, Mumps, and Rubella (MMR) Vaccine | #2 |

# ANTICIPATORY GUIDANCE FOR THE FAMILY

In addition to providing anticipatory guidance, many health professionals give families handouts
at an appropriate reading level or a videotape that they can review or study at home.[3]

## Promotion of healthy habits

Be a role model for the child by having a healthy lifestyle.

Ensure that the child gets adequate sleep. For children through 5 years of age, the suggested bedtime is 7–8 P.M.; for those ages 6–10, it is 8–9 P.M.

Encourage regular physical activity.

Limit television watching to an average of one hour per day of appropriate programs. Watch the programs together and discuss them.

Teach the child about personal care and hygiene.

## Injury prevention

Establish and enforce consistent, explicit, and firm rules for safe behavior.

Ensure that the child wears a seat belt in the car at all times.

Teach the child about safety rules for swimming pools. Teach the child how to swim.

Ensure that swimming pools in the child's community, in her apartment complex, or at her home have a four-sided fence with a self-closing, self-latching gate. Children should be supervised by an adult whenever they are in or near water.

Continue to put sunscreen on the child before she goes outside to play or swim.

Continue to keep the child's environment free of smoke.

Test smoke detectors to ensure that they work properly. Change batteries yearly.

Teach the child about safety rules for the home. Conduct fire drills at home. Lock up poisons, matches, and electrical tools.

Ensure that guns, if in the home, are locked up and that ammunition is stored separately. A trigger lock is an additional important precaution.

Teach the child about safety rules for getting to and from school. Teach pedestrian and neighborhood safety skills.

Teach the child about safety rules for bicycles. Teach the correct signals for traffic safety (e.g., right turn, left turn, and stop). Ensure that the child always wears a helmet when riding a bicycle.

Discuss playground safety with the child.

Ensure that the child is supervised before and after school in a safe environment.

Choose caregivers carefully. Discuss with them their attitudes about and behavior in relation to discipline. Prohibit corporal punishment.

Teach the child about safety rules for interacting with strangers (e.g., answering the telephone or the door, never getting into a stranger's car). Ensure that the child's school curriculum includes information on how to deal with strangers.

## Nutrition

Serve the child three regular meals and two nutritious snacks per day.

Make mealtimes pleasant and companionable. Encourage conversation.

Provide nutritious snacks rich in complex carbohydrates. Limit high-fat or low-nutrient foods and beverages such as candy, chips, or soft drinks.

Model and encourage good eating habits. Serve a variety of healthy foods.

Encourage the child to eat a balanced breakfast or ensure that the school provides one.

Ensure that the child eats a nutritious lunch at school, either through the school lunch program or by packing a balanced lunch.

## Oral health

Ensure that the child brushes her teeth twice a day with a pea-size amount of fluoridated toothpaste. Regularly supervise tooth brushing.

Give the child fluoride supplements as recommended by the health professional based on the level of fluoride in the child's drinking water.

Learn how to prevent dental injuries and handle dental emergencies.

If the child regularly sucks her fingers or thumb, begin to intervene gently to get her to discontinue.

Schedule a dental appointment for the child every six months, unless her dentist determines otherwise based on her individual needs/susceptibility to disease.

As the child's permanent molars erupt, ensure that her dentist evaluates them for application of dental sealants.

## Sexuality education

Recognize that a child's sexual curiosity and exploration are normal.

Use correct terms for all body parts, including genitalia.

Obtain picture books on sexuality for family reading.

## Promotion of social competence

Praise the child for cooperation and accomplishments.

Encourage the child to talk with you about her school or friends. Answer her questions.

Encourage the child to express her feelings.

Encourage interactive reading with the child.

Spend individual time with the child, doing something you both enjoy.

Enhance the child's experiences through trips and visits to parks, libraries, and other places of interest.

Provide opportunities for the five year old to interact with other children.

Help the child learn how to get along with her peers.

Promote physical activity in a safe environment.

Set limits. Use time out and establish consequences for unacceptable behavior.

Encourage self-discipline and impulse control.

Expect the child to follow family rules, such as those for bedtime, television viewing, and chores.

Teach the child to respect authority.

Teach the child the difference between right and wrong.

Teach the child how to manage anger and resolve conflicts without violence.

Assign age-appropriate chores.

## Promotion of constructive family relationships and parental health

Serve as a positive ethical and behavioral role model.

Listen to and show respect for the child.

Show interest in school and after-school activities.

Set reasonable expectations.

Show affection in the family.

Spend some individual time with each child.

Participate in games and other physical activities with the child.

Encourage the development of good sibling relationships. Acknowledge conflicts between siblings. Whenever possible, attempt to resolve conflicts without taking sides. Do not allow hitting, biting, or other violent behavior.

Share meals as a family whenever possible. Spend time talking to each other.

Handle anger constructively in the family.

Discuss with the health professional your own preventive and health-promoting practices (e.g., using seat belts, avoiding tobacco, eating properly, exercising and doing breast self-exams or testicular self-exams).

## Promotion of community interactions

If you need financial assistance to help pay for health care expenses, ask about resources or for referrals to the state Medicaid programs or other state medical assistance programs.

Ask about resources or referrals for food, housing, or transportation if needed.

Discuss with the health professional possible programs for the child: schools; swimming, soccer, or other exercise programs; or other community programs.

Participate as a family in school and community organizations and activities.

Contribute regularly to school or community activities that require adult supervision.

Explore or continue to participate in social, religious, cultural, volunteer, and recreational organizations.

Find out what you can do to make your community safer. Advocate for and participate in a neighborhood watch program.

Advocate for adequate housing and play spaces/playgrounds.

Recommend that schools provide early and regular comprehensive health education that encourages healthy lifestyles.

## Promotion of successful school entry

Meet with the child's teachers.

Prepare the child for school. Talk about new opportunities, friends, and activities at school.

Tour the child's school with her.

Be involved with the child's school, perhaps as a volunteer.

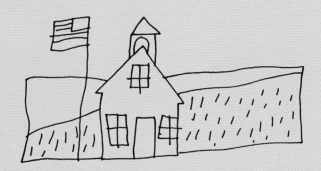

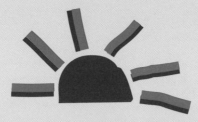

# Is the Family Prepared for Health Supervision?

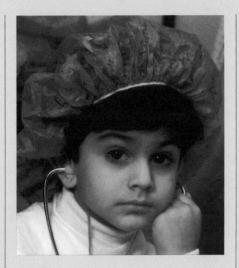

Michael is about to turn five. His mother makes an appointment with the pediatrician because the school has sent home a note explaining that Michael must have a second measles vaccination before he enters school in the fall. He will also be attending a day camp this summer, and the camp requires a physical exam.

During the health supervision visit, Dr. Hillborough asks Michael about his interests, how he likes his child care provider, and how he gets along with his little brother. Michael has not been prepared for the interview and seems bewildered by the questions. Michael's mother assures Dr. Hillborough that things are fine but provides little specific information about Michael. The health supervision visit is short, and Michael and his mother leave with little more than a measles vaccination and a completed camp physical form.

Lin Shu is also about to turn five. His father makes an appointment with Dr. Gomez. Prior to the day of the visit, Lin Shu's father does a few things in preparation. The father asks Lin Shu if he has any questions he would like to ask the doctor. He also spends time thinking about the questions he wants to ask and makes a list of them to bring to the doctor's office. He also brings Lin Shu's record, which he has had since his

son's birth, as well as Lin Shu's latest progress report from preschool.

During the visit Dr. Gomez asks how things are going for Lin Shu and asks his father if he has any questions. The father responds with several questions: Is it time for the parents to try to help Lin Shu stop sucking his thumb? What should they do? How much "silly behavior" is appropriate for a five year old? What can be done about the constant fighting between Lin Shu and his older sister? Can Lin Shu play soccer despite having asthma? Dr. Gomez addresses their concerns during the health supervision visit, and he gives Lin Shu and his father some tips on how to handle the changes elementary school will bring. Lin Shu and his father leave half an hour later feeling encouraged and satisfied. Lin Shu's father has some strategies to handle behavior that has been bothering him. He also has the information he needs to feel comfortable enrolling Lin Shu in a soccer program.

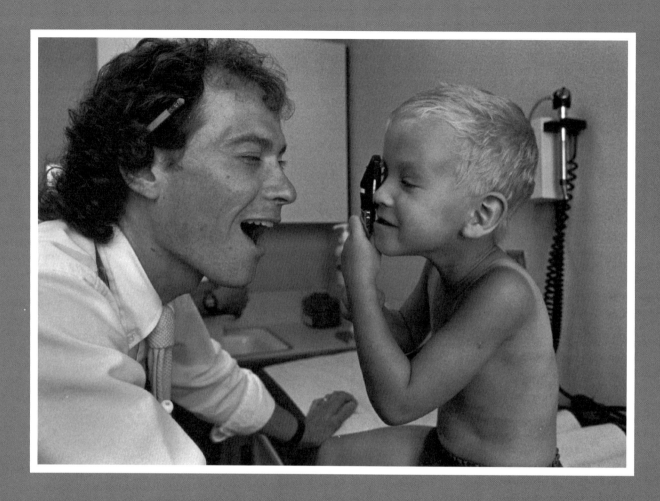

*Since the six year old shows increasing social maturity
and growing understanding, the health professional can use
health supervision visits to foster a therapeutic alliance
directly with him.*

# Six Year Visit

A six year old is eager to act independently, but he is not yet able to make wise decisions consistently. He likes to climb trees or fire escapes, and he plays in the yard or on the sidewalk with other children. He is learning about safety—crossing streets, riding a bicycle, and dealing with strangers. Before he begins going out into the community on his own, the child must be able to remember safety rules and understand them well enough to interpret them and adapt them for different situations. His parents should continue to set appropriate boundaries and other limits while encouraging and promoting the growth of his independence.

Friends and others outside of the home become increasingly important to the six year old. His parents need to encourage his friendships and respect the growing influence of new peers, but family rules should remain consistent. It is important for parents to meet their child's friends and their families.

A six year old is interested in testing the limits of his body. How fast can he run? How far can he throw? As he learns about how his body works, he gains the confidence and skills needed to participate in activities such as soccer or dancing. Bicycles must match the child's size and level of ability, and he should always wear an approved helmet while riding. Adult supervision is needed for swimming and other water sports. The child should wear appropriate protective equipment for organized sports. Parents should ensure that coaches' demands upon children are reasonable and that children are not overscheduled.

Discussing the child's school progress is an important part of health supervision. School systems are required by law to evaluate children who are experiencing learning or developmental difficulties. Health professionals can remind parents of their child's right to an appropriate public education and assist parents in understanding special education programs and services. They should also identify community resources to help the family.

Since the six year old shows increasing social maturity and intellectual skills, the health professional can use health supervision visits to foster a therapeutic alliance directly with him. The child may look forward to being included in the interview. The health professional can encourage the child to begin to assume responsibility for his clothes, toys, or other belongings; selected chores; and good health habits. This self-reliance will help promote autonomy, independence, and a sense of mastery.

This material is also appropriate for a Seven Year Visit.

**MIDDLE CHILDHOOD • 6 YEARS**

# HEALTH SUPERVISION INTERVIEW

## TRIGGER QUESTIONS

To be used selectively by the health professional. Discuss any issues or concerns of the family.

### For the Parent(s)

How are you?

How are things going at home?

What questions or concerns do you have today?

What are you especially proud of about Lashonda?

Have there been any major changes or stresses in your family since your last visit?

What do you and Roberto like to do together?

How is school going for Jo?

Does Tita talk to you about what's happening in school?

What does Bonnie eat for an after-school snack?

How many hours a day does Max sleep? Does he seem rested when he wakes up?

What have you done to prepare Cathy for crossing the street on the way to school or for taking a school bus? Is her bus stop safe?

Does Noreen participate in any after-school sports?

What are the child care arrangements for Darryl before and after school?

Have you ever been in a relationship where you have been hurt, threatened, or treated badly?

Have you ever been worried that someone was going to hurt your child?
Has your child ever been abused?

## For the Child

How is school going? What do you like the most about school? The least?

Tell me some of the things you are best at.

If you had three wishes, what would they be?

What do you like to do after school?

What are your favorite TV shows? Toys? Movies? Food?

Do you have a best friend? Tell me about your best friend.

Draw me a picture of your family. Tell me a story about them.

Do you wear a bicycle helmet?

Do kids you know get into trouble at school sometimes? Do you ever get into trouble?

When you have a problem, who do you talk to about it?

Do you have chores to help your parents around the house?

How do you get along with your brothers and sisters? With your parents?

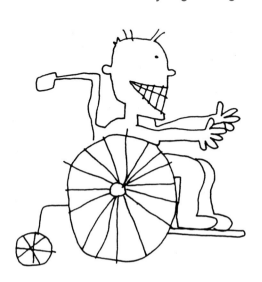

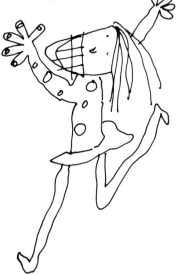

# Developmental Surveillance and School Performance

Review copy of child's report card.
Review copy of Individualized Education Program (IEP) if child has special needs.

**Do you have any specific concerns about Jackson's development or behavior?**

**How do you think Jackson is performing in school?**

**How is his attendance?**

**Does Jackson seem to be able to follow the rules at school?**

**When he plays with other children, can he keep up with them?**

**Is he proud of his achievements at school?**

**How do you acknowledge and praise Jackson's achievements at school?**

**Have you visited Jackson's classroom?**

**Do you participate in activities at his school?**

**Does Jackson talk to you about what goes on in school?**

**What did the teacher say about Jackson during your parent-teacher conference?**

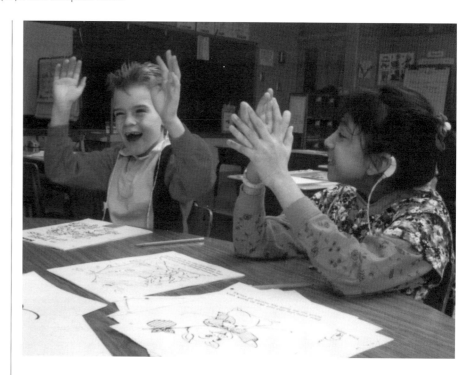

## Observation of Parent-Child Interaction

Does the child sit with the parent or in his own chair? When the health professional asks the child a question, does the parent answer or does the child? Is the child active in the reception room or the examination room? How does the parent respond to this activity? How does the parent discipline the child? What is the child's reaction to the discipline?

## Physical Examination

Measure and plot on a standard chart the height, weight, and weight for height. Share the information with the parent.

As part of the complete physical examination, the following should be noted:

Caries, developmental anomalies, malocclusion, pathologic conditions, or dental injuries

Evidence of neglect or abuse

### ADDITIONAL SCREENING PROCEDURES

Assessment of risk of high-dose lead exposure[1]

Vision screening
(Vision screening guidelines appear in appendix F, page 265)

Hearing screening

Assessment of risk for hyperlipidemia[2]

Annual tuberculin test (PPD) if any of the following risk factors are present:

Low socioeconomic status
Residence in areas where tuberculosis is prevalent
Exposure to tuberculosis
Immigrant status

Blood pressure screening

Perform tuberculin test (PPD) once before school entry at four to six years of age

### IMMUNIZATIONS

Ensure that immunization status is up to date

Administer once before school entry at four to six years of age:

| | |
|---|---|
| Diphtheria, Tetanus, Pertussis (DTP) Vaccine (The acellular DTaP Vaccine may be substituted) | #5 |
| Oral Poliovirus (OPV) Vaccine | #4 |
| Measles, Mumps, and Rubella (MMR) Vaccine | #2 |

# ANTICIPATORY GUIDANCE FOR THE FAMILY

In addition to providing anticipatory guidance, many health professionals give families handouts
at an appropriate reading level or a videotape that they can review or study at home.[3]

## Promotion of healthy habits

Be a role model for the child by having a healthy lifestyle.

Ensure that the child gets adequate sleep. For children 6–10 years of age, the suggested bedtime is 8–9 P.M.

Encourage regular physical activity.

Limit television watching to an average of one hour per day of appropriate programs. Watch the programs together and discuss them.

Reinforce with the child personal care and hygiene.

## Injury prevention

Enforce consistent, explicit, and firm rules for safe behavior.

Continue to ensure that the child wears a seat belt in the car at all times.

Reinforce with the child safety rules for swimming pools. Teach the child how to swim.

Ensure that swimming pools in the child's community, in his apartment complex, or at his home have a four-sided fence with a self-closing, self-latching gate. Children should be supervised by an adult whenever they are in or near water.

Teach the child how to put on sunscreen before he goes outside to play or swim.

Continue to keep the child's environment free of smoke.

Test smoke detectors to ensure that they work properly. Change batteries yearly.

Reinforce with the child safety rules for the home. Conduct fire drills at home. Lock up poisons, matches, and electrical tools.

Ensure that guns, if in the home, are locked up and that ammunition is stored separately. A trigger lock is an additional important precaution.

Reinforce with the child safety rules for getting to and from school. Reinforce with the child pedestrian and neighborhood safety skills.

Reinforce with the child safety rules for bicycles, including use of proper traffic signals. Ensure that the child always wears a helmet when riding a bicycle.

Reinforce playground safety.

Ensure that the child is supervised before and after school in a safe environment.

Reinforce with the child safety rules for interacting with strangers (e.g., answering the telephone or the door, never getting into a stranger's car). Ensure that the child's school curriculum includes information on how to deal with strangers.

Teach the child about sports safety, including the need to wear protective sports gear such as a mouth guard or a face protector.

## Nutrition

Ensure that the child eats three regular meals and two nutritious snacks per day.

Make mealtimes pleasant and companionable. Encourage conversation.

Provide nutritious snacks rich in complex carbohydrates. Limit high-fat or low-nutrient foods and beverages such as candy, chips, or soft drinks.

Model and encourage good eating habits. Serve a variety of healthy foods.

Help the child learn to choose appropriate foods, including five servings of fruits and vegetables daily.

Encourage the child to eat a balanced breakfast or ensure that the school provides one.

Ensure that the child eats a nutritious lunch at school, either through the school lunch program or by packing a lunch.

## Oral health

Ensure that the child brushes his teeth twice a day with a pea-size amount of fluoridated toothpaste. Regularly supervise tooth brushing.

Give the child fluoride supplements as recommended by the health professional based on the level of fluoride in the child's drinking water.

Learn how to prevent dental injuries and handle dental emergencies, especially the loss or fracture of a tooth.

If the child regularly sucks his fingers or thumb, begin to intervene gently to get him to discontinue.

Schedule a dental appointment for the child every six months, unless his dentist determines otherwise based on his individual needs/susceptibility to disease.

As the child's permanent molars erupt, ensure that his dentist evaluates them for application of dental sealants.

## Sexuality education

Answer questions at a level appropriate to the child's understanding.

Have age-appropriate sexual education books in the home that will answer some questions and encourage the child to ask others.

## Promotion of social competence

Praise the child for cooperation and accomplishments.

Encourage the child to talk with you about his school, friends, or observations. Answer his questions.

Encourage the child to express his feelings.

Encourage reading.

Spend individual time with the child, doing something you both enjoy.

Enlarge the child's experiences through family trips.

Provide opportunities for the six year old to interact with other children, including team or group activities.

Help the child learn how to get along with his peers.

Help the child learn how to follow group rules.

Promote physical activity in a safe environment.

Set limits and establish consequences for unacceptable behavior.

Encourage self-discipline and impulse control.

Expect the child to follow family rules, such as those for bedtime, television viewing, and chores.

Teach the child to respect authority.

Foster the child's ability to communicate with parents, teachers, and other adults.

Ensure that the child understands the difference between right and wrong.

Teach the child how to manage anger and resolve conflicts without violence.

Assign age-appropriate chores, including responsibility for own belongings.

Provide personal space for the child at home, even if limited.

## Promotion of constructive family relationships and parental health

Serve as a positive ethical and behavioral role model.

Contribute to the child's self-esteem through praising him and showing affection toward him.

Show interest in school and after-school activities.

Set reasonable expectations.

Promote self-responsibility.

Show affection in the family.

Spend some individual time with each child.

Participate in games and physical activities with the child.

Encourage the development of good sibling relationships.

Share meals as a family whenever possible. Spend time talking to each other.

Know the child's friends and their families.

Handle anger constructively in the family.

Discuss with the health professional your own preventive and health-promoting practices (e.g., using seat belts, avoiding tobacco, eating properly, exercising and doing breast self-exams or testicular self-exams).

## Promotion of community interactions

If you need financial assistance to help pay for health care expenses, ask about resources or for referrals to the state Medicaid programs or other state medical assistance programs.

Ask about resources or referrals for food, housing, or transportation if needed.

Discuss with the health professional possible programs for the child: schools; before- and after-school programs; swimming, soccer, or other exercise programs; or other community programs.

Participate as a family in school and community organizations and activities.

Contribute regularly to school or community activities that require adult supervision.

Explore or continue to participate in social, religious, cultural, volunteer, and recreational organizations.

Advocate for community programs and facilities for children (recreational, sports, and educational activities).

Promote social connections with friends and neighbors and ties with extended family members.

Participate in activities that reflect cultural diversity (e.g., holidays, festivals, musical events, dance performances), and teach the child about his own culture.

Find out what you can do to make your community safer. Advocate for and participate in a neighborhood watch program.

Recommend that schools provide early and regular comprehensive health education that encourages healthy lifestyles.

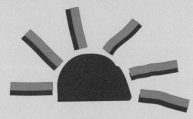

# I Am Mommy's Best Friend

*Ms. Goldstein senses that something is troubling Penny. After chatting with Penny for a few minutes, Ms. Goldstein asks her directly, "Are you worried about something?"*

Penny, a first-grade student, has not been participating in class activities all morning. Walking around the room and staring out the window, she is obviously preoccupied. After trying several times to get Penny to join her classmates, the teacher takes her to see the school nurse, Ms. Goldstein. "Please find out what is going on," she asks. "Penny has come to the health room often and she trusts you. Something isn't right."

Ms. Goldstein has seen Penny four times in the past month. Each time Penny had a vague complaint, and Ms. Goldstein determined that the complaint did not indicate a serious physical illness. Now the nurse begins to ask Penny questions to get her talking about her life. Penny talks about her little sister Wanda, her dog Kiki, and her favorite television show. Ms. Goldstein senses that something is troubling Penny. After chatting with Penny for a few minutes, Ms. Goldstein asks her directly, "Are you worried about something?" Penny responds,

"I'm supposed to be taking care of Mommy. I'm her best friend and Daddy hurts her when I'm not home." The nurse, questioning Penny further, finds out that Penny's mother was treated in the emergency room the night before and then released. Penny is terrified by the continued violence at home and feels that she must protect her mother.

Ms. Goldstein arranges an emergency meeting with the principal and Penny's mother. Penny's mother confirms the story. Ms. Goldstein helps the mother contact the local social services department. Penny, her mother, and her sister get into a shelter that afternoon. Ms. Goldstein's probing questions to Penny and her knowledge of community resources were essential in getting help for this family.

**MIDDLE CHILDHOOD • 6 YEARS**

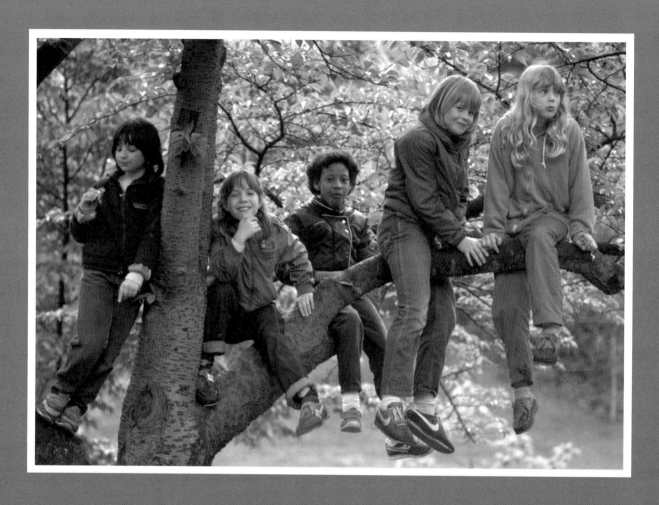

The growing influence of peers may present a
challenge to the family, and the child now begins to
view her parents as ordinary people.

# Eight Year Visit

The eight year old in charge of such tasks as making her own bed, bathing herself, putting her clothes in the hamper, or setting the table develops a sense of personal competence. The sense of accomplishment and pride she feels makes her confident and interested in attempting activities requiring more responsibility. The child is able to focus on multiple aspects of a problem, establish hierarchies, and use logic. Busy with school projects, book reports, and collections, the eight year old is interested in how things work and has many questions. She also begins to recognize that the viewpoints of others may differ from her own.

The eight year old is looking outside the family for new ideas and activities. Her peer group becomes important; she identifies with children of the same gender and with similar interests and abilities. She often has a best friend, a milestone in interpersonal development. The growing influence of peers may present a challenge to the family, and the child now begins to view her parents as ordinary people.

The health professional should speak directly with the child throughout the health supervision visit. How does she feel about her school work and friends? What are her other interests? How and when does she expect her body to change? Does she have a best friend, and what do they like to do after school? This is an opportunity for the health professional to build a stronger relationship with the child. As she gets older she will need to feel comfortable asking questions and discussing concerns.

Parents should be encouraged to discuss with the health professional their own perspective of the child's school progress, other activities and accomplishments, and friends. What are their attitudes regarding family life education? What aspects of sexuality have they discussed with the child?

Since the eight year old is developing health habits—including those related to diet, exercise, and safety—this is an excellent time to foster self-responsibility for health behaviors. Personal health education should help the child make wise choices. She should learn to floss her teeth and brush twice a day, participate in sports or exercise programs as opposed to engaging in passive activities such as watching television, eat a balanced diet rather than "junk food," use seat belts in the car, and wear a helmet while bicycling. As she acquires confidence in making good choices, she is developing the sense of personal competence that will help her withstand future peer pressure and make wise decisions.

This material is also appropriate for a Seven or Nine Year Visit.

**MIDDLE CHILDHOOD • 8 YEARS**

# HEALTH SUPERVISION INTERVIEW

## TRIGGER QUESTIONS

To be used selectively by the health professional. Discuss any issues or concerns of the family.

### For the Parent(s)

How are you?

How are things going at home?

What questions or concerns do you have today?

Have there been any major changes or stresses in your family since your last visit?

What are some of the things you do together as a family?

How is Janice doing in school?

How many hours a day does Georgina sleep? Does she seem rested when she wakes up?

Does Suri bring friends home? Does she go to friends' homes?

What does Peter do when he is stressed, angry, or frustrated?

Is Ashley involved in sports? If so, does she get along with the coaches?

Do you talk to your child about sensitive subjects such as sex, drugs, or drinking?

What are the rules at home in relation to food, movies, toys, language, and makeup?

Do you enforce the use of bicycle helmets and seat belts?

What are the child care arrangements for Colin before and after school?

Have you ever been in a relationship where you have been hurt, threatened, or treated badly?

Have you ever been worried that someone was going to hurt your child?
Has your child ever been abused?

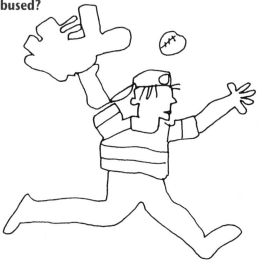

**For the Child**

**How is school going?**

**What are you the best at? What are you really proud of?**

**Tell me about your friends.**

**What do you do for fun?**

**What kinds of clubs are there at your school?**

**What kinds of school and after-school activities are you involved in?**

**Do you stay home by yourself, either before or after school?**

**Tell me about your neighborhood. Do you feel safe there?**

**Does your school/neighborhood have gangs?**

**Do you get picked on by other kids at school?**

**Have you ever been pressured to do things you didn't want to do?**
**Have you ever been tempted to do things you knew you shouldn't do?**

**Has anyone ever touched you in a way you didn't like?**

**Has anyone ever tried to harm you physically?**

**When you are riding your bicycle, do you wear a helmet?**

**If you could change your life, school, family, or home, what changes would you make?**

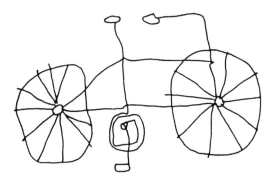

# Developmental Surveillance and School Performance

Review copy of child's report card.
Review copy of Individualized Education Program (IEP) if child has special needs.

**Do you have any specific concerns about Claire's school work or behavior?**

**How is her attendance?**

**Is she reading at grade level? Doing math at grade level?**

**Is she in any special classes?**

**Does Claire follow the rules at school and during after-school activities?**

**Is she proud of her achievements at school?**

**How do you acknowledge and praise Claire's achievements at school?**

**Have you visited Claire's classroom?**

**Do you participate in activities at her school?**

**Does Claire talk to you about what goes on in school?**

**What did the teacher say about Claire during your parent-teacher conference?**

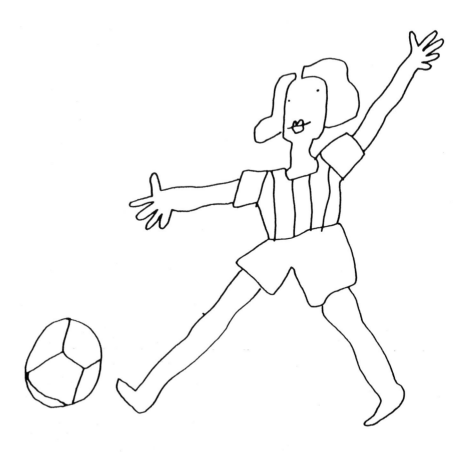

## Observation of Parent-Child Interaction

Do both the parent and the child ask questions? Does the parent let the child speak directly to the health professional, or does the parent interrupt? Is the child playful or serious with the health professional? Do the parent and child make eye contact with each other and with the health professional?

## Physical Examination

Respect the child's privacy by using appropriate draping during the examination.

Measure and plot on a standard chart the height, weight, and weight for height. Share the information with the parent.

As part of the complete physical examination, the following should be noted:

Scoliosis (Make orthopedic referral for curves greater than 15°–20°)

Early puberty (girls)

Caries, developmental dental anomalies, malocclusion, pathologic conditions, or dental injuries

Evidence of neglect or abuse

**ADDITIONAL SCREENING PROCEDURES**

Vision screening
(Vision screening guidelines appear in appendix F, page 265)

Hearing screening

Assessment of risk for hyperlipidemia[2]

Annual tuberculin test (PPD) if any of the following risk factors are present:

Low socioeconomic status
Residence in areas where tuberculosis is prevalent
Exposure to tuberculosis
Immigrant status

Blood pressure screening

**IMMUNIZATIONS**

Ensure that immunization status is up to date

# ANTICIPATORY GUIDANCE FOR THE FAMILY

In addition to providing anticipatory guidance, many health professionals give families handouts
at an appropriate reading level or a videotape that they can review or study at home.[3]

## Promotion of healthy habits

Supervise the child's activities with peers.

Be a role model for the child by having a healthy lifestyle.

Ensure that the child gets adequate sleep. For children 6–10 years of age, the suggested bedtime is 8–9 P.M.

Encourage regular physical activity.

Limit television watching to an average of one hour per day of appropriate programs.

Supervise the child's personal care and hygiene.

Counsel the child about avoiding the use of alcohol, tobacco, and drugs. Ensure that the child's school curriculum includes information about substance abuse.

## Injury prevention

Reinforce important safety considerations. Anticipate that the child may make errors in judgment because she is trying to imitate peers.

Anticipate providing less direct supervision.

Continue to ensure that the child wears a seat belt in the car at all times.

Reinforce with the child safety rules for swimming pools. Teach the child how to swim.

Ensure that swimming pools in the child's community, in her apartment complex, or at her home have a four-sided fence with a self-closing, self-latching gate. Children should be supervised by an adult whenever they are in or around water.

Ensure that the child puts on sunscreen before she goes outside for long periods of time.

Continue to keep the child's environment free of smoke.

Test smoke detectors to ensure that they work properly. Change batteries yearly.

Reinforce with the child safety rules for the home, including what to do when home alone. Discuss visitors, not tying up the telephone for long periods of time, and what to do in case of fire or other emergencies. Conduct fire drills at home. Lock up poisons, matches, and electrical tools.

Ensure that guns, if in the home, are locked up and that ammunition is stored separately.

Reinforce the child's knowledge of neighborhood safety rules.

Reinforce with the child safety rules for bicycles, including use of proper traffic signals. Ensure that the child always wears a helmet when riding a bicycle.

Ensure that the child is supervised before and after school in a safe environment.

Reinforce with the child safety rules for interacting with strangers (e.g., answering the telephone or the door, never getting into a stranger's car). Ensure that the child's school curriculum includes information on how to deal with strangers.

Reinforce sports safety with the child, including the need to wear protective sports gear such as a mouth guard or a face protector.

Do not allow the child to operate a power lawn mower or motorized farm equipment.

## Nutrition

Encourage the child to eat three regular meals per day and nutritious snacks.

Share meals as a family on a regular basis. Make mealtimes pleasant and companionable. Encourage conversation.

Model and encourage good eating habits. Serve a variety of healthy foods.

Teach the child how to choose nutritious snacks rich in complex carbohydrates. Limit high-fat or low-nutrient foods and beverages such as candy, chips, or soft drinks.

Teach the child how to eat a balanced diet. Teach her to choose plenty of fruits and vegetables; breads, cereals, and other grain products; low-fat dairy products; lean meats; and foods prepared with little or no fat.

Teach the child how to eat a nutritious lunch at school, either through the school lunch program or by packing a balanced lunch.

## Oral health

Ensure that the child brushes her teeth twice a day with a pea-size amount of fluoridated toothpaste. Teach her how to floss.

Give the child fluoride supplements as recommended by the health professional based on the level of fluoride in the child's drinking water.

Schedule a dental appointment for the child every six months, unless her dentist determines otherwise based on her individual needs/susceptibility to disease.

As the child's permanent molars erupt, ensure that her dentist evaluates them for application of dental sealants.

Teach the child how to handle dental emergencies, especially the loss or fracture of a tooth.

Teach the child not to smoke or use smokeless tobacco.

## Sexuality education

Have age-appropriate sexual education books in the home that will answer some questions and encourage the child to ask other questions.

If the child receives family life education at school or in the community, discuss it with her.

Answer questions at a level appropriate to the child's understanding.

For parents of girls: Prepare your daughter for menstruation.

## Promotion of social competence

Praise the child for personal successes.

Encourage the child to talk with you about her school, friends, or feelings. Answer her questions.

Encourage reading and hobbies.

Spend individual time with the child, doing something you both enjoy.

Enhance the child's experiences through family trips.

Promote interaction and allegiance with peers through participation in social activities, community groups, and team sports.

Help the child learn how to get along with her peers. Discuss her awareness of differences among peers.

Set limits and establish consequences for unacceptable behavior.

Expect the child to follow family rules, such as those for bedtime, television viewing, and chores.

Promote positive interactions between the child and her teachers and other adults.

Help the child learn appropriate and reasonable behavior.

Help the child develop an ability to deal constructively with conflict and anger in the family, at school, and in the neighborhood.

Assign age-appropriate chores.

Provide personal space for the child at home, even if limited.

## Promotion of constructive family relationships and parental health

Serve as a positive ethical and behavioral role model.

Contribute to the child's self-esteem by praising her and showing affection toward her.

Show interest in the child's school performance and after-school activities.

Set reasonable but challenging expectations.

Promote self-responsibility.

Show affection in the family.

Spend some individual time with each child.

Participate in games and physical activities with the child.

Encourage positive interactions between the child and her parents and siblings.

Share meals as a family whenever possible. Spend time talking to each other.

Know the child's friends and their families.

Handle anger constructively in the family.

Discuss with the health professional your own preventive and health-promoting practices (e.g., using seat belts, avoiding tobacco, eating properly, exercising and doing breast self-exams or testicular self-exams).

## Promotion of community interactions

If you need financial assistance to help pay for health care expenses, ask about resources or for referrals to the state Medicaid programs or other state medical assistance programs.

Ask about resources or referrals for food, housing, or transportation if needed.

Discuss with the health professional possible programs for the child: before- and after-school programs; swimming, soccer, or other exercise programs; or other community programs.

Participate as a family in school and community organizations and activities.

Contribute regularly to school or community activities that require adult supervision.

Explore or continue to participate in social, religious, cultural, volunteer, and recreational organizations.

Advocate for community programs and facilities for children (recreational, sports, and educational activities).

Encourage the child to participate in organized groups.

Discuss current events and social responsibility.

Promote social connections with neighbors and ties with extended family members.

Participate in activities that reflect cultural diversity (e.g., holidays, festivals, musical events, dance performances), and teach the child about her own culture.

Find out what you can do to make your community safer. Advocate for and participate in a neighborhood watch program.

Encourage peer-mediated conflict management in schools from third grade through high school.

Recommend that schools provide early and regular comprehensive health education that encourages healthy lifestyles.

# Can the Dentist Fix My Broken Tooth?

**K**evin is eight years old, and he isn't happy. He broke his front tooth playing softball with his friends. Now his dad is taking him to see Dr. Wilson, his dentist. Kevin is really upset about a lot of things. He wonders if his tooth will ever look the same again. It is jagged and sharp and looks terrible. But even if it does look the same, his front teeth stick out and some of the boys in his third-grade class call him "Dracula." Most of the time he doesn't even want to smile and show his teeth in front of the other kids. He is afraid that it will hurt to have his teeth treated.

At Dr. Wilson's office, the dental assistant immediately takes Kevin and his dad back to the treatment room. Kevin has known Dr. Wilson for years. In fact, Dr. Wilson says that he was barely walking when he came in for his first visit. He has always been nice to him. He has had his teeth cleaned many times, has had fluoride applied to them, and has even had plastic sealants painted on

his back teeth. But coming to the dentist has always been easy because he has never had a cavity or a filling. Kevin is worried that it might be harder today.

Kevin is surprised at how upset his father is now that they are in the treatment room. But he begins to feel better when Dr. Wilson comes in and calmly asks him about the injury. How did it happen? Does he have any other injuries? But Dr. Wilson puts them both at ease by answering their questions and telling them exactly what he is going to do. First he will take an x-ray of Kevin's tooth to make sure it is not injured beneath the gum. Then he will put the tooth to sleep and use a tooth-colored material to make it look like new again. The best part is that it won't hurt.

The visit lasts about 45 minutes and doesn't hurt a bit. Not only does Kevin's tooth look great, but Dr. Wilson talks to his dad about braces to align his teeth. This will help him look and feel better and will reduce the risk that his teeth will be injured

again. Next month, at Kevin's follow-up visit, Dr. Wilson will make him a mouth guard to wear every time he plays softball. Kevin leaves the office much relieved.

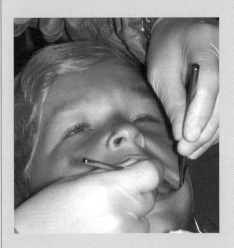

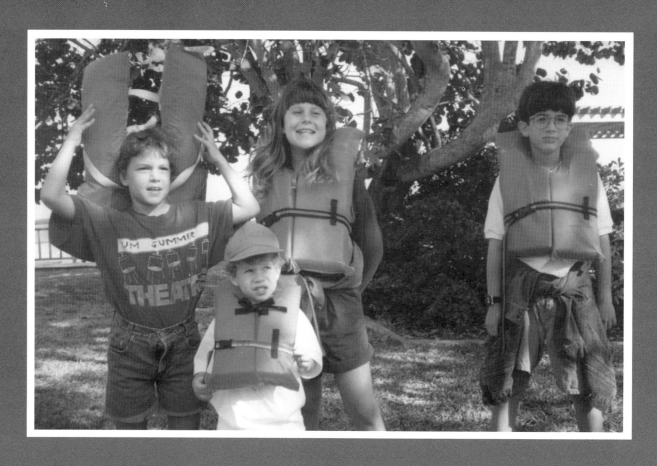

*Children who feel good about themselves*
*are better equipped to withstand peer pressure.*

# Ten Year Visit

By the age of 10, children have informally chosen the leader of their peer group, whether it is the child who plays baseball well, the one who can run fast, or the one with new ideas for games. At the same time, those who fail to fit in are often reminded of their faults and pushed aside. Ten year olds have primarily same-sex friends. Friends assume greater importance, and the child's independence from the family is now obvious.

For some families, conflict appears if the parents misinterpret the normal realignment of allegiance toward peers as a rejection of their values, past support, and guidance. Parents can acknowledge the child's evolving desire for independence by offering increasing responsibility. For example, parents may identify certain tasks as appropriate chores, while allowing the child to decide himself when to complete them. An allowance may also promote the child's growing sense of independence.

Injury prevention should be stressed with the 10 year old. The child may engage in dangerous risk-taking behaviors (e.g., dares, drinking, smoking) as a result of peer pressure. Some children are able to influence their peers to engage in dangerous or illegal activities against their better judgment. If the peer group includes older children, the child may encounter pressure to perform acts and take risks for which he is not developmentally competent. Recognizing this possibility may help parents teach their children about dealing with peer pressure.

Supporting and enhancing the child's self-esteem and self-confidence is critical during this period. Children who feel good about themselves are better equipped to withstand peer pressure. Parents need to spend time with the child, talk to him, and praise him for his achievements. Health professionals can help by identifying the child's strengths and promoting communication between him and his parents.

School progress, achievements, or problems can be an issue for many children and families. Learning problems may not become evident until the later elementary school years, as classroom expectations for performance increase. Some children and parents are apprehensive about the transition into middle school.

Health professionals can help parents and children prepare for the major changes that take place in adolescence. Parents can ask about problems that may arise in adolescence and strengths that adolescents are likely to have. With the physical changes of puberty approaching—and already present for some children—information regarding physical development and pubertal changes is a crucial component of health supervision.

This material is also appropriate for a Nine Year Visit.

**MIDDLE CHILDHOOD • 10 YEARS**

# HEALTH SUPERVISION INTERVIEW

## TRIGGER QUESTIONS

To be used selectively by the health professional. Discuss any issues or concerns of the family.

### For the Parent(s)

How are you?

How are things going at home?

What questions or concerns do you have today?

What about Karina makes you most proud?

Have there been any major changes or stresses in your family since your last visit?

What are some of the things you do together as a family?

How is Nasser doing in school?

Tell me about Afi's relationships with other children.

Does Sanjay share his feelings and his school experiences with you?

How does Rory express his feelings?

How much television does Kamal watch?

What is Calvin's bedtime?

Is Laurie involved in sports? If so, how does she get along with the coaches?

Do you talk to your child about sensitive subjects such as sex, drugs, or drinking?

What family life education has Nani received? Who provided it? Did you discuss it with her? Does she know about menstruation?

Does Patrick know about wet dreams?

What are the rules at home in relation to food, movies, toys, language, and makeup?

What do you and your partner do when you disagree or argue about limits for Jeremy?

Have you ever been in a relationship where you have been hurt, threatened, or treated badly?

Have you ever been worried that someone was going to hurt your child? Has your child ever been abused?

## For the Child

How is school going? How are your grades?

What are you best at? What are you really proud of?

Tell me about your friends. Do you have a best friend?
What do you like to do together?

Do your friends pressure you to do things you don't want to do?

What education have you had about sex?
What are some of the questions that I can answer for you?

Have you ever been pressured to have sex?

If you could, how would you change your life? Your home? Your family?

How are you getting along with your parents? Your brother(s)? Your sister(s)?

What kind of activities are you involved in at school? After school?

Do you get any of your own meals? What do you like to eat?

Are you concerned about your weight? Are you trying to change it?

How much time do you spend watching television every day?

Do you belong to a gang? Have you thought about joining one?

Do your friends smoke? Drink? Take drugs? Have sex?

Do you smoke? Drink? Take drugs? Have sex?

Do you stay home by yourself, either before or after school?

Is there anyone in the family whose health worries you?

What are some of the other things that worry you?

What are some of the things that make you happy?

What do you do to have fun?

What are some of the things that make you sad? Angry? How do you handle that?

Has anyone ever touched you in a way you didn't like?

Has anyone ever tried to harm you physically?

# Developmental Surveillance and School Performance

Review copy of child's report card.
Review copy of Individualized Education Program (IEP) if child has special needs.

**Do you have any specific concerns about Pablo's grades?**

**How is his attendance?**

**Is he reading at grade level? Doing math at grade level?**

**Is he in any special classes?**

**Does Pablo follow the rules at school?**

**Is he proud of his achievements at school?**

**How do you acknowledge and praise Pablo's achievements at school?**

**Have you visited Pablo's classroom?**

**Do you participate in activities at his school?**

**Does Pablo talk to you about what goes on in school?**

**Has he identified certain interests he wants to pursue or talents he would like to develop?**

**What did the teacher say about Pablo during your parent-teacher conference?**

**Is Pablo ready for middle school?**

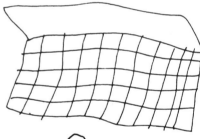
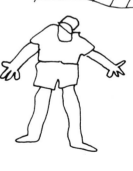
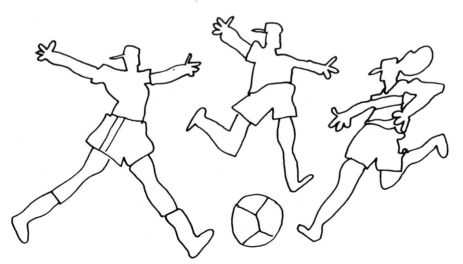

## Observation of Parent-Child Interaction

Do both the parent and the child ask the questions? Does the parent let the child speak directly to the health professional, or does the parent interrupt? Is the child playful or serious with the health professional? Do the parent and child make eye contact with each other and with the health professional? If the health professional speaks with the child alone, how comfortable is the child? How does the parent react to being asked to wait outside?

## Physical Examination

Respect the child's privacy by using appropriate draping during the examination.

Measure and plot on a standard chart the child's height and weight. Determine the body mass index (BMI) (see chart in appendix G, page 266). If a child has a BMI ≥ 95th percentile for age and gender, or ≤ 5th percentile, refer for dietary assessment and counseling. Children with a BMI between the 85th and 95th percentile need initial evaluation and counseling for obesity.[4]

As part of the complete physical examination, the following should be noted:

Scoliosis (Make orthopedic referral for curves greater than 15°–20°)

Tanner stage or Sexual Maturity Rating (SMR)

Caries, developmental anomalies, malocclusion, pathologic conditions, or dental injuries

Evidence of neglect or abuse

**ADDITIONAL SCREENING PROCEDURES**

Vision screening
(Vision screening guidelines appear in appendix F, page 265)

Hearing screening

Assessment of risk for hyperlipidemia[2]

Annual tuberculin test (PPD) if any of the following risk factors are present:

Low socioeconomic status
Residence in areas where tuberculosis is prevalent
Exposure to tuberculosis
Immigrant status

Blood pressure screening

**IMMUNIZATIONS**

Ensure that immunization status is up to date

# ANTICIPATORY GUIDANCE FOR THE FAMILY

In addition to providing anticipatory guidance, many health professionals give families handouts
at an appropriate reading level or a videotape that they can review or study at home.[3]

## Promotion of healthy habits

Supervise the child's activities with peers.

Be a role model for the child by having a healthy lifestyle.

Ensure that the child gets adequate sleep.

Encourage regular physical activity.

Enforce reasonable television/music standards.

Supervise the child's personal care and hygiene.

Counsel the child about avoiding the use of alcohol, tobacco, and drugs. Ensure that the child's school curriculum includes information about substance abuse.

## Injury prevention

Reinforce important safety considerations. Anticipate that the child may make errors in judgment due to increased risk-taking behavior.

Anticipate providing less direct supervision.

Continue to ensure that the child wears a seat belt in the car at all times.

Reinforce with the child safety rules for swimming pools. Teach the child how to swim.

Ensure that the child puts on sunscreen before he goes outside for long periods of time.

Continue to keep the child's environment free of smoke.

Test smoke detectors to ensure that they work properly. Change batteries yearly.

Reinforce with the child safety rules for the home, including what to do when home alone. Discuss visitors, not tying up the telephone for long periods of time, and what to do in case of fire or other emergencies. Conduct fire drills at home.

Ensure that guns, if in the home, are locked up and that ammunition is stored separately.

Reinforce safety rules for bicycles. Ensure that the child always wears a helmet when riding a bicycle.

Reinforce sports safety with the child, including the need to wear protective sports gear such as a mouth guard or a face protector.

Teach the child to avoid high noise levels, especially when using music headsets.

## Nutrition

Encourage the child to eat three regular meals per day and nutritious snacks.

Share meals as a family on a regular basis. Make mealtimes pleasant and companionable. Encourage conversation.

Model and encourage good eating habits. Serve a variety of healthy foods.

Teach the child how to choose nutritious snacks rich in complex carbohydrates. Limit high-fat or low-nutrient foods and beverages such as candy, chips, or soft drinks.

Teach the child how to eat a balanced diet. Teach him to choose plenty of fruits and vegetables; breads, cereals, and other grain products; low-fat dairy products; lean meats; and foods prepared with little or no fat.

Teach the child how to eat a nutritious lunch at school, either through the school lunch program or by packing a balanced lunch.

## Oral health

Ensure that the child brushes his teeth twice a day with a pea-size amount of fluoridated toothpaste and flosses.

Give the child fluoride supplements as recommended by the health professional based on the level of fluoride in the child's drinking water.

Schedule a dental appointment for the child every six months, unless his dentist determines otherwise based on his individual needs/susceptibility to disease.

As the child's permanent molars erupt, ensure that his dentist evaluates them for application of dental sealants.

Reinforce with the child how to handle dental emergencies, especially the loss or fracture of a tooth.

Reinforce with the child the dangers of smoking and smokeless tobacco.

## Sexuality education

Assess the child's preparation for puberty and sexual development.

If the child receives family life education at school or in the community, discuss it with him. Provide additional information as needed.

For parents of girls: Prepare your daughter for menstruation.

For parents of boys: Prepare your son for wet dreams.

Begin to teach the child that delaying sexual behavior is the surest form of protection against disease and pregnancy.

Explore the child's understanding of sexually transmitted diseases, including AIDS.

## Promotion of social competence

Praise the child for achievements.

Help the child choose activities in which he can be successful.

Encourage the child to talk with you about his school, friends, or feelings. Answer his questions.

Encourage reading and hobbies.

Spend individual time with the child, doing something you both enjoy.

Enhance the child's experiences through family trips (e.g., to parks, museums, or cultural events) or vacations.

Promote interaction and allegiance with peers through participation in social activities, community groups, and team sports.

Help the child learn how to get along with his peers. Discuss his awareness of differences among peers.

Promote independence by encouraging developmentally appropriate decision-making.

Set limits and establish consequences for unacceptable behavior. Expect the child to follow family rules, such as those for bedtime, television viewing, and chores.

Promote positive interactions between the child and his teachers and other adults.

Help the child learn appropriate or reasonable behavior.

Help the child develop an ability to withstand peer pressure. Discuss strategies and try role-playing.

Help the child develop an ability to deal constructively with conflict and anger in the family, at school, and in the neighborhood.

Assign age-appropriate chores, including responsibility for some household or yard tasks.

Provide personal space for the child at home, even if limited.

Teach a sense of social responsibility and acceptance of diversity.

## Promotion of constructive family relationships and parental health

Anticipate the normal range of adolescent behaviors, including the pervasive influence of peers, a change in the communication pattern between adolescents and parents, sudden challenges to parental rules and authority, conflicts over issues of independence, adolescents' refusal to participate in some family activities, their moodiness, and their risk taking.

Serve as a positive ethical and behavioral role model.

Contribute to the child's self-esteem by praising him and showing affection toward him.

Show interest in the child's school performance and after-school activities. Set reasonable but challenging expectations.

Promote self-responsibility.

Show affection in the family.

Spend some individual time with each child.

Participate in games and physical activities with the child.

Share meals as a family whenever possible.

Foster conversation and open communication in the family.

Know the child's friends and their families.

Encourage the development of good sibling relationships.

Acknowledge the conflicts between siblings. Whenever possible, attempt to resolve conflicts without taking sides. Do not allow violence. Handle anger constructively in the family.

Discuss with the health professional your own preventive and health-promoting practices (e.g., using seat belts, avoiding tobacco, eating properly, exercising and doing breast self-exams or testicular self-exams).

## Promotion of community interactions

If you need financial assistance to help pay for health care expenses, ask about resources or for referrals to the state Medicaid programs or other medical assistance programs.

Ask about resources or referrals for food, housing, or transportation if needed.

Discuss with the health professional possible programs for the child: before and after-school programs; swimming, soccer, or other exercise programs; or other community programs.

Participate as a family in school and community organizations and activities.

Contribute regularly to school or community activities that require adult supervision.

Encourage the child to participate in social, religious, cultural, volunteer, and recreational organizations.

Advocate for community programs and facilities for children (recreational, sports, and educational activities).

Discuss current events and social responsibility.

Promote social connections with neighbors and ties with extended family members.

Participate in activities that reflect cultural diversity (e.g., holidays, festivals, musical events, dance performances), and teach the child about his own culture.

Find out how to make your community safer. Advocate for and participate in a neighborhood watch program.

Encourage peer-mediated conflict management in schools from third grade through high school.

Advocate for after-school supervision for all children.

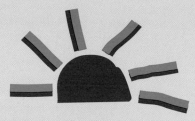

# A Visit to the School Health Room

Dahlia Petrovic, a fourth grader, has moved several times in the past few months. She moved to a new country, a new town, and a new home. Now she is starting a new school. As she walks down the hallways of the large elementary school building to the principal's office, she clutches her father's hand tightly.

Mr. Petrovic discusses Dahlia's new teacher and classmates with the school principal. In the school health room, the principal introduces them to the school nurse, Ms. Maxwell, who has just begun working there herself.

Dahlia is surprised when she walks into the health room. The walls are painted a soft yellow with white trim, and they are covered with pictures students have drawn about healthy foods, bicycle safety, how to say no to strangers, and how to keep a healthy smile. In a corner of the room are posters, books, and games related to staying healthy.

"It's nice to meet you, Dahlia," Ms. Maxwell says as she takes Dahlia's hand. "Let me show you what we have here. There are coloring books about how to brush your teeth and cookbooks for making healthy snacks." Ms. Maxwell walks with Dahlia to another room with a door. "Here is a scale that you can get on so I can weigh you, and then I'll measure your height."

"Is that your bed?" Dahlia asks Ms. Maxwell, pointing to a cot in a corner of an adjoining room.

"We use that cot for girls and boys who aren't feeling well and need a quiet place to lie down and rest," replies Ms. Maxwell.

Ms. Maxwell leads Dahlia and Mr. Petrovic to her desk in the corner of the health room. She takes out a form from her desk and attaches it to a clipboard. She asks both Dahlia and her father questions about Dahlia's health history, including questions about whether Dahlia has a chronic condition, uses medications, requires any special treatments during the school day, or might need emergency care to manage any special health conditions. She reviews Dahlia's address and records the emergency contact numbers for her family members, doctor, and dentist. Ms. Maxwell also receives Mr. Petrovic's permission to contact Dahlia's primary care providers for further information.

Dahlia leaves the health room holding her father's hand and carrying a sticker she received from Ms. Maxwell. The sticker says: "I'm happy because I'm healthy!"

# MIDDLE CHILDHOOD HEALTH SUPERVISION SUMMARY

## What else should we talk about?

### Summarize findings of the visit

Emphasize the strengths of both the child and the parents. Compliment the child for efforts and achievements. Commend the parents on their efforts to care for the child. Give suggestions, reading materials, and resources to promote health and reinforce good health practices.

### Arrange continuing care

### Next visit

Give the parents materials to prepare them for the next health supervision visit.

Recommend that the parents make an appointment for the next regularly scheduled visit.

If indicated, ask the parents to make an appointment for a supplementary health supervision visit.

### Other care

Ensure that the parents make an appointment to return to the health facility for follow-up on problems identified during the health supervision visit, or refer the child for secondary or tertiary medical care.

Consult with the school as necessary, especially if school progress is unsatisfactory or teacher evaluations are needed. (Obtain the parents' permission.)

Refer the family to appropriate community resources for help with problems identified during the visit (e.g., food programs, parenting classes, marital counseling, mental health services, special education programs). Make arrangements to follow up on referrals and coordinate care.

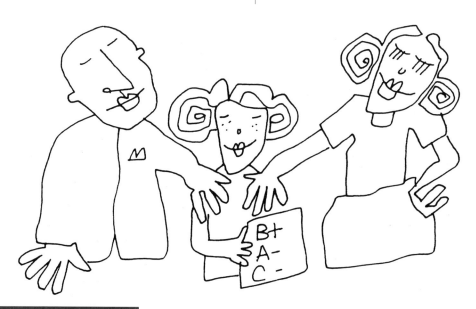

## Middle Childhood Endnotes

1.  To assess the risk of high-dose lead exposure, ask:

    Does your child live in or regularly visit a house (or a preschool or child care center) built before 1960? Does it have peeling or chipping paint? Has there been recent renovation or remodeling, or is any planned?

    Does your home's plumbing have lead pipes or copper with lead solder joints?

    Does your child live near a heavily travelled major highway where soil and dust may be contaminated with lead?

    Does your child frequently come in contact with an adult who works with lead (e.g., in construction, welding, pottery, or other trades)?

    Does your child live near a lead smelter, battery recycling plant, or other industrial site likely to release lead?

    Do you give your child any home remedies that may contain lead?

    Have any of your children or any of their playmates had lead poisoning?

    If any answer is positive, the child is considered at high risk for high-dose lead exposure. Administer a blood lead screening test immediately and at every health supervision visit through six years of age.

    If any blood test result is ≥10 µg/dL, the health professional should refer to the Centers for Disease Control and Prevention (CDC) guidelines and develop a management/treatment plan. (The CDC guidelines are subject to change, so consult the latest edition.)

    U.S. Department of Health and Human Services, Public Health Service, Centers for Disease Control. 1991. Preventing lead poisoning in young children: A statement by the Centers for Disease Control—October 1991. N.p.: Centers for Disease Control.

2.  Hyperlipidemia screening if any of the following risk factors are present:

    Parents or grandparents with a history of coronary or peripheral vascular disease before 55 years of age (Obtain a fasting serum lipid profile that includes determination of the low-density lipoprotein [LDL] cholesterol value.)

    Parents with a blood cholesterol level ≥240 mg/dL (Obtain a nonfasting total blood cholesterol level; perform at least once.)

    Hyperlipidemia screening at the discretion of the health professional if family history cannot be ascertained and any of the following risk factors are present in the family:

    > Smoking
    > Hypertension
    > Physical inactivity
    > Obesity
    > Diabetes mellitus
    > (Obtain a nonfasting total blood cholesterol.)

    American Academy of Pediatrics. 1989. Indications for cholesterol testing in children. *Pediatrics* 83(1):141–142.

    American Academy of Pediatrics, Committee on Nutrition. 1992. Statement on cholesterol. *Pediatrics* 90(3):469–473.

    National Cholesterol Education Program (NCEP) Expert Panel on Blood Cholesterol Levels in Children and Adolescents. 1992. NCEP: Highlights of the report of the Expert Panel on Blood Cholesterol Levels in Children and Adolescents. *Pediatrics* 89(3):495–500.

3.  The Injury Prevention Program (TIPP) of the American Academy of Pediatrics produces parent information sheets that highlight injury prevention priorities at each age, as well as parent information sheets on specific issues such as water safety. Community-based prevention groups, such as SAFE KIDS, also produce injury prevention materials.

4.  BMI

A child with a BMI ≥ the 95th percentile for age and gender is overweight. A child with a BMI ≤ the 5th percentile for age and gender is underweight. Both overweight and underweight children should be referred for in-depth dietary and health assessment.

Children with a BMI between the 85th and 95th percentiles are at risk for becoming overweight. A dietary and health assessment should be performed if:

-   The BMI has increased by two or more units during the previous 12 months;

-   There is a family history of premature heart disease, obesity, hypertension, or diabetes mellitus;

-   The child expresses concern about his or her weight; or

-   The child has elevated serum cholesterol levels or blood pressure.

If this assessment is negative, the child should be given general dietary and exercise counseling and should be monitored annually.

Assess children with low BMIs (especially female children) for eating disorders. If the eating pattern does not change promptly with intervention, referral is indicated.

Himes JH, Dietz WH. 1994. Guidelines for overweight in adolescent preventive services: Recommendations from an expert committee. *American Journal of Clinical Nutrition* 94(59):307–316.

## Bibliography

American Academy of Pediatrics, Committee on School Health. 1992, February. The role of the physician in school; Policy Statement. *AAP News*.

Carnegie Council of Adolescent Development, Task Force on Education of Young Adolescents. 1989. *Turning Points: Preparing American Youth for the 21st Century*. Washington, DC: Carnegie Council on Adolescent Development.

Center for the Future of Children. 1992. School Linked Services. *The Future of Children* 2(1):1–144. Los Altos, CA: David and Lucille Packard Foundation.

DiGuiseppi CG, Rivara FP, Koepsell TD, Polissar L. 1989. Bicycle helmet use by children: Evaluation of a community-wide helmet campaign. *Journal of the American Medical Association* 262(16):2256–2261.

DuRant RH, Pendergrast RA, Seymore C, Gaillard G, Donner J. 1992. Findings from the preparticipation athletic examination and athletic injuries. *Sports Medicine* 146:85–91.

Dworkin PH. 1989. Behavior during middle childhood: Developmental themes and clinical issues. *Pediatric Annals* 18(6):347–355.

Fergusson DM, Horwood J, Lynskey MT. 1993. Maternal smoking before and after pregnancy: Effects on behavioral outcomes in middle childhood. *Pediatrics* 92(6):815–822.

Frankowski BL, Weaver SO, Secker-Walker RH. 1993. Advising parents to stop smoking: Pediatricians' and parents' attitudes. *Pediatrics* 91(2):296–300.

Lauer RM, Clarke WR. 1990. Use of cholesterol measurements in childhood for the prediction of adult hypercholesterolemia: The Muscatine study. *Journal of the American Medical Association* 264(23):3034–3038.

Marsh JS. 1993. Screening for scoliosis. *Pediatrics in Review* 14(8):297–298.

Palfrey JS, McDowell M, Ciborowski J. 1992. Children's services in health and education. *Current Opinion in Pediatrics* 4(5):763–769.

Palfrey JS, Rappaport L, DeGraw C. 1989. The school-age child: Putting it all together. *Current Problems in Pediatrics* 19(6):290–322.

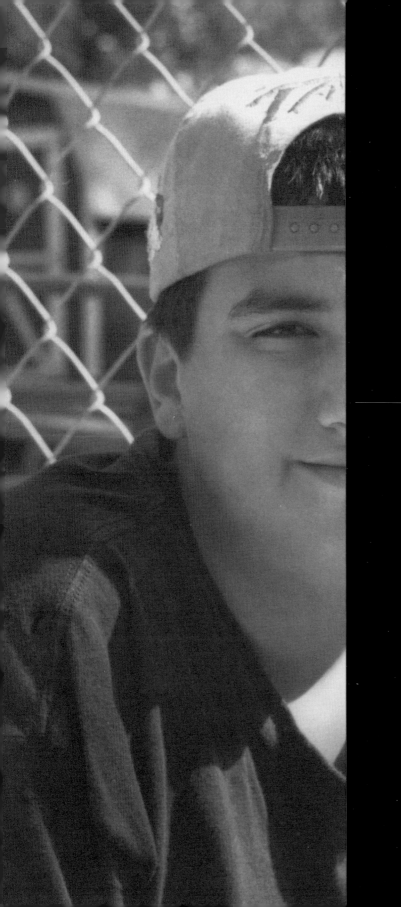

# 11–21 Years
# Adolescence

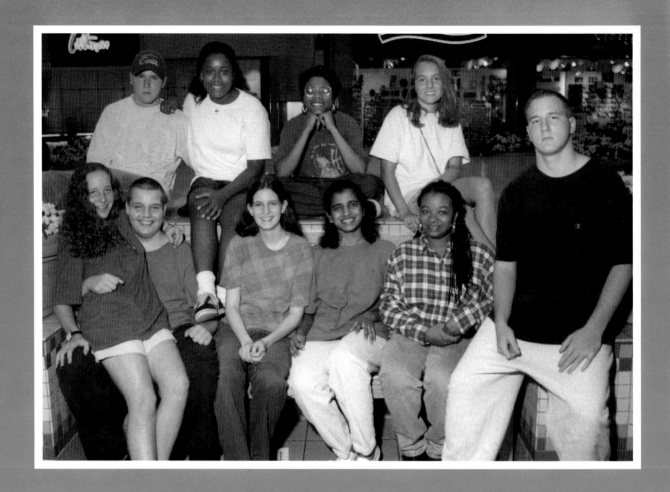

*The health system must adapt to the needs of adolescents
and their needs reside as much in preventative medicine
as they do in curative medicine.*

—Michael I. Cohen, M.D.
Professor and Chairman, Department of Pediatrics,
Albert Einstein College of Medicine

# Adolescence

Adolescence, the transition between childhood and adult life, is one of the most dynamic stages of human development. Adolescence is accompanied by dramatic physical, cognitive, social, and emotional changes that present both opportunities and challenges for adolescents, families, health professionals, teachers, and communities. While prior life experiences form the foundation of adolescence, current experiences continuously contribute to the maturation and differentiation of the young person. The health professional must also be sensitive to the changes that must occur in the health supervision relationship as the adolescent becomes increasingly capable of making autonomous decisions about health.

Adolescence is generally a period characterized by good health. For millions of adolescents, however, these years are accompanied by considerable preventable morbidity, mortality, and poor health habits. Unintentional injuries, homicide, and suicide are leading causes of death, while sexually transmitted diseases, substance abuse, adolescent pregnancy, antisocial behavior, and school dropout are important causes of physical, emotional, and social morbidity.

Adolescence is a time when childhood health disorders either resolve or persist into adulthood, new issues emerge, and risks for some long-term adult problems become detectable. Thus, this pivotal developmental period offers special opportunities for preventive and health-promoting services. A major role of health supervision is the periodic assessment and support of the adolescent's adaptation to new roles and risks that accompany growth and development. Providing adolescents with a sense of self-assurance, knowledge of what to do, and the belief that they can do it, and encouraging and reinforcing healthy choices, helps them develop the social competence and self-responsibility needed for personal health, school achievement, and job performance.

## Physical

The most noticeable physical changes during adolescence are those of somatic and sexual growth and development, including the appearance of secondary sexual characteristics and the capacity to reproduce. Young adolescents in particular are preoccupied with these physical changes and how they are perceived by others. Anticipatory guidance can help prepare adolescents and their parents for these changes. For example, many families are reassured to learn about the variability in the onset of these changes.

## Cognitive

The changes in cognitive development during adolescence are, in their own way, as dramatic as those in the physical domain. During this period, the adolescent may advance from concrete operational to formal operational thinking. What initially was a primary focus on the present should mature into an ability to consider the future implications of current actions. This shift obviously has enormous implications for health supervision; for the first time, adolescents may begin to have the cognitive capacity to comprehend the impact of their present behaviors on their future health. It is important to note, however, that this emerging way of thinking is still limited and occurs erratically throughout much of adolescence.

The limited capacity to see beyond simple solutions to complex problems evolves into a tolerance for ambiguity and the growing recognition that many issues have multiple causes and interrelationships. These psychological developments help account for the frequent questions posed by adolescents, their sometimes argumentative behavior, and their recurring challenges to parental authority.

## Social/emotional

Peer relationships during adolescence play a major role in the adolescent's emotional separation and individuation. Research suggests that adolescents often seek out peers whose beliefs, values, and even behaviors are similar to those of their families. While peer and other social influences often reinforce familial values, some influences may expose the adolescent to values that differ significantly from the family's. Thus the need to balance peer pressure and family expectations creates both new challenges and family tensions as adolescents begin to make independent decisions. In their struggle to gain autonomy while retaining interdependence, they may be understandably ambivalent about replacing their familiar comfort with and dependence on their parents with the uncertainty of relationships with others. The health professional is in a key position to offer guidance and support for families as they adapt to these changes.

The ability to integrate emotional and physical intimacy in a love relationship is an important developmental task for the older adolescent. Health supervision must address the sexual experimentation and concomitant risks that accompany this aspect of development.

## Health behaviors

Adolescence is a time of trying out all sorts of new behaviors. While this experimentation is essential for development, it may also lead to an increase in risky behaviors. The potential negative health consequences are likely to be underestimated by the adolescent. For example, nontraditional eating patterns, such as fad diets, may be adopted. Continued, periodic health supervision during adolescence is imperative in order to provide anticipatory guidance, support health-promoting behaviors, and help the adolescent apply increasingly sophisticated thinking in evaluating the consequences of new behaviors and roles.

## Family

The dramatic changes that have occurred in the American family are particularly significant for adolescents. The decrease in the time that many parents, extended family members, and neighbors are able to spend with children leads to less communication with, support from, and supervision by adults at a crucial period in development. At the very time when they are most likely to experiment with behaviors that can have serious health consequences, adolescents have more unsupervised time concurrent with less parental involvement. Parents should maintain a regular interest in their adolescents' daily activities and concerns. Adolescents are more likely to become successful young adults if their families remain actively involved with them, providing authoritative parenting in a democratic fashion. As the nature of family relationships changes, the health professional plays an important role in helping families negotiate the most useful balance between supervision and promotion of the adolescent's growing independence.

Continued parental involvement is enhanced when families receive useful information about the physical, cognitive, social, and emotional changes that occur in adolescence. Health professionals should emphasize that families serve as the major ethical and behavioral role models for adolescents and should communicate their expectations to them. The adolescent also needs the family's praise, support, availability, and unconditional positive regard.

## Community

Success in school contributes greatly to an adolescent's self-esteem and progress toward becoming a socially competent adult. Health promotion programs in schools can foster the establishment of good health habits and the avoidance of those that may lead to morbidity and mortality. Health promotion curricula can include family life education and social skills training, and information on pregnancy prevention, abstinence, conflict resolution, healthy nutritional practices, and avoidance of unhealthy habits such as smoking, drinking, and substance abuse. On-site integrated health services in the schools—with referrals to primary care physicians and community agencies (including mental health centers) for supplementary services—are evolving as an effective way to deliver adolescent health care in medically underserved areas.

Community recreational programs and facilities are important resources for adolescents. Opportunities for meaningful work experiences, community service, and participation in local governmental activities relating to adolescence contribute to an adolescent's sense of being included and valued. Community regulations and legislation that control the sale of alcohol, cigarettes, and guns and mandate seat belt/helmet use are important

health supervision measures, as is the availability of contraceptives and family planning services.

## Health supervision is a partnership

Health supervision efforts are most likely to succeed when they foster the joint participation and shared responsibility of adolescents, parents, health professionals, teachers, and others who have a personal, professional, or supervisory relationship with adolescents. Requirements for success in health supervision include a respect for individual differences, support of the adolescent's emerging autonomy, a developmental approach, and a focus on the adolescent's strengths. The health professional should have an ability to establish a therapeutic alliance, an expertise in health matters that the adolescent can respect and trust, and an enjoyment of the rewards that come from helping adolescents achieve their full potential.

Adolescents may need special efforts to help them engage in regular health supervision. They are often more comfortable with health professionals who have the special training and experience to deal with their particular issues. Different types of settings, such as community or school health clinics, may also be more successful in encouraging adolescents to participate in regular health supervision.

# ADOLESCENCE DEVELOPMENTAL CHART

Health professionals should assess the achievements of the adolescent and provide guidance to the family on anticipated tasks. The effects are demonstrated by health supervision outcomes.

## DEVELOPMENTAL ACHIEVEMENTS

Responsibility for good health habits

Somatic and sexual growth and development

Social and conflict resolution skills

Good peer relationships with the same and opposite sex

Capacity for intimacy

Responsible sexual behavior and a sexual identity

Coping skills and strategies

Appropriate level of autonomy

Personal value system

Progression from concrete to formal operational thinking

Academic and career goals

Educational or vocational competence

## TASKS FOR THE ADOLESCENT

Maintain good eating habits and dental hygiene

Exercise regularly and maintain appropriate weight

Use seat belt and helmet

Avoid alcohol, tobacco, and other drugs

Practice abstinence or safer sex

Engage in safe and age-appropriate experimentation

Manage negative peer pressure

Learn conflict resolution skills

Protect self from physical, emotional, and sexual abuse

Develop self-confidence, self-esteem, and own identity

Develop ability to interact with peers, siblings, and adults

Continue process of separating from family

Develop sense of responsibility for others

Be responsible for school performance

Develop good oral and written language skills

## HEALTH SUPERVISION OUTCOMES

Self-efficacy and mastery

Independence

Active role in health supervision and promotion

Optimal nutrition

Satisfactory growth and development

Good health habits

Reduction of high-risk behavior

Injury prevention

Promotion of developmental potential

Prevention of behavioral problems

Sense of responsibility and morality

Promotion of family strengths

Enhancement of parental effectiveness

Educational/vocational success

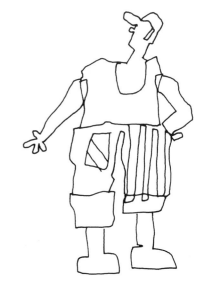

# FAMILY PREPARATION FOR ADOLESCENCE HEALTH SUPERVISION

Instructions to be provided to the family by the health professional.

Be prepared to give updates on the following at your next visit:

Illnesses and infectious diseases
Injuries
Visits to other health facilities or providers
Use of the emergency department
Hospitalizations or surgeries
Immunizations
Food and drug allergies
Eating habits
Medications
Supplementary fluoride and vitamins
Dental care
Vision and hearing
Chronic health conditions
Growth and development
Sexual activity

Update the adolescent's personal health record.

Be prepared to provide the following information on your family:

Health of and location of each significant family member

Genetic disorders

Depression or other mental health problems in the immediate or extended family

Alcoholism or other substance abuse (including use of tobacco) in the immediate or extended family

Family transitions (e.g., birth, death, marriage, divorce, loss of income, move, frequently absent parent, incarceration)

Home environment/neighborhood

Hazardous exposures (e.g., violence, asbestos, tuberculosis)

Prepare and bring in questions, concerns, and observations about issues such as:

Physical and mental health
Substance abuse
Sexuality
Interactions (family and peer)
School concerns
Increasing independence and new challenges
Achievements

Bring in reports from school and results of parent-teacher conferences. Bring in the Individualized Education Program (IEP) if the adolescent has special needs.

Complete special questionnaires on psychosocial topics (e.g., family, peers, school, dating, sexual activity, recreation, employment, future plans), health-related issues (e.g., nutrition, sleep patterns, sports and physical activity, substance use, moods, vehicle safety), or other areas.

Fill out and bring in health forms (camp, sports participation) for completion by the health professional.

Talk to the adolescent about the health supervision visit, including the general physical exam, the genital/gynecological exam, immunizations, and other procedures.

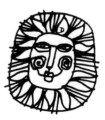

**ADOLESCENCE • 11–21 YEARS**

# STRENGTHS DURING ADOLESCENCE

Health professionals should remind families of their strengths during the health supervision visit.
Strengths and issues for adolescent, family, and community are interrelated and interdependent.

## ADOLESCENT

Has good physical health and nutritional status

Maintains an appropriate weight

Develops a positive body image

Develops responsibility for own health and engages in healthy behaviors

Has regular dental care

Maintains own physical fitness

Engages in safe, age-appropriate experimentation

Has positive, cheerful, friendly temperament

Has confidants and develops capacity for intimacy

Is socially competent

Experiences hope, joy, success, love

Has high self-esteem and expects personal success

Practices stress management

Establishes appropriate level of independence

Develops own identity

Respects rights and needs of others

Establishes educational and vocational goals

## FAMILY

Meets basic needs (food, shelter, clothing, safety, health care)

Accepts lability of feelings and moods during adolescence

Supports activities that enhance adolescent's self-image

Spends individual time with adolescent

Praises and takes pride in adolescent's achievements

Reinforces adolescent's feeling of being loved

Encourages the adolescent's development of close friendships

Recognizes changing role of parent(s) and adolescent

Serves nutritious family meals on a regular basis

Provides sexuality education at home

Encourages adolescent's increasing independence and responsibility

Develops balance between support, acceptance, and appropriate limits

Supports adolescent's educational and vocational goals

Provides value system and role models

## COMMUNITY

Provides quality educational and vocational opportunities for all adolescents and families

Provides activities for adolescents (recreational, sports, educational, social)

Provides support for families with special needs

Passes and enforces legislation to protect adolescents (drunk driving, gun control, tobacco, seat belt/helmet use)

Provides comprehensive health education and services (mental health, nutrition, oral health, physical health and fitness, sexuality, substance use, injury and violence prevention)

Recognizes increasing autonomy of adolescents (legal rights, confidential care)

Provides an environment free of hazards (violence, pollution, asbestos, radiation)

Ensures that neighborhoods are safe

Provides affordable housing and public transportation

Develops integrated systems of adolescent health care, with multiple ways that adolescents can access care

Fluoridates drinking water

Promotes positive ethnic/cultural milieu

# ISSUES DURING ADOLESCENCE

Health professionals should address issues—problems, stressors, and concerns—that families raise during health supervision.
Strengths and issues for adolescent, family, and community are interrelated and interdependent.

## ADOLESCENT

School concerns (poor grades, underachievement, disinterest, truancy)

Vocational concerns

Behavioral concerns (disobedience, aggression, violence, homicide)

Social concerns (lack of friends, negative peer influence, withdrawal from family)

Emotional concerns (depression, anxiety, schizophrenia, confusion about sexual orientation, low self-esteem, threat of suicide, suicide)

Early sexual activity, inappropriate sexual behavior, pregnancy, sexually transmitted diseases, HIV infection

Substance abuse (alcohol, drugs, tobacco, steroids)

Poor safety behaviors (drunk driving, failure to use seat belts or helmets)

Medical concerns (acne, myopia, scoliosis, problems with menstruation, hyperlipidemia, hypertension)

Weight and height concerns, poor nutrition, eating disorders (obesity, anorexia, bulimia)

Failure to exercise

Multiple somatic complaints

Chronic illness or disability

## FAMILY

Dysfunctional parents or other family members (depressed, mentally ill, abusive, disinterested, overly critical, overprotective, incarcerated)

Marital problems

Domestic violence (verbal, physical, or sexual abuse)

Frequently absent parent

Rotating "parents" (parents' girlfriends or boyfriends)

Family health problems (illness, siblings or parents with chronic illness or disability)

Substance use (alcohol, drugs, tobacco)

Financial insecurity/homelessness

Family transitions (move, divorce, remarriage, incarceration, death)

Lack of knowledge about adolescent development

Lack of parental self-esteem and self-efficacy

Poor family communication

Social isolation and lack of support

Rejection of adolescent

## COMMUNITY

Poverty

Inadequate housing

Environmental hazards

Unsafe neighborhood

Community violence

Poor opportunities for vocational training and employment

Low-quality or unsafe schools

Lack of supervised programs before and after school

Lack of programs for families with special needs

Isolation in a rural community

Lack of social, educational, cultural, and recreational opportunities

Discrimination and prejudice

Lack of access to medical/dental services

Inadequate public services (transportation, garbage removal, lighting, repair of public facilities, police and fire protection)

Inadequate fluoride levels in community drinking water

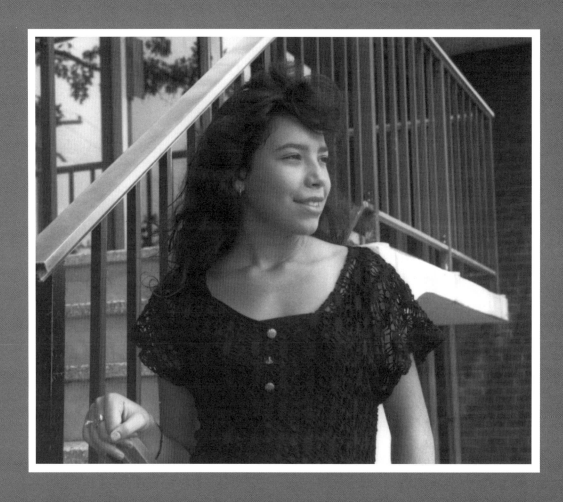

*Dramatic physical changes are the hallmark of early adolescence. Generally, girls begin puberty an average of two years earlier than boys.*

# 11, 12, 13, and 14 Year Early Adolescence Visits

Dramatic physical changes are the hallmark of early adolescence. Generally, girls begin puberty an average of two years earlier than boys. During early adolescence, most girls experience a rapid growth spurt, changes in fat distribution, and the development of secondary sexual characteristics such as pubic hair and breasts. For most boys, the early adolescent period marks only the beginning of the biological changes of puberty, with increased abdominal fat deposits, testicular growth, voice changes, and the development of acne, pubic hair, and nocturnal emissions. Since many young adolescents are unaware that the onset and rate of puberty vary greatly, they need reassurance that their own growth and development are normal, and they will benefit from learning about the progression of physiological changes.

The profound biological changes of puberty engender feelings of extreme vulnerability and sensitivity to physical appearance. Young adolescents are very egocentric, intensely preoccupied with the question "Who am I, physically?" and feelings of being "on stage." Many teens spend seemingly endless hours grooming in front of the mirror. Because of their sensitivity and modesty about their bodies, young adolescents have a heightened need for privacy. Families must learn to respect a "closed-door policy."

Many young adolescents, preoccupied with their attractiveness, will try to change their appearance through dieting or consumer fad food products. Anorexia and bulimia may occur especially among females. Some males use supplements and steroids for bodybuilding. While some teens exercise regularly and develop bodies that are extremely fit, others remain sedentary and have poor physical fitness. These behaviors are often predictors of fitness habits later in life.

While young adolescents have increasing potential for abstract thought, their cognition still tends to be concrete and present oriented. Their sense of morality, also concrete, is driven by rules. Young adolescents see people and their behaviors as good or bad, right or wrong.

The transition to middle school often makes the young adolescent anxious, as she learns to cope with less adult support and more anonymity. While the elementary school child stays in one classroom in a relatively small school and is usually taught by a single teacher, youth in middle schools often find themselves in large institutions where they have a new teacher and classroom for each subject. Scholastic demands also increase, requiring the student to be more organized and efficient. A decrease in a student's academic performance is not uncommon. Girls' math and science scores in particular often suffer, due in part to teachers' attitudes and their low expectations. Truancy and school dropout can also begin to occur. Participation in sports encourages some teens to stay in school by providing positive group recognition and adult mentors.

School is the primary place where peer norms are communicated. Friendships are often with same-sex peers, and the seductiveness of peer conformity is a powerful phenomenon. Preparing the young adolescent to deal with increasing peer pressure is an important part of health supervision. Although parents' modeling of healthy behaviors remains the largest influence, the attitudes of schoolmates can greatly influence adolescents' perceptions of health-promoting behaviors. Middle schools offer new and greater possibilities for poor health choices (e.g., candy and chips available in vending machines).

Some adolescents belong to organizations such as the Girl Scouts, Boy Scouts, or Girls and Boys Clubs, and participate in cultural and religious youth groups. Unfortunately, to reduce costs, many public schools have cut back on after-school clubs and activities. Many youth lack recreational opportunities. They may come under intense pressure to join gangs or feel endangered by gang activities or other types of violence. Some youth carry weapons as a means of protection or intimidation. Young adolescents may be lured into making money by selling drugs, stealing, or engaging in other illegal activities.

Communities have become more transient and impersonal, offering less support and supervision to young adolescents. Many communities lack visible positive adult role models. The media compound this problem, since most of the videos, music, films, and television programs that fascinate adolescents do not promote healthy behaviors. Communities also vary in creating and enforcing regulations that affect the health and safety of adolescents (e.g., prohibiting access to cigarette machines or alcohol and mandating helmet use).

Exploration—usually in the company of peers—serves important developmental purposes. Unfortunately, many of the behaviors that adolescents experiment with can have serious health consequences. By ninth grade, 82 percent of students have already experimented with alcohol, and almost one quarter report at least one occasion of heavy drinking (i.e., having five or more drinks) during the preceding month. Over half of ninth graders have tried cigarette smoking, and 17 percent report smoking regularly. One fifth of ninth graders report having used marijuana, and 4 percent have used cocaine.[1] Inhalant abuse is another problem among young adolescents.

Sexual exploration also increases during early adolescence. By ninth grade, almost 40 percent of students report having had sexual intercourse, although the frequency is low.[1] For the majority of young adolescents, however, masturbation and petting are the most common sexual behaviors. Young adolescents are not likely to use either contraception or methods to prevent sexually transmitted diseases, especially during first encounters. Many adolescents have experienced sexual victimization or nonconsensual sexual intercourse.

Young adolescents harbor much misinformation about sexuality. Issues related to the menstrual cycle, fertility, and sexually transmitted diseases should be explored and clarified by the adolescents' parents and the health professional. Virgins can be supported in their decision to defer intercourse. Those who are sexually active can be helped to understand and practice protective behaviors.

Injuries from sports, other physical activities, work, or operation of farm machinery are common causes of morbidity for young adolescents. More than half of injury-related deaths involve motor vehicles, with the adolescent as a passenger or pedestrian or on a bicycle. Few early adolescents take measures to reduce their risk of injury. Less than one-fourth of eighth graders state that they always wear seat belts, and only 1 percent report wearing bicycle helmets consistently.[1]

Ambivalent about their impending emotional independence, young adolescents often display erratic, moody behavior. The young adolescent may be extremely opinionated, challenging family rules, values, and behaviors. Families need to keep supervising the adolescent and setting appropriate limits. At the same time, they must promote the youth's increasing autonomy in decision-making. Parents are still important role models for the adolescent, especially now that she is exposed to increasingly varied behavior. Families need support since they often feel sad and anxious as they try to negotiate new understandings with their teenager.

While the early adolescent's mind and body are becoming more capable and adultlike, she still lacks the experience and judgment to use these increasing capabilities wisely. The challenge for the health professional is to support the adolescent and the family so that opportunities for exploration and continued growth and autonomy are presented in a safe and nurturing context.

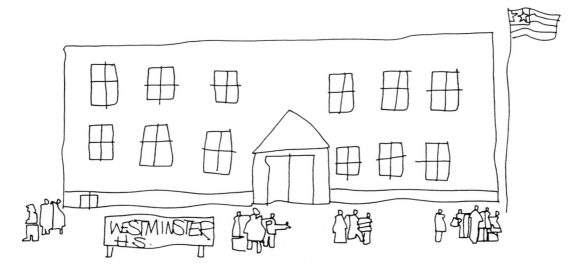

**EARLY ADOLESCENCE • 11, 12, 13, 14 YEARS**

# HEALTH SUPERVISION INTERVIEW

## TRIGGER QUESTIONS

To be used selectively by the health professional. Discuss any issues or concerns of the family.

### For the Parent(s)

**How are you?**

**How are things going now that Angela is becoming/is a teenager?**

**What about Sonja makes you most proud?**

**What questions or concerns do you have today?**

(e.g., the adolescent's growth; eating patterns; weight gain/loss; use of diet pills, tobacco, alcohol, drugs, or inhalants; frequent physical complaints; depression; loneliness; or sexual activity)

**Have there been any major changes or stresses in your family since your last visit?**

**What are some of the things you do together as a family? How often?**

**How is Lichua doing in school?**

**What does Maya do after school?**

**Are you concerned about Jacob's choice of music?**

**Are you happy with Jeremy's friends?**

**What has Rose been taught in school or at home about drugs, sex, or other health topics?**

**Do you think that smoking, drinking, or drug use is a problem for anyone in your family?**

**Does Ted understand what you consider appropriate behavior?**
**Have you clearly stated rules about how you want him to act?**

**Does Eduardo exercise on a regular basis (three times per week)?**

**Do you remind Carrie to wear a seat belt in the car or a helmet if riding a bicycle or motorcycle? Do you always wear a seat belt yourself?**

# Developmental Surveillance and School Performance

## For the Adolescent

### Social and Emotional Development

Who is your best friend? What do you do together? About how many friends do you have? What do you and your friends do outside of school? How old are your friends?

Tell me some of the things you're really good at.

What do you do for fun?

What are some of the things that worry you? Make you sad? Make you angry? What do you do about these things? Who do you talk to about them?

Do you ever have bad dreams? How often?

Do you often feel sad or alone at a party?

Have you ever thought about running away?

Do you know if any of your friends or relatives have tried to hurt or kill themselves?

Have you ever thought about hurting yourself or killing yourself?[2]

Have you ever been in trouble at school or with the law?

### Physical Development and Health Habits

Has anyone talked with you about what to expect as your body develops? Have you read about it?

Do you think you are developing pretty much like the rest of your friends?

How do you feel about the way you look?

What kind of exercise or organized sports do you do? Have you been injured in sports? How hard does the coach push you? Is the training about right?

How much time each week do you spend watching television or videos? Playing video games?

Do you use a sunscreen when in the sun?

How do you feel about your weight? Are you trying to change your weight? How?

What do you usually eat in the morning? At noon? In the afternoon? In the evening?

How many servings of milk products did you have in the last 24 hours? Is that a typical amount?

Do your friends smoke? Chew tobacco? Drink? Take drugs?

What do you think about smoking? Chewing tobacco? Drinking? Taking drugs?

Did you smoke any cigarettes in the last month? Chew tobacco? How often?

Have you drunk alcohol in the last month? How much? What is the most you have ever had to drink?

Have you ever tried other drugs? How often have you taken them in the past month?

Have you ever been in a car where the driver was drinking or on drugs?

What education have you had about smoking or chewing tobacco? Drinking? Drugs?

Are you worried about any friends or family members and how much they drink or use drugs?

Do your friends try to pressure you to do things that you don't want to do? How do you handle that?

Do you wear a seat belt when riding in a car? Do you wear a helmet when riding on a motorcycle? On a bicycle? In an all-terrain vehicle?

Do you own a gun? Do any of your friends? Where is it kept? Is there a gun in your house?

Have you ever been frightened by violent or sexual things someone has said to you?

Have you ever witnessed violence? Been threatened with violence? Been a victim of violence?

Has anyone ever tried to harm you physically?

## Sexual Development

Have you started having wet dreams? Your period? Is it regular?

Do your friends date? Have sex?

Have you started dating? How often do you date?

Do you date one person or a lot of people?

Do you have any worries or questions about sex?

Are you worried about having sexual feelings for someone of your own sex?

Have you begun having sexual intercourse? Circumstances?

Do you feel support from your family, friends, and community to delay sexual intercourse?

Have you thought about what you might do if you ever felt pressure to have sex?

Have you ever been pregnant (or gotten someone pregnant)?

Would you like to have a baby? What do you think it means to have a baby?

Have you ever had any sexually transmitted diseases such as gonorrhea, chlamydia, herpes, syphilis, or genital warts?

Do you use a kind of birth control? What kind?

Do you use condoms?

Has anyone ever touched you in a way you didn't like? Forced you to have sex?

## Family Functioning

Who do you live with?

How do you get along with family members?

If teenager lives with one parent:
How often do you see the parent who does not live with you? What do you do together? How do you feel about this arrangement?

Are the rules in your family clear and fair?

Do the adults in your family talk about decisions and make decisions fairly?

What types of responsibilities do you have at home?

Do you feel that your family listens to you? Do you feel that they spend enough time with you?

What would you like to change about your family if you could?

## School Performance

Compared with others in your class (not just your friends), how well do you think you are doing? Average? Better than average? Below average?

How often do you miss school? How often are you late for school?

What activities are you involved in?

## Observation of Parent-Adolescent Interaction

In the joint interview, does the parent allow the adolescent to answer some of the questions? Is the parent supportive of the adolescent? How does the adolescent react to being interviewed alone? How does the parent react to being asked to wait outside? Is the parent able to discuss sensitive topics?

## Physical Examination

Measure and plot on a standard chart the adolescent's height and weight. Determine the body mass index (BMI) (see appendix G, page 266). If an adolescent has a BMI ≥ 95th percentile for age and gender, or ≤ 5th percentile, refer for dietary assessment and counseling. Adolescents with a BMI between the 85th and 95th percentile need initial evaluation and counseling for obesity.[3]

As part of the complete physical examination, the following should be noted:

Scoliosis
(Make orthopedic referral for curves greater than 15°–20° if spinal growth is not completed. Adolescent girls usually complete spinal growth 18–24 months after menarche.)

Acne and common dermatoses

Caries, developmental dental anomalies, malocclusion, gingivitis, pathologic conditions, or dental injuries

Evidence of abuse

Evaluate for Tanner stage or Sexual Maturity Rating (SMR).

For females: Provide instruction in breast self-examination. Inspect genitalia externally for condyloma/lesions. If teenager is sexually active, perform pelvic exam annually.

For males: Evaluate for gynecomastia. Examine for hernias, condyloma/lesions, and testicular cancer (high-risk group is those with a history of undescended testes, single testicle). Provide educational testicular examination.

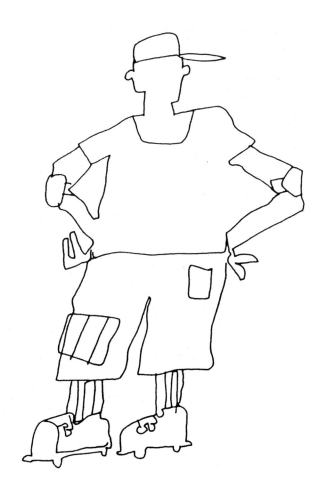

## ADDITIONAL SCREENING PROCEDURES

Vision screening if adolescent is not tested at school or reports problems
(Vision screening guidelines appear in appendix F, page 265)

Hearing screening if adolescent is exposed to loud noises regularly, has recurring ear infections, or reports problems

Annual tuberculin test (PPD) if any of the following risk factors are present:

   Low socioeconomic status
   Residence in areas where tuberculosis is prevalent
   Exposure to tuberculosis
   Immigrant status
   Homelessness
   History of incarceration
   Employment or volunteer work in health care setting

Tuberculin test (PPD) once at 14–16 years of age if no risk factors are present

Annual blood pressure screening

Annual hematocrit or hemoglobin screening for females if any of the following risk factors are present:

   Moderate to heavy menses
   Chronic weight loss
   Nutritional deficit
   Athletic activity

Hyperlipidemia screening[4] if any of the following risk factors are present:

   Parents or grandparents with a history of coronary or peripheral vascular disease before 55 years of age

   Parents with a blood cholesterol level ≥240 mg/dL

Hyperlipidemia screening at the discretion of the health professional if family history cannot be ascertained and any of the following risk factors for future coronary vascular disease are present:

   Smoking
   Hypertension
   Physical inactivity
   Obesity
   Diabetes mellitus

Annual pap smear for sexually active females (Females with a history of condyloma or previous abnormal pap smears may need more frequent screening)

Annual screening for sexually active adolescents:

   Gonorrhea

   Chlamydia
   (For asymptomatic males, urine dipstick for leukocytes may be sufficient)

Syphilis screening (VDRL/RPR) if the adolescent asks to be tested or if any of the following risk factors are present:

- History of sexually transmitted diseases
- More than one sexual partner in the past six months
- Intravenous drug use
- Sexual intercourse with a partner at risk
- Sex in exchange for drugs or money
- For males: Sex with other males
- Homelessness
- Residence in areas where syphilis is prevalent

HIV screening if the adolescent asks to be tested or if any of the following risk factors are present:

- Blood transfusion before 1985
- History of sexually transmitted diseases
- More than one sexual partner in the past six months
- Intravenous drug use
- Sexual intercourse with a partner at risk
- Sex in exchange for drugs or money
- For males: Sex with other males
- Homelessness
- (HIV screening should be done with informed consent and pretest and posttest counseling.)

Annual screening for behaviors or emotions that may indicate:

- Multiple stressors
- Use of tobacco products, alcohol, or other drugs
- Sexual behavior
- Recurrent or severe depression or risk of suicide
- History of emotional, physical, or sexual abuse
- Learning or school problems (see Developmental Surveillance for suggested questions)

## IMMUNIZATIONS

Ensure that immunization status is up to date

Hepatitis B Virus (HBV) Vaccine      #1, #2, and/or #3
(If not administered previously.
Use series of three doses: First dose at
elected date, second dose one month later,
third dose six months after first dose.)

Measles, Mumps, and Rubella (MMR) Vaccine      #2
(If not administered previously or if immunization status is uncertain. Administer at
11–12 years of age. Do not administer if
adolescent is pregnant.)

Tetanus and Diphtheria (Td) Vaccine      #6
(Administer 10 years after previous DTP
or Td booster, usually at 14–16 years of age.)

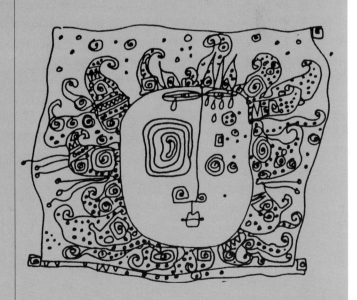

# ANTICIPATORY GUIDANCE FOR THE ADOLESCENT

In addition to providing anticipatory guidance, many health professionals give adolescents and families handouts at an appropriate reading level or a videotape that they can review or study at home.[5]

## Promotion of healthy habits

Get adequate sleep.

Exercise vigorously at least three times per week. Encourage friends and family members to exercise.

Discuss with the health professional or your coach athletic conditioning, weight training, fluids, and weight gain or loss.

Limit television viewing to an average of one hour per day.

## Injury and violence prevention

Wear a seat belt in the car.

Learn how to swim.

Do not drink alcohol, especially while boating or swimming.

Protect yourself from skin cancer by putting sunscreen on before you go outside for long periods of time.

Ask your parents to test smoke detectors to ensure that they work properly and to change batteries yearly.

Discuss with your parents safety rules for the home, including those about visitors, use of the telephone, and what to do in case of fire or other emergencies. Conduct fire drills at home.

Always wear a helmet when on a motorcycle, in an all-terrain vehicle, or riding a bicycle. Even with a helmet, motorcycles and ATVs are very dangerous.

Wear protective sports gear such as a mouth guard or a face protector.

Wear appropriate protective gear at work and follow job safety procedures.

Avoid high noise levels, especially in music headsets.

Do not carry or use a weapon of any kind.

Develop skills in conflict resolution, negotiation, and dealing with anger constructively.

Learn techniques to protect yourself from physical, emotional, and sexual abuse, including rape by either strangers or acquaintances.

Seek help if you are physically or sexually abused or fear that you are in danger.

## Mental health

Take on new challenges that will increase your self-confidence.

Continue learning about yourself—e.g., what you believe in, what is important to you.

Recognize that you are growing and changing.

Learn to feel good about yourself through learning what your strengths are and listening to what good friends and valued adults say about you.

Talk with the health professional or another trusted adult if you are often sad or nervous or feel that things are just not going right.

Learn to recognize and deal with stress.

Understand the importance of your religious and spiritual needs and try to fulfill them.

## Nutrition

Eat three meals per day. Breakfast is especially important. Eat meals with your family on a regular basis.

Choose a variety of healthy foods.

Choose nutritious snacks rich in complex carbohydrates. Limit high-fat or low-nutrient foods and beverages such as candy, chips, or soft drinks.

Choose plenty of fruits and vegetables; breads, cereals, and other grain products; low-fat dairy products; lean meats; and foods prepared with little or no fat. Include foods rich in calcium and iron in your diet.

Select a nutritious meal from the school cafeteria or pack a balanced lunch.

Achieve and maintain a healthy weight. Manage weight through appropriate eating habits and regular exercise.

## Oral health

Brush your teeth twice a day with a pea-size amount of fluoridated toothpaste, and floss daily.

Take fluoride supplements as recommended by the health professional based on the level of fluoride in your drinking water.

Ask the health professional any questions you have about how to handle dental emergencies, especially the loss or fracture of a tooth.

Schedule a dental appointment every six months, unless your dentist determines otherwise based on your individual needs/susceptibility to disease.

As your permanent molars erupt, ensure that your dentist evaluates them for application of dental sealants.

Do not smoke or use chewing tobacco.

## Sexuality[6]

Identify a supportive adult who can give you accurate information about sex.

Ask the health professional any questions you have about body changes during puberty, including variations from individual to individual.

Ask any questions you have about birth control or sexually transmitted diseases.

Having sexual feelings is normal, but you should wait to have sex until you and your partner want to.

Not having sexual intercourse is the safest way to prevent pregnancy and sexually transmitted diseases, including HIV infection/AIDS.

Learn about ways to say no to sex.

If you are engaging in sexual activity, including intercourse, ask the health professional for an examination and discuss methods of birth control. Learn about safer sex.

Practice safer sex. Limit the number of partners and use latex condoms and other barriers correctly.

## Prevention of substance use/abuse

Do not smoke, use smokeless tobacco, drink alcohol, or use drugs, diet pills, or steroids. Do not become involved in selling drugs.

If you smoke, discuss smoking cessation with the health professional.

If you use drugs or alcohol, discuss this with the health professional or other trusted adult.

Avoid situations where drugs or alcohol are easily available.

Support friends who choose not to use tobacco, alcohol, drugs, steroids, or diet pills.

Become a peer counselor to prevent substance abuse.

## Promotion of social competence

Spend time with your family doing something you all enjoy.

Participate in social activities, community groups, and team sports.

Make sure you understand your parents' limits and the consequences they have established for unacceptable behavior.

Learn to get along with, respect, and care about your peers and siblings.

Discuss with the health professional and your family and friends your strategies and coping mechanisms for handling negative peer pressure. Practice peer refusal skills.

Continue your progress in separating from your family, making independent decisions, and understanding the consequences of your behavior.

## Promotion of responsibility

Respect the rights and needs of others.

Serve as a positive ethical and behavioral role model.

Follow family rules, such as those for curfews, television viewing, and chores.

Share in household chores.

Learn about how you can take on new responsibility for your family, peers, and community.

Learn new skills that may be useful with your friends, family, or community (e.g., cardiopulmonary resuscitation [CPR]).

## Promotion of school achievement

If you are anxious about the transition to middle school or high school, discuss it with the health professional.

Become responsible for your own attendance, homework, and course selection.

If you feel frustrated with school or are thinking about dropping out, discuss your feelings and options with a trusted adult.

Participate in school activities.

Identify talents and interests that you might want to pursue as a career or for enjoyment.

Begin to think about college options, vocational training, the military, or other career choices.

## Promotion of community interactions

If you need financial assistance to help pay for health care expenses, ask about resources or for referrals to the state Medicaid programs or other state medical assistance programs.

Ask for help with food, housing, or transportation if needed.

Participate in social, religious, cultural, volunteer, or recreational organizations or activities.

Discuss current events and social responsibility with friends, family, and others.

Learn about your cultural heritage and that of others. Participate in activities that reflect cultural diversity (e.g., holidays, festivals, musical events, dance performances).

Find out what you can do to make your community safer.

Participate in peer-mediated conflict management training if it is offered through your school.

Join community campaigns to prevent substance abuse. Advocate for smoke-free environments and smoking cessation programs in your school, workplace, and community.

# ANTICIPATORY GUIDANCE FOR THE PARENT(S)

Understand that the adolescent may be unwilling to participate in some family activities and may suddenly challenge parental authority.

Decide with the adolescent when she can do things on her own, including staying at home alone.

Establish realistic expectations for family rules, with increasing autonomy and responsibility given to the adolescent.

Establish and communicate clear limits and consequences for breaking rules. Demonstrate interest in the adolescent's school activities and emphasize the importance of school.

Enhance the adolescent's self-esteem by providing praise and recognizing positive behavior and achievements.

Minimize criticism, nagging, derogatory comments, and other belittling or demeaning messages.

Spend time with the adolescent.

Respect the adolescent's need for privacy.

Discuss with the health professional your own preventive and health-promoting practices (e.g., using seat belts, avoiding tobacco, eating properly, exercising and doing breast self-exams or testicular self-exams).

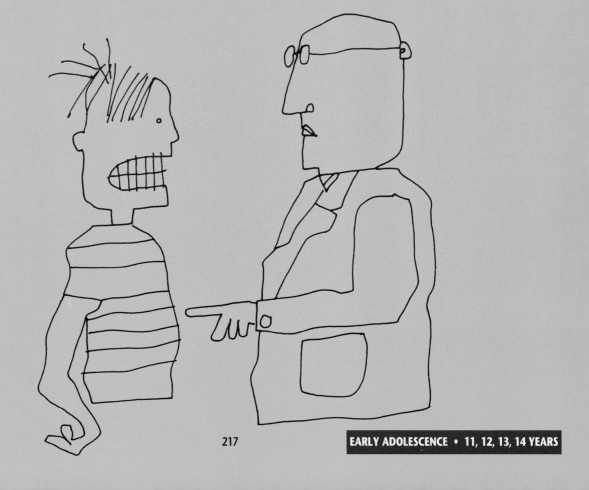

217

# Olympic Dreams

Thomas Galinsky is 11 years old and full of energy. He anxiously awaits the tryouts for his elementary school's soccer team. His 13-year-old sister, Nicole, plays on the basketball and softball teams at her junior high school. Both Thomas and Nicole are extremely active and interested in being the best at the sports in which they participate. Thomas even has dreams of playing professional soccer and keeps pictures of World Cup soccer players on his bedroom wall. Nicole wants to go to a Division One college someday and play basketball. Her coach, Sarah, played on a college team and encourages Nicole to keep working on her skills. Both Thomas and Nicole dream of Olympic stardom.

Thomas and Nicole's parents take them to Dr. Jackson's office to have their school preparticipation physical evaluation forms filled out. Meeting with the whole family at the conclusion of the visit, she asks the family if they have any questions or concerns they would like to talk about. Mrs. Galinsky says, "I know that exercise is important, but I'm worried that Thomas and Nicole are too young to be spending so much time practicing for their sports teams every day and playing games every weekend. They hardly have time for anything else."

Dr. Jackson tells the parents, "Specializing in just one sport can give children a competitive edge. But sometimes they feel too much pressure and lose their special drive early, before they have a chance to contribute much to their sport. At Nicole's age, she can start to focus on the sports that interest her, but Thomas should still be trying out lots of activities. A fifth grader shouldn't be treated like a high school athlete."

Mr. Galinsky is concerned about sports injuries. "I'm worried that Thomas or Nicole might get hurt. And I don't think they would be able to get the same medical attention and treatment as high school and college athletes receive from their sports programs."

Dr. Jackson explains, "A sports injury might seem trivial, but you should still have it checked out. If it's more than a very minor injury, you should see a doctor who knows about sports injuries, or a certified trainer."

Turning to Thomas and Nicole, Dr. Jackson asks, "Have your coaches talked to you about how to prevent injuries?"

"A little," says Nicole.

"We learned that you have to warm up," Thomas volunteers.

"That's right," Dr. Jackson says. "You should always stretch both before and after you exercise, and make sure that you drink a lot of water. You should also wear a mouth guard. If you do get hurt, and you get the right treatment, you can return to your sport when you have healed."

Turning back to Mr. and Mrs. Galinsky, Dr. Jackson says, "Coaches are really important. They have a lot of influence, just like teachers and doctors. Good coaches will help your children prevent sports-related injuries."

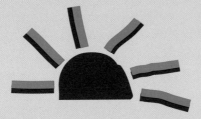

# William's Temper

Two months after William begins junior high school, his mother takes him to their family physician's office for his 12 year health supervision visit. Before the visit, William's mother indicates on his personal health record that his school work is satisfactory. She notes, however, that he is having some problems with his behavior in the classroom and on the school grounds.

During the health supervision visit, Dr. Stedman learns that William has been sent home from school four times for fighting. Although he wasn't suspended, his mother had to go to his school for conferences following the last two episodes. William and his younger brother also seem to "play rough" and often get into fistfights to resolve their differences. William had been in an after-school program at a local church, but he dropped out, complaining that the walk to the program was too far.

As Dr. Stedman interviews William, he finds that he is very nonchalant about his school behavior. While acknowledging that he has some trouble controlling his temper, William doesn't see this as a problem.

Dr. Stedman asks William and his mother about any experiences he may have had with guns. His mother replies that they don't have a gun at home. William states that he has never used or carried a gun, nor have any of his friends. He has never been threatened, and he feels safe where he lives and where he goes with his friends. William also denies using alcohol or other drugs.

Dr. Stedman stresses that although William has not been involved in any "serious" offenses, he does appear to have a problem controlling his temper when he gets into conflicts. Without some attempt to work with William's temper at this point, says Dr. Stedman, the violence could escalate over time, or he could be seriously injured by someone if he picks a fight. Dr. Stedman urges William and his mother to give the church program another try—they are familiar with the program, and it provides individual counseling, tutoring, and group sessions on issues such as conflict resolution. The program also offers a support group for single mothers, and Dr. Stedman encourages William's mother to join. They discuss some options for transportation to the program. Maybe William's grandmother can give him a ride there two or three days a week.

With the consent of William and his mother, Dr. Stedman calls the school principal to discuss school resources that might be helpful. The school does have a class that teaches conflict resolution skills, including peer mediation. The principal agrees to meet with William to discuss whether he wants to join the class. Dr. Stedman also suggests a follow-up visit after six weeks to discuss progress in William's behavior. If William continues to have problems controlling his impulses, Dr. Stedman, William, and his mother will discuss the possibility of a more intensive mental health intervention.

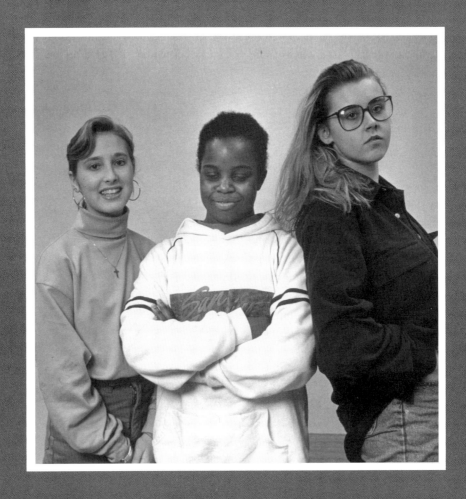

*Whenever possible, the health professional should
try to use peer influence in adolescent health promotion efforts.*

# 15, 16, and 17 Year Middle Adolescence Visits

By the age of 15, most girls have completed the changes associated with puberty and have menstrual periods, and most boys are well on their way to finishing pubertal development, having gained muscle mass and strength as well as secondary sexual characteristics. Questions about identity center on "Who am I?" as middle adolescents sort out values and beliefs in their quest for a clearer sense of self. Most middle adolescents are increasingly comfortable with their sexual identity, but for gay and lesbian youth, recognition of their sexual orientation may precipitate feelings of depression and ideas of suicide.

Most 15 and 16 year olds remain concrete in their thinking. Some middle adolescents, however, begin to make the transition from concrete to formal operational thinking, becoming more capable in abstractions, problem solving, and future-oriented thinking. They are better able to understand complexities in causality and appreciate the perspectives of others.

Changes in moral development also continue. As adolescents broaden their perspective, they often become concerned about community and societal issues such as homelessness, crime, or environmental degradation. This concern can lead to involvement in community service.

As friends assume greater importance, middle adolescents spend less time with their families. Youth of this age are extremely sensitive to the social norms of the peer group, including choices in dress, hairstyle, vocabulary, and music. They tend to have a small group of friends who share similar values and behaviors.

As adolescents deal with issues of independence, they test rules and question authority. With gains in cognition and increasing autonomy, adolescents often become extremely opinionated and challenging, which frequently results in family conflict, especially over issues such as dress, music, and social etiquette. New activities such as driving and dating require negotiating additional family rules. When at home, adolescents often seek privacy in their rooms. While parental frustration may be common, continued communication within the family is crucial and should be supported during health supervision.

Adolescents' academic decisions during high school have major implications for future educational and career choices, so it is not surprising that many middle adolescents are anxious about their academic performance. Adolescents often use their capabilities to excel and to enhance their skills. Too many youth, however, are consigned to underachievement by truancy and school dropout.

Middle adolescents can obtain work permits for paid employment. When earning a salary, adolescents may gain some skills in money management. Excessive time spent in after-school jobs, however, can bring down academic performance. About 20 hours per week appears to be a cutoff. Unfortunately, the money some adolescents earn is spent on drugs.

**MIDDLE ADOLESCENCE • 15, 16, 17 YEARS**

Adolescent safety has become a major concern, especially in many urban schools where violence is more common. Fear of physical harm is often uppermost in adolescents' minds. Almost one out of four high school students reports carrying a weapon at least once during the prior month.[1] The potential for sexual and physical victimization—especially date rape—is also a concern.

Middle adolescents have reached the legal age to drive, gaining a mobility that offers risks as well as new opportunities and choices. Adolescents who enjoy sports are usually involved with school and/or community athletics. Recreational opportunities geared specifically toward middle adolescents are minimal, especially in low-income neighborhoods and rural communities. Shopping malls and fast food restaurants, popular adolescent gathering places, offer potential opportunities for creative health promotion programs.

With their increasing cognitive and psychosocial capacities, middle adolescents are able to assume significant responsibility for their health. There is, however, potential for exploration of risky behaviors. Substance use and sexual activity increase with each successive year of high school. By 12th grade, almost 87 percent of students have used alcohol, with 39 percent reporting at least one episode of heavy drinking the previous month.[1] Just over 40 percent of seniors report having used marijuana, and over 8 percent report having used cocaine.

By 12th grade, 30 percent of students report occasional use of tobacco, with almost 16 percent smoking frequently.[1] Many regular smokers report some failed efforts to quit. Chewing or smokeless tobacco poses the risk of oral cancer. Alcohol and drugs are major factors in deaths among adolescents, contributing to motor vehicle crashes, homicides, and suicides.

By 12th grade, 67 percent of students have had sexual intercourse. Among 12th grade students who have had sexual intercourse in the last 30 days, 58 percent did not use a condom. Nearly 25 percent of 12th graders have had sexual intercourse with four or more partners.[1] Unless safer sex is practiced, sexual intercourse leads to high rates of unplanned pregnancies and sexually transmitted diseases, and increases the risk of acquiring HIV. Out-of-school youth who are not sampled in surveys of high school youth are likely to have an even higher rate of risk-taking behavior.

Feelings of sadness and depression should not be dismissed as "normal" moodiness during this period. Situational losses— including the death of a pet, problems with girlfriends or boyfriends, school failure, and parental disappointment—can lead to depression and even suicide. Over one-fourth of high school students have thought seriously during the past year about committing suicide, and more than eight percent have actually attempted it.

By this stage of development, adolescents may have formulated attitudes and values that will affect their future behavior and quality of life. Their increasingly sophisticated cognitive capability offers the health professional the opportunity to relate to them in a new way. Whenever possible, the health professional should try to use peer influence in adolescent health promotion efforts.

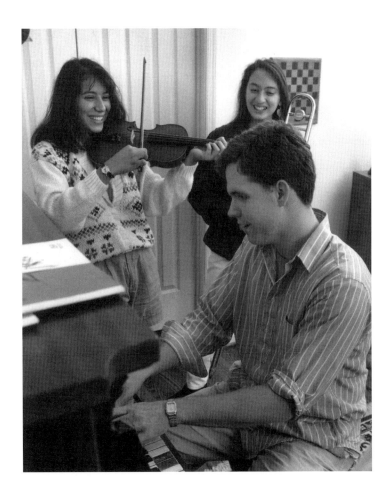

# HEALTH SUPERVISION INTERVIEW

## TRIGGER QUESTIONS

To be used selectively by the health professional. Discuss any issues or concerns of the family.

### For the Parent(s)

**How are you?**

**What about Jiang makes you proud?**

**What questions or concerns would you like to discuss today?**

(e.g., the adolescent's growth; eating patterns; weight gain/loss;
use of diet pills, tobacco, alcohol, drugs, or inhalants; frequent physical complaints; depression; loneliness; or sexual activity)

**Have there been any major changes or stresses in your family since your last visit?**

**What are some of the things you do together as a family? How often?**

**Have you talked with Alida about sexuality and your values about sex?**

**Do you feel that Isabel's school performance matches her future goals?
Does it match your goals for her?**

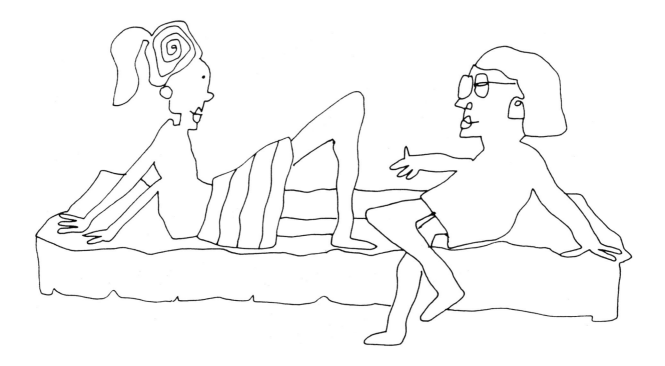

# Developmental Surveillance and School Performance

## For the Adolescent

### Social and Emotional Development

Who is your best friend? What do you do together? How many friends do you have? Is it easy or hard for you to make friends?

What do you and your friends do outside of school? How old are your friends?

Tell me some of the things you're really good at.

What do you do for fun?

Do you feel you'll be successful and achieve what you would like to do?

What are some of the things that worry you? Make you sad? Make you angry? What do you do about these things? Who do you talk to about them?

Do you often feel sad or alone at a party?

Have ever you thought about leaving home?

Do you ever feel really down and depressed?

Have any of your friends or relatives tried to hurt or kill themselves?

Have you ever thought about hurting yourself or killing yourself?[2]

Have you ever been in trouble at school or with the law?

If you could change anything in your life, what would you change?

### Physical Development and Health Habits

Do you think you have developed pretty much like the rest of your friends?

How do you feel about the way you look?

What kind of exercise or organized sports do you do? Have you been injured in sports? How hard does the coach push you? Is the training about right?

How much time each week do you spend watching television or videos? Playing video games?

Do you work? How many hours per week?

Do you use a sunscreen when in the sun?

How do you feel about your weight? Are you trying to change your weight? How?

What do you usually eat in the morning? At noon? In the afternoon? In the evening?

How many servings of milk products did you have in the last 24 hours? Is that a typical amount?

Did you smoke any cigarettes in the last month? Chew tobacco? How often?

Have you drunk alcohol in the last month? How much? What is the most you have ever had to drink?

Have you ever tried other drugs? How often have you taken them in the past month?

Have you ever been in a car where the driver was drinking or on drugs?

What education have you had about smoking or chewing tobacco? Drinking? Drugs?

Are you worried about any friends or family members and how much they drink or use drugs?

Do your friends try to pressure you to do things that you don't want to do? How do you handle that?

Do you wear a seat belt when riding in or driving a car? Do you wear a helmet when riding on a motorcycle? On a bicycle? In an all-terrain vehicle? Are you aware of the hazards involved with the use of motorcycles and ATVs?

Do you own a gun? Do any of your friends? Where is it kept? Is there a gun in your home?

Have you ever been frightened by violent or sexual things someone has said to you?

Have you witnessed violence? Been threatened with violence? Been a victim of violence?

Has anyone ever tried to harm you physically?

## Sexual development

Do you date? Do you have a steady partner? Are you happy with dating/this relationship?

Do you have any worries or questions about sex?

Are you worried about having sexual feelings for someone of your own sex?

Have you begun having sex?

On what will/do you base your decision to have sex?

Have you ever been pregnant (or gotten someone pregnant)?

Would you like to have a baby? What do you think it means to have a baby?

Have you ever had any sexually transmitted diseases such as gonorrhea, chlamydia, herpes, syphilis, or genital warts?

Do you use a kind of birth control? What kind?

Do you use condoms?

Has anyone ever touched you in a way you didn't like? Forced you to have sex?

## Family functioning

Who do you live with?

How do you get along with family members?

If teenager lives with one parent:
How often do you see the parent who does not live with you? What do you do together? How do you feel about this arrangement?

Are the rules in your family clear and reasonable?

What types of responsibilities do you have at home?

What would you like to change about your family if you could?

## School performance

Compared with others in your class (not just your friends), how well do you think you are doing? Average? Better than average? Below average?

How often do you miss school?

What activities are you involved in?

## Observation of Parent-Adolescent Interaction

In the joint interview, does the parent allow the adolescent to answer some of the questions? Is the parent supportive of the adolescent? Does the adolescent's attitude change when the parent is not in the room? How does the parent react to being asked to wait outside? Is the parent able to discuss sensitive topics?

## Physical Examination

Measure and plot on a standard chart the adolescent's height and weight. Determine the body mass index (BMI) (see chart in appendix). If an adolescent has a BMI ≥ 95th percentile for age and gender, or ≤ 5th percentile, refer for dietary assessment and counseling. Adolescents with a BMI between the 85th and 95th percentile need initial evaluation and counseling for obesity.[3]

As part of the complete physical examination, the following should be noted:

Scoliosis
(Make orthopedic referral for curves greater than 15°–20° if spinal growth is not completed. Adolescent girls usually complete spinal growth 18–24 months after menarche.)

Acne and common dermatoses

Caries, developmental dental anomalies, malocclusion, gingivitis, pathologic conditions, or dental injuries

Evidence of abuse

Evaluate for Tanner stage or Sexual Maturity Rating (SMR). If puberty is delayed, consider obtaining consultation.

For females: Provide instruction in breast self-examination. Inspect genitalia externally for condyloma/lesions. If teenager is sexually active, perform pelvic exam annually.

For males: Evaluate for gynecomastia. Examine for hernias, condyloma/lesions, and testicular cancer (high-risk group is those with a history of undescended testes, single testicle). Provide educational testicular examination.

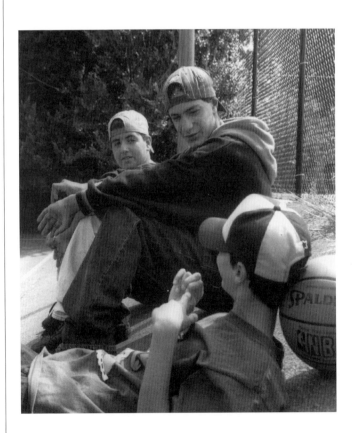

## ADDITIONAL SCREENING PROCEDURES

Vision screening if adolescent is not tested at school or reports problems
(Vision screening guidelines appear in appendix F, page 265)

Hearing screening if adolescent is exposed to loud noises regularly (e.g., rock music, occupational noise, gunshots in hunting), has recurring ear infections, or reports problems

Annual tuberculin test (PPD) if any of the following risk factors are present:

Low socioeconomic status
Residence in areas where tuberculosis is prevalent
Exposure to tuberculosis
Immigrant status
Homelessness
History of incarceration
Employment or volunteer work in health care setting

Tuberculin test (PPD) once at 14–16 years of age if no risk factors are present

Annual blood pressure screening

Annual hematocrit or hemoglobin screening for females if any of the following risk factors are present:

Moderate to heavy menses
Chronic weight loss
Nutritional deficit
Athletic activity

Hyperlipidemia screening if any of the following risk factors are present:[4]

Parents or grandparents with a history of coronary or peripheral vascular disease before 55 years of age

Parents with a blood cholesterol level ≥240 mg/dL

Hyperlipidemia screening at the discretion of the health professional if family history cannot be ascertained and any of the following risk factors for future coronary vascular disease are present:

Smoking
Hypertension
Physical inactivity
Obesity
Diabetes mellitus

Annual pap smear for sexually active females
(Females with a history of condyloma or previous abnormal pap smears may need more frequent screening)

Annual screening for sexually active adolescents:

Gonorrhea
Chlamydia
(For asymptomatic males, urine dipstick for leukocytes may be sufficient)

Syphilis screening (VDRL/RPR) if the adolescent asks to be tested or if any of the following risk factors are present:

History of sexually transmitted diseases
More than one sexual partner in the past six months
Intravenous drug use
Sexual intercourse with a partner at risk
Sex in exchange for drugs or money
For males: Sex with other males
Homelessness
Residence in areas where syphilis is prevalent

HIV screening if the adolescent asks to be tested or if any of the following risk factors are present:

Blood transfusion before 1985
History of sexually transmitted diseases
More than one sexual partner in the past six months
Intravenous drug use
Sexual intercourse with a partner at risk
Sex in exchange for drugs or money
For males: Sex with other males
Homelessness
(HIV screening should be done with informed consent and pretest and posttest counseling)

Annual screening for behaviors or emotions that may indicate:

Multiple stressors
Use of tobacco products, alcohol, or other drugs
Sexual behavior
Recurrent or severe depression or risk of suicide
History of emotional, physical, or sexual abuse
Learning or school problems (see Developmental Surveillance for suggested questions)

## IMMUNIZATIONS

Ensure that immunization status is up to date

Hepatitis B Virus (HBV) Vaccine     #1, #2, and/or #3
(If not administered previously.
Use series of three doses: First dose at
elected date, second dose one month later,
third dose six months after first dose.)

Measles, Mumps, and Rubella (MMR) Vaccine     #2
(If not administered previously or if immunization status is uncertain. Do not administer
if adolescent is pregnant.)

Tetanus and Diphtheria (Td) Vaccine     #6
(Administer 10 years after previous DTP
or Td booster, usually at 14–16 years of age)

# ANTICIPATORY GUIDANCE FOR THE ADOLESCENT

In addition to providing anticipatory guidance, many health professionals give adolescents and families handouts at an appropriate reading level or a videotape that they can review or study at home.[5]

## Promotion of healthy habits

Get adequate sleep.

Exercise vigorously at least three times per week. Encourage friends and family members to exercise.

Discuss with the health professional or your coach athletic conditioning, weight training, fluids, and weight gain or loss.

Limit television viewing to an average of one hour per day.

## Injury and violence prevention

Wear a seat belt while driving or riding in the car. If you are driving, insist that your passengers wear seat belts. Follow the speed limit.

Learn how to swim.

Do not drink alcohol, especially while driving, boating, or swimming. Plan to have a designated driver if drinking.

Protect yourself from skin cancer by putting sunscreen on before you go outside for long periods of time. Avoid tanning salons.

Test smoke detectors in your home to ensure that they work properly. Change batteries yearly.

Always wear a helmet when on a motorcycle, in an all-terrain vehicle, or riding a bicycle. Even with a helmet, motorcycles and ATVs are very dangerous.

Wear protective sports gear such as a mouth guard or a face protector.

Wear appropriate protective gear at work and follow job safety procedures.

Avoid high noise levels, especially in music headsets.

Do not carry or use a weapon of any kind.

Develop skills in conflict resolution, negotiation, and dealing with anger constructively.

Learn techniques to protect yourself from physical, emotional, and sexual abuse, including rape by either strangers or acquaintances.

Seek help if you are physically or sexually abused or fear that you are in danger.

## Mental health

Take on new challenges that will increase your self-confidence.

Continue to develop your sense of identity, clarifying your values and beliefs.

Explore new roles without hurting yourself or others.

Accept who you are and enjoy both the adult and the child in you.

Trust your own feelings as well as listening to the ideas of good friends and valued adults.

Seek help if you often feel angry, depressed, or hopeless.

Learn how to deal with stress.

Set reasonable but challenging goals.

Understand the importance of your spiritual and religious needs and try to fulfill them.

## Nutrition

Eat three meals per day. Breakfast is especially important. Eat meals with your family or residential group on a regular basis.

Choose and prepare a variety of healthy foods.

Choose nutritious snacks rich in complex carbohydrates. Limit high-fat or low-nutrient foods and beverages such as candy, chips, or soft drinks.

Choose plenty of fruits and vegetables; breads, cereals, and other grain products; low-fat dairy products; lean meats; and foods prepared with little or no fat. Include foods rich in calcium and iron in your diet.

Select a nutritious meal from the school cafeteria or pack a balanced lunch.

Achieve and maintain a healthy weight. Manage weight through appropriate eating habits and regular exercise.

## Oral health

Brush your teeth twice a day with a pea-size amount of fluoridated toothpaste, and floss daily.

Take fluoride supplements as recommended by the health professional based on the level of fluoride in your drinking water.

Ask the health professional any questions you have about how to handle dental emergencies, especially the loss or fracture of a tooth.

Schedule a dental appointment every six months, unless your dentist determines otherwise based on your individual needs/susceptibility to disease.

As your permanent molars erupt, ensure that your dentist evaluates them for application of dental sealants.

Do not smoke or use chewing tobacco.

## Sexuality[6]

Identify a supportive adult who can give you accurate information about sex.

Get accurate information about birth control and sexually transmitted diseases.

Having sexual feelings is normal, but having sex should be a well thought out decision. Do not have sex if you do not want to.

Not having sexual intercourse is the safest way to prevent pregnancy and sexually transmitted diseases, including HIV infection/AIDS.

Learn about ways to say no to sex.

If you are engaging in sexual activity, including intercourse, ask the health professional for an examination and discuss methods of birth control. Learn about safer sex.

Practice safer sex. Limit the number of partners, and use latex condoms and other barriers correctly.

If you are confused or concerned about your sexual feelings (for the same sex or opposite sex), talk to a trusted adult or the health professional.

## Prevention of substance use/abuse

Do not smoke, use smokeless tobacco, drink alcohol, or use drugs, diet pills, or steroids. Do not become involved in selling drugs.

If you smoke, find out about smoking cessation programs.

If you use drugs or alcohol, ask for help (e.g., a substance abuse treatment program).

Avoid situations where drugs or alcohol are easily available.

Support your friends who choose not to use tobacco, alcohol, drugs, steroids, or diet pills.

Become a peer counselor to prevent substance abuse.

## Promotion of social competence

Spend time with your family doing something you all enjoy.

Participate in social activities, community groups, and team sports.

Make sure you understand your parents' limits and the consequences they have established for unacceptable behavior.

Develop satisfying peer and sibling relationships.

Discuss with the health professional and your family and friends your strategies and coping mechanisms for handling negative peer pressure. Practice peer refusal skills.

Continue your progress in separating from your family, making independent decisions, and understanding the consequences of your behavior.

## Promotion of responsibility

Respect the rights and needs of others.

Serve as a positive ethical and behavioral role model.

Follow family rules, such as those for curfews or driving.

Share in household chores.

Learn about how you can take on new responsibility for your family, peers, and community.

Learn new skills that may be useful with your friends, family, or community (e.g., CPR).

Discuss with the health professional becoming a health care consumer. Practice a healthy lifestyle.

## Promotion of school achievement

Be responsible for your own attendance, homework, course selection, and extracurricular activities.

If you feel frustrated with school or are thinking about dropping out, discuss your feelings and options with a trusted adult.

Identify talents and interests that you want to pursue.

Make plans for what you will do after high school—e.g., college options (including financing), vocational training, the military, or other career choices.

## Promotion of community interactions

If you need financial assistance to help pay for health care expenses, ask about resources or for referrals to the state Medicaid programs or other state medical assistance programs.

Ask for help with food, housing, or transportation if needed.

Participate in social, religious, cultural, volunteer, or recreational organizations or activities.

Advocate for community programs (recreational, sports, educational).

Discuss current events and social responsibility with friends, family, and others.

Learn about your cultural heritage and that of others. Participate in activities that reflect cultural diversity (e.g., holidays, festivals, musical events, dance performances).

Find out what you can do about community problems such as unemployment, lack of housing, violence, crime, environmental issues, or poor public services.

# ANTICIPATORY GUIDANCE FOR THE PARENT(S)

Decide with the adolescent when he can do things on his own, including staying at home alone.

Establish realistic expectations for family rules, with increasing autonomy and responsibility given to the adolescent.

Reach agreement with the adolescent about limits, consequences for breaking rules, and appropriate disciplinary actions.

Enhance the adolescent's self-esteem by providing praise and recognizing positive behavior and achievements.

Minimize criticism, nagging, derogatory comments, and other belittling or demeaning messages.

Spend time with the adolescent.

Respect the adolescent's need for privacy.

Discuss with the health professional your own preventive and health-promoting practices (e.g., using seat belts, avoiding tobacco, eating properly, exercising and doing breast self-exams or testicular self-exams).

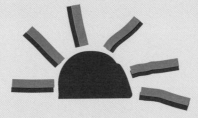

# Vicki's Close Call

Fifteen-year-old Vicki goes to see Ms. Harris, the nurse at her high school's health center. Vicki is worried that she is pregnant. She has missed a few menstrual periods, although she can't remember exactly how many. She has been dating her present boyfriend for five months and has been sexually active for the past year. She has had a total of three sexual partners. Since she feels that she "hasn't had sex enough times to get pregnant," Vicki has never used birth control. She has not discussed birth control methods with her boyfriend, and he has never brought up the issue. Vicki does not talk with her mother about her sexual activity because she is afraid that her mother would be very angry.

Ms. Harris reviews reproductive information with Vicki and learns that she does not have an adequate understanding of how pregnancy occurs. In addition to going over the menstrual cycle and conception, the nurse also talks with Vicki about the risk of sexually transmitted diseases. They discuss birth control methods as well as methods to prevent infection.

Ms. Harris tries to find out more about Vicki to determine if she has other risk factors for becoming pregnant. During their conversation, Vicki tells her, "I don't really like school—I don't care if I graduate or not. My sister Dawn had a baby when she was 16. My family was mad at first, but they stuck with her. My niece is really cute. My mom helps with babysitting for her." Ms. Harris finds out that Vicki's boyfriend is 17 years old and attends school sporadically. He has already fathered one child and has mentioned to Vicki that he'd like to have a baby with her. When asked if she would like to have a baby, Vicki responds that she is not sure if she is ready to be a mother.

Vicki's pregnancy test is negative. Ms. Harris is concerned, however, about her high risk of becoming pregnant. She refers Vicki to the nearby health department for birth control counseling and sexually transmitted disease testing. She encourages Vicki to ask her boyfriend to go with her. Ms. Harris makes a return appointment for Vicki so that she can follow up on Vicki's visit to the health department, and also explore more fully her family relationships, her home environment, and her dissatisfaction with school.

# Coming Into His Own

After his 16th birthday, John calls his family physician's office to make an appointment for his health supervision visit. Dr. Lewin has known John since he was born. John's medical history has been uneventful, except for a serious bicycle injury at age 12, from which he has fully recovered.

At the health supervision visit, as is routine in Dr. Lewin's office, John and his parents first spend some time talking with Dr. Lewin together. Dr. Lewin notices that John seems impatient with his parents during the family interview. "John, I know you might be more comfortable talking about some issues without your parents. That's understandable, and we'll do that in a few minutes. However, it's also useful for all of us to talk together."

John replies, "I don't think my parents understand what's going on today. How are they going to help me?" John's mother acknowledges that they don't understand everything John is going through, but says that she and John's father went through some of the same things when they were his age.

"It's helpful for us to know what you're feeling, and we might be able to help you out on some things," John's father says. "You'll also know how we feel so you can understand where we're coming from." John's mother adds, "We want to help you become more independent, but we don't want anything to happen to you."

After they all discuss John's school performance and goals for the future, John and Dr. Lewin move to the examining room. As well as doing a physical exam, Dr. Lewin asks John a series of questions. One of the questions is: "Do your friends ever try to pressure you to drink alcohol or use drugs?" John admits that they sometimes do and that he isn't happy about this. He doesn't want to drink or use drugs, but he doesn't want to lose his friends. Dr. Lewin and John discuss some strategies he can use to resist the pressure from his friends.

Dr. Lewin also stresses the importance of communication between John and his parents, especially regarding difficult issues such as alcohol and drug use, sex and sexuality, and violence. He says that although John's parents have signed a statement acknowledging his right to seek care without parental permission or notification—unless there is a threat of serious harm to John or others—they can still offer helpful advice as he becomes more independent. Dr. Lewin mentions that in subsequent visits he will spend more time with John and less with his parents.

**MIDDLE ADOLESCENCE • 15, 16, 17 YEARS**

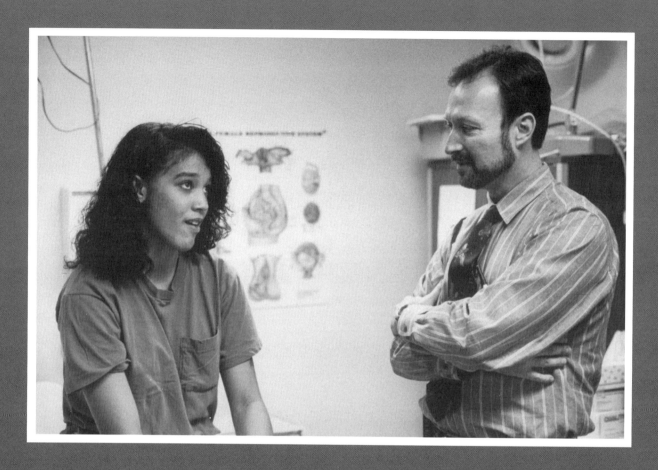

*The older adolescent and the health professional
should develop an adult-to-adult relationship.
Health supervision can be influential and supportive
in easing the young person's transition to adulthood.*

# 18, 19, 20, and 21 Year Late Adolescence Visits

With pubertal development complete, the older adolescent focuses on achieving autonomy and creating an adult sense of self, while maintaining emotional ties to the family. Vocational and personal options are paramount. Older adolescents are also working to develop a capacity for mature emotional intimacy. Late adolescents usually have the potential for formal operational thinking, though they may not use it in daily life. They can draw upon more life experiences to generate options and make decisions. Many—though not all—late adolescents have sophisticated moral reasoning, and they can formulate and follow abstract ethical principles.

Most 18 year olds have decided whether they will go on to college, join the workforce, or enter the military. While late adolescence should be a time of choice and empowerment, it can also bring intense frustration to youth with restricted options. Some may be expected to begin working to help support their families financially. For others, the cost of college tuition may place higher educational opportunities out of reach. Those who have not concentrated on academic performance now confront severely curtailed choices. High unemployment rates among youth—especially those who are unskilled or belong to minority groups—underscore the fact that vocational options are limited. This harsh reality diminishes the young person's sense of hope for the future unless some positive intervention is offered.

As older adolescents become more comfortable with themselves and their emotional independence, their relationships with family members become more accepting and harmonious. As parents cope with the adolescent's transition to adulthood, they must also come to terms with their own sense of loss. For youth with disabilities, the transition to adulthood precipitates complex new issues, such as whether independent living is realistic.

Legally responsible for themselves, many older adolescents are physically separated from their families. They may live at college, on their own, or with a spouse. Often residing in new communities, they are viewed as autonomous individuals rather than extensions of their family of origin. Many high-risk behaviors peak at this time, and older adolescents are now in the novel position of confronting behavioral consequences without the benefit of parental support. Along with alcohol and drug use, eating disorders such as bulimia and anorexia can be particular problems.

Youth 18–24 years of age are the most infrequent users of health care services. They are also the age group most likely to be uninsured. Many are no longer covered by their parents' insurance plan, and those who work often have entry-level jobs that offer no health insurance benefits.

During late adolescence, gains in autonomy, identity formation, and cognitive development are consolidated. It is also a time of transition and vulnerability, as adolescents rely less on family and community supports and ever more on their own resources. Pressures resulting from independent living and changing relationships create new issues for health supervision. The older adolescent and the health professional should develop an adult-to-adult relationship. Health supervision can be influential and supportive in easing the young person's transition to adulthood.

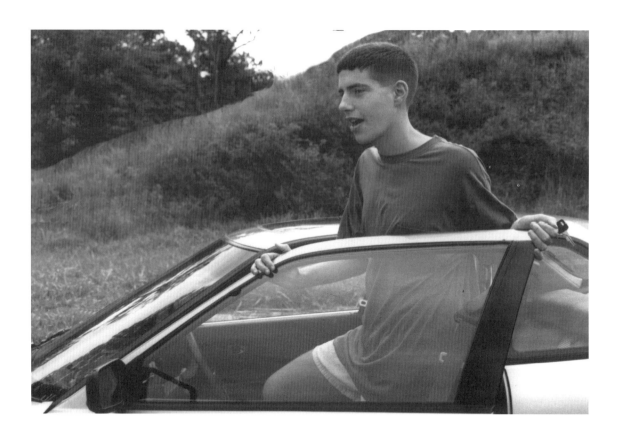

# HEALTH SUPERVISION INTERVIEW

## TRIGGER QUESTIONS

### For the Adolescent

To be used selectively by the health professional. Discuss any issues or concerns of the adolescent.

# Developmental Surveillance and School/Vocational Performance

How are you?

What questions or concerns would you like to discuss today?

**Social and Emotional Development**

Is it easy or hard for you to make friends?

What do you usually do with your friends?

Tell me some of the things you're really good at.

What do you do for fun?

Do you feel you'll be successful and achieve what you would like to do?

What are some of the things that worry you? Make you sad? Make you angry? What do you do about these things? Who do you talk to about them?

Do you ever feel really down and depressed?

Have any of your friends or relatives tried to hurt or kill themselves?

Have you ever thought about hurting yourself or killing yourself?[2]

Have you ever been in trouble with the law?

If you could change anything in your life, what would you change?

**Physical Development and Health Habits**

What kind of exercise or organized sports do you do? Have you been injured in sports? How hard does the coach push you? Is the training about right?

How much time each week do you spend watching television or videos? Playing video games?

Do you use a sunscreen when in the sun?

How do you feel about your weight? Are you trying to change your weight? How?

What do you usually eat in the morning? At noon? In the afternoon? In the evening?

239

Do you smoke cigarettes? Chew tobacco? How often?

Have you drunk alcohol in the past month? How much? What is the most you have ever had to drink?

Do you use other drugs? If so, how often in the past month?

Have you ever been in a car where the driver was drinking or on drugs?

Are you concerned about the alcohol or drug use of anyone you know?

Do you wear a helmet when riding a motorcycle, on a bicycle, or in an all-terrain vehicle? Are you aware of the hazards involved with the use of motorcycles and ATVs?

Do you wear a seat belt when driving or riding in a car?

Do you own a gun? Do any of your friends? Where is it kept? Is there a gun in your home?

Have you ever been frightened by violent or sexual things someone has said to you?

Have you ever witnessed violence? Been threatened with violence? Been a victim of violence?

Has anyone ever tried to harm you physically?

## Sexual Development

Do you date? Do you have a steady partner? Are you happy with dating/this relationship?

Do you have any worries or questions about sex or sexual orientation?

Have you begun having sexual intercourse? If so, do you have sex with men, women, or both?

On what will/do you base your decision to have sex?

Have you ever been pregnant (or gotten someone pregnant)?

Have you ever had any sexually transmitted diseases such as gonorrhea, chlamydia, herpes, syphilis, or genital warts?

Do you use a kind of birth control? What kind?

Do you use condoms?

Has anyone ever touched you in a way you didn't like? Forced you to have sex?

## Family Functioning

Who do you live with? How do you get along with family members?

What does your family do together?

What would you like to change about your family if you could?

How are you and your parent(s) dealing with your living away from home/preparing to do so? If you are already living away from home, what is it like?

## School/Vocational Performance

Are you going to school? Are you working?

How are you doing in school?

What activities are you involved in?

What do you like to do when you're not in class or working?

How is school or your job search going?

How is your job? Are you satisfied with it?

Have you thought about getting additional education or training?

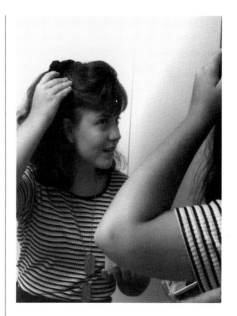

241

## For Parent(s) If Accompanying the Adolescent

**How are things going?**

**What questions or concerns would you like to discuss today?** (e.g., the adolescent's growth; eating patterns; weight gain/loss; use of diet pills, tobacco, alcohol, drugs, or inhalants; frequent physical complaints; depression; loneliness; or sexual activity)

**Have you discussed your concerns with Leila?**

**For parent(s) of adolescents who will be living away from home:**

**How do you think Desiree's living away will affect things at home? How prepared is she to live away? What help will she need?**

**Are you prepared for changes in Andy when he returns home to visit?**

**Have you made plans for Jodie's health insurance coverage when she is at school/living on her own?**

**For parent(s) of adolescent with special health needs, include discussion of health care, medications, living arrangements, diet, and social support.**

# Physical Examination

Measure and plot on a standard chart the adolescent's height and weight. Determine the body mass index (BMI) (see chart in appendix G, page 266). If an adolescent has a BMI ≥ 95th percentile for age and gender, or ≤ 5th percentile, refer for dietary assessment and counseling. Adolescents with a BMI between the 85th and 95th percentile need initial evaluation and counseling for obesity.[3]

As part of the complete physical examination, the following should be noted:

Scoliosis
(Make orthopedic referral for curves greater than 15°–20° if spinal growth is not completed. Adolescent girls usually complete spinal growth 18–24 months after menarche.)

Acne and common dermatoses

Caries, developmental dental anomalies, malocclusion, gingivitis, pathologic conditions, or dental injuries

Evidence of abuse

Evaluate for Tanner stage or Sexual Maturity Rating (SMR). If puberty is delayed, consider obtaining consultation.

For females: Provide instruction in breast self-examination and encourage the adolescent to do an exam at home each month. Inspect genitalia externally for condyloma/lesions. Perform annual pelvic exam.

For males: Evaluate for gynecomastia. Examine for hernias, condyloma/lesions, and testicular cancer (high-risk group is those with a history of undescended testes, single testicle). Provide educational testicular examination.

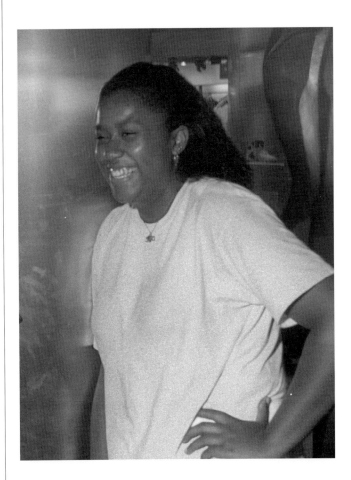

## ADDITIONAL SCREENING PROCEDURES

Vision screening if adolescent is not tested at school or reports problems
(Vision screening guidelines appear in appendix F, page 265)

Hearing screening if adolescent is exposed to loud noises regularly (e.g., rock music, occupational noise, gunshots in hunting), has recurring ear infections, or reports problems

Annual tuberculin test (PPD) if any of the following risk factors are present:

Low socioeconomic status
Residence in areas where tuberculosis is prevalent
Exposure to tuberculosis
Immigrant status
Homelessness
History of incarceration
Employment or volunteer work in health care setting

Annual blood pressure screening

Annual hematocrit or hemoglobin screening for females if any of the following risk factors are present:

Moderate to heavy menses
Chronic weight loss
Nutritional deficit
Athletic activity

Hyperlipidemia screening if any of the following risk factors are present:[4]

Parents or grandparents with a history of coronary or peripheral vascular disease before 55 years of age

Parents with a blood cholesterol level ≥240 mg/dL

Hyperlipidemia screening at the discretion of the health professional if family history cannot be ascertained and any of the following risk factors for future coronary vascular disease are present:

Smoking
Hypertension
Physical inactivity
Obesity
Diabetes mellitus

Obtain a nonfasting total blood cholesterol level for adolescents over the age of 19 (do at least once)

Hyperlipidemia screening[2] for adolescents over age 19 to obtain baseline information

Annual pap smear for sexually active females (Females with a history of condyloma or previous abnormal pap smears may need more frequent screening)

Annual screening for sexually active adolescents:

Gonorrhea
Chlamydia
(For asymptomatic males, urine dipstick for leukocytes may be sufficient)

Syphilis screening (VDRL/RPR) if the adolescent asks to be tested or if any of the following risk factors are present:

Blood transfusion before 1985
History of sexually transmitted diseases
More than one sexual partner in the past six months
Intravenous drug use
Sexual intercourse with a partner at risk
Sex in exchange for drugs or money
For males: Sex with other males
Homelessness
Residence in areas where syphilis is prevalent

HIV screening if the adolescent asks to be tested or if any of the following risk factors are present:

History of sexually transmitted diseases
More than one sexual partner in the past six months
Intravenous drug use
Sexual intercourse with a partner at risk
Sex in exchange for drugs or money
For males: Sex with other males
Homelessness
(HIV screening should be done with informed consent and pretest and posttest counseling)

Annual screening for behaviors or emotions that may indicate:

Multiple stressors
Use of tobacco products, alcohol, or other drugs
Sexual behavior
Recurrent or severe depression or risk of suicide
History of emotional, physical, or sexual abuse
Learning or school problems (see Developmental Surveillance for suggested questions)

## IMMUNIZATIONS

Ensure that immunization status is up to date

Hepatitis B Virus (HBV) Vaccine    #1, #2, and/or #3
(If not administered previously.
Use series of three doses: First dose at
elected date, second dose one month later,
third dose six months after first dose.)

Measles, Mumps, and Rubella (MMR) Vaccine    #2
(If not administered previously or if immunization status is uncertain. Do not administer
if adolescent is pregnant.)

Tetanus and Diphtheria (Td) Vaccine    #6
(Administer 10 years after previous DTP or
Td booster, usually at 14–16 years of age)

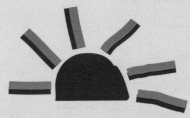

# Taking Health to Heart

Eighteen-year-old Alex visits his new primary care provider, Dr. Rosen, for a college entrance physical. During the health history, Dr. Rosen asks Alex if he has a family history of cardiovascular disease (CVD). Alex replies that his mother recently found out that she had "high cholesterol." "I think she said it was 280," he says. Alex's physical exam is normal, and he has no CVD risk factors such as obesity, smoking, or elevated blood pressure.

Following the National Cholesterol Education Program recommendations on cholesterol screening, Dr. Rosen orders a total blood cholesterol test. The results indicate an elevated blood cholesterol level (205 mg/dl), so a lipoprotein analysis is ordered. The initial and repeat lipoprotein analyses indicate borderline low-density lipoprotein (LDL) cholesterol (120 mg/dl).

"Alex, because of this borderline count, it is important that you do not put yourself at further risk for heart disease or stroke," Dr. Rosen advises Alex. "You need to keep exercising regularly and stay away from cigarettes or other tobacco products." She refers Alex to a dietitian for therapeutic dietary instruction. "Would you be free to come see me in a month or two so we can check on how you're doing and follow up on what you and the dietitian talk about?"

The dietitian explains to Alex that the goal of diet therapy is to lower LDL and total cholesterol levels while maintaining a nutritionally adequate diet. She provides basic principles for healthy, low-fat eating and guidelines for making healthier eating an enjoyable part of Alex's lifestyle. The dietitian meets several times with Alex to provide information and encourage him to follow the recommendations.

In follow-up with Dr. Rosen, Alex's total blood cholesterol (170 mg/dl) and LDL cholesterol (90 mg/dl) are at acceptable levels. He has reached his goal. Dr. Rosen tells Alex that she will continue to check how well he is following his diet and will evaluate his lipid levels just once a year as long as they remain within normal range.

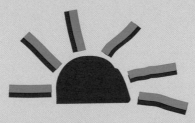

# I'm Not Skinny Enough!

Janet, a 19-year-old student, has just completed her first year at college. She has started dating only recently, and she is very concerned about her appearance.

Since Janet returned home for the summer, her mother has noticed a dramatic change in Janet's eating habits. She refuses to eat many of the foods served at meals—especially meats, main dishes, and desserts. Her diet consists mostly of salads, vegetables, pasta, and cereal. She refuses to eat breakfast and often skips other meals. Janet's mother is concerned that she is not getting enough calories. She has also noticed that Janet is constantly commenting on how fat she feels, despite the fact that she jogs almost every day and does not appear overweight. When her mother mentions her concerns, Janet brushes her off, saying, "Mom, don't worry about me."

Janet's mother encourages her to consult the family physician about whether or not she needs to lose weight, and Janet arranges an appoint-ment while she is home. During the interview, the nurse practitioner measures Janet's height and weight and asks her questions about her eating and exercise patterns. Using the Body Mass Index (BMI) tables, the nurse practitioner determines that Janet is at the lower end of the normal range for her age. When she asks Janet to tell her about her weight loss, Janet replies, "I've lost about four pounds over the past six weeks. My boyfriend tells me I'm skinny, but I feel fat."

After assuring Janet that she is not overweight but at a healthy weight, the nurse practitioner discusses with her the hazards of unhealthy weight loss diets. She also talks to Janet about anorexia nervosa and bulimia nervosa. "Society says that women have to be thin to be attractive. This can make women diet too much or not eat well because they're trying so hard to lose weight. These ideals aren't realistic—they can even be dangerous," she explains. Janet still seems uncomfortable with the suggestion that she increase her food intake and eat regular meals, so she is referred to a dietitian.

During the consultation, the dietitian obtains a dietary assessment and nutrition, exercise, and weight history. She asks Janet to tell her about her eating habits at college and with her friends. "My room-mates order out all the time. All the food they order is so high in fat and calories. I usually study late at the library so I don't have to feel weird about not eating anything."

Janet and the dietitian go over the daily recommended servings of food using the Food Pyramid Guidelines and discuss how to incor-porate them into Janet's lifestyle. The dietitian helps Janet plan several fast food meals that will fit into a healthy eating plan. This way she will be able to enjoy eating out with her friends. The dietitian also gives Janet sugges-tions to share with her parents on how to purchase and prepare healthy low-fat meals at home. Janet's weight stabilizes, and on her follow-up visits to her family physician, she has normal weight and Body Mass Index values.

# ANTICIPATORY GUIDANCE FOR THE ADOLESCENT

In addition to providing anticipatory guidance, many health professionals give adolescents and families handouts
at an appropriate reading level or a videotape that they can review or study at home.[5]

## Promotion of healthy habits

Get adequate sleep.

Exercise vigorously at least three times per week. Encourage
friends and family members to exercise.

Discuss with the health professional or your coach athletic
conditioning, weight training, fluids, and weight gain or loss.

Limit television viewing to an average of one hour per day.

## Injury and violence prevention

Wear a seat belt while driving or riding in the car. If you are
driving, insist that your passengers wear seat belts. Follow
the speed limit.

Learn how to swim.

Do not drink alcohol, especially while driving, boating, or
swimming. Plan to have a designated driver if drinking.

Protect yourself from skin cancer by putting sunscreen on
before you go outside for long periods of time. Avoid tanning
salons.

Test smoke detectors in your home to ensure that they work
properly. Change batteries yearly.

Always wear a helmet when on a motorcycle, in an all-terrain
vehicle, or riding a bicycle. Even with a helmet, motorcycles
and ATVs are very dangerous.

Wear protective sports gear such as a mouth guard or a face
protector.

Wear appropriate protective gear at work and follow job safety
procedures.

Avoid high noise levels, especially in music headsets.

Do not carry or use a weapon of any kind.

Develop skills in conflict resolution, negotiation, and dealing
with anger constructively.

Learn techniques to protect yourself from physical, emotional,
and sexual abuse, including rape by either strangers or
acquaintances.

Seek help if you are physically or sexually abused or fear that
you are in danger.

## Mental health

Take on new challenges that will increase your self-confidence.

Continue to develop your sense of identity, clarifying your
values and beliefs.

Accept who you are and enjoy both the adult and the child
in you.

Trust your own feelings as well as feedback from friends
and adults.

Seek help if you often feel angry, depressed, or hopeless.

Learn how to deal with stress.

Set reasonable but challenging goals.

Understand the importance of your spiritual and religious
needs and try to fulfill them.

## Nutrition

Eat three meals per day. Breakfast is especially important.

Eat at regularly scheduled times in a pleasant environment.

Eat meals with your family or residential group on a regular
basis.

Choose, purchase, and prepare a variety of healthy foods.

Choose nutritious snacks rich in complex carbohydrates. Limit high-fat or low-nutrient foods and beverages such as candy, chips, or soft drinks.

Choose plenty of fruits and vegetables; breads, cereals, and other grain products; low-fat dairy products; lean meats; and foods prepared with little or no fat. Include foods rich in calcium and iron in your diet.

Select a nutritious lunch from the cafeteria at your school or workplace, or pack a balanced lunch.

Achieve and maintain a healthy weight. Manage weight through appropriate eating habits and regular exercise.

## Oral health

Brush your teeth twice a day with a pea-size amount of fluoridated toothpaste, and floss daily.

Ask the health professional any questions you have about how to handle dental emergencies, especially the loss or fracture of a tooth.

Schedule a dental appointment every six months, unless your dentist determines otherwise based on your individual needs/susceptibility to disease.

As your permanent molars erupt, ensure that your dentist evaluates them for application of dental sealants.

Do not smoke or use chewing tobacco.

## Sexuality[6]

Educate yourself about birth control, sexually transmitted diseases, gay and lesbian issues, celibacy, and other issues related to sexuality.

Having sexual intercourse should be a well thought out decision. Do not have sex if you do not want to.

Not having sexual intercourse is the safest way to prevent pregnancy and sexually transmitted diseases, including HIV infection/AIDS.

Learn about ways to say no to sex.

If you are engaging in sexual activity, including intercourse, ask the health professional for an examination and discuss methods of birth control. Learn about ways to negotiate safer sex and to share your feelings about sexuality with your partner.

Practice safer sex. Limit the number of partners, and use latex condoms and other barriers correctly.

If you are confused or concerned about your sexual feelings (for the same sex or opposite sex), talk to a trusted adult or the health professional.

## Prevention of substance use/abuse

Do not smoke, use smokeless tobacco, drink alcohol, or use drugs, diet pills, or steroids. Do not become involved in selling drugs.

If you smoke, find out about smoking cessation programs.

If you use drugs or alcohol, ask for help (e.g., a substance abuse treatment program).

Support friends who choose not to use tobacco, alcohol, drugs, steroids, or diet pills.

Become a peer counselor to prevent substance abuse.

## Promotion of social competence

Participate in social activities, community groups, and team sports.

Develop satisfying peer and sibling relationships.

Identify social support systems.

Practice peer refusal skills to handle negative peer pressure.

Continue your progress in separating from your family, making independent decisions, and understanding the consequences of your behavior.

## Promotion of responsibility

Respect the rights and needs of others.

Serve as a positive ethical and behavioral role model.

Discuss with the health professional your plans for the future (e.g., employment, education, housing, marriage). Discuss lifetime reproductive plans.

Learn about how you can take on new responsibility for your family, peers, and community.

Learn new skills that may be useful with your friends, family, or community (e.g., CPR).

Discuss with the health professional becoming a health care consumer (e.g., health insurance coverage, responsibility for a healthy lifestyle).

Ask for assistance with entering the adult health care system if your care has been provided by a pediatrician or pediatric nurse practitioner.

## Promotion of school/vocational achievement

Identify talents and interests that you want to pursue.

Plan for the future (e.g., college, graduate school, vocational training, the military, job/career).

## Promotion of community interactions

If you need financial assistance to help pay for health care expenses, ask about resources or for referrals to the state Medicaid programs or other state medical assistance programs.

Ask for help with food, housing, or transportation if needed.

Participate in social, religious, cultural, volunteer, or recreational organizations or activities.

Advocate for community programs (recreational, sports, educational).

Discuss current events and social responsibility with friends, family, and others.

Learn about your cultural heritage and that of others. Participate in activities that reflect cultural diversity (e.g., holidays, festivals, musical events, dance performances).

Find out what you can do about community problems such as unemployment, lack of housing, violence, crime, environmental issues, or poor public services.

Join community campaigns to prevent substance abuse. Advocate for smoke-free environments and smoking cessation programs in your school, workplace, and/or community.

# ANTICIPATORY GUIDANCE FOR THE PARENT(S)

Encourage the adolescent's independent decision-making when appropriate.

Discuss with the adolescent her plans for independent living (money management, health care, food preparation, education, job/career).

Establish joint expectations with the adolescent regarding family rules and responsibilities.

Enhance the adolescent's self-esteem by providing praise and recognizing positive behavior and achievements.

Minimize criticism, nagging, derogatory comments, and other belittling or demeaning messages.

Spend time with the adolescent.

Respect the adolescent's need for privacy.

Discuss with the health professional your own preventive and health-promoting practices (e.g., using seat belts, avoiding tobacco, eating properly, exercising and doing breast self-exams or testicular self-exams).

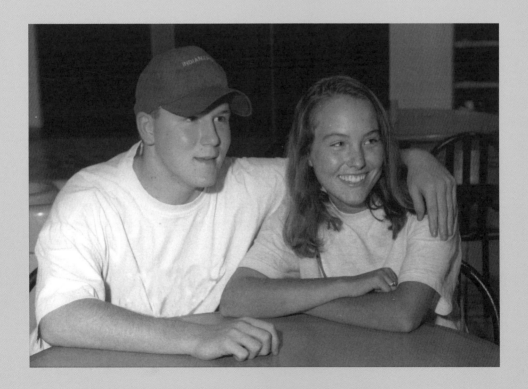

# ADOLESCENCE HEALTH SUPERVISION SUMMARY

## What else should we talk about?

### Summarize findings of the visit

Emphasize the strengths of both the adolescent and the parents. Compliment the adolescent for efforts and achievements. Commend the parents on their efforts to guide the adolescent. Remind the adolescent that you are available for further confidential discussion and additional care. Give suggestions, reading materials, and resources to promote health and reinforce good health practices.

### Arrange continuing care

#### Next visit

Give the adolescent/family materials to prepare them for the next health supervision visit.

Recommend that the adolescent/family make an appointment for the next regularly scheduled visit.

If indicated, ask the family to make an appointment for a supplementary health supervision visit.

#### Other care

Ensure that the adolescent/family make an appointment to return to the health facility for follow-up on problems identified during the health supervision visit, or refer the adolescent for secondary or tertiary medical care.

Consult with the school as necessary, especially if school progress is unsatisfactory or teacher evaluations are needed. (Obtain the permission of the parents/adolescent.)

Refer the family to appropriate community resources for help with problems identified during the health supervision visit (e.g., food programs, parenting classes, marital counseling, mental health services, special education programs, vocational training). Make arrangements to follow up on referrals and coordinate care.

### For older adolescents

Discuss arrangements for interim or independent health care if the adolescent is living away from home. Explore options for the transition to the adult health care system and health insurance, especially if the adolescent has special health needs.

### For pregnant or parenting adolescents

Discuss prenatal care with the adolescent. Refer her to a facility with an adolescent pregnancy program if available. Discuss pregnancy prevention/birth control with both pregnant and parenting adolescents, and provide family planning services or make a referral.

Refer the adolescent to resources for child care, education programs, parenting classes, housing, insurance coverage for pregnancy-related services, and other entitlement benefits such as WIC.

Refer the adolescent for dental care.

Plan for a return appointment after the birth of the child—or within three to six months for parenting adolescents—to follow up on referrals and coordinate care. Discuss health supervision for the adolescent's child. Recommend an appointment or refer the child for care.

## Adolescence Endnotes

1.  U.S. Department of Health and Human Services, Public Health Service, Centers for Disease Control and Prevention. 1991. *1991 Youth Risk Behavior Surveillance System (YRBSS)*. Atlanta, GA: Centers for Disease Control and Prevention.

2.  If the adolescent indicates that he or she has thought about suicide, ask, "How would you do it?" or "Do you have a plan?"

    If there is a plan, stop the regular health supervision visit to address this issue. The parents should be contacted and a psychiatric referral made.

    If there is no plan, ask, "Would you see a counselor if I made a referral for you right now?"

    Behavioral warning signs of suicide include:

    > Making statements like "I want to die" or "I feel dead inside"

    > Previous suicide attempts

    > Abuse of alcohol or drugs

    > Giving away prized possessions, writing a will, or making other "final" arrangements

    > Preoccupation with themes of death or expression of suicidal thoughts

    > Changes in sleeping patterns (too much or too little)

    > Withdrawal from friends or family, or other major behavioral changes

    > Changes in school performance (lower grades, cutting classes, dropping out of activities)

    > Frequent complaints of physical symptoms such as stomachaches, headaches, or fatigue

    > Sudden and extreme changes in eating habits, or loss or gain of unusual amounts of weight

    > Depression

    > Sudden cheerfulness after a prolonged period of depression

    Authier KJ, Mott MA, Peterson JL. 1993. *Suicidal Behavior Among Abused and Neglected Children: A Multidisciplinary Approach*. Boys Town, NE: Father Flanagan's Boys Home.

    Blumenthal SJ. 1990. Youth suicide: The physician's role in suicide prevention. *Journal of the American Medical Association* 264(24):3194.

3.  BMI

    An adolescent with a BMI ≥ the 95th percentile for age and gender is overweight. An adolescent with a BMI ≤ the 5th percentile for age and gender is underweight.  Both overweight and underweight adolescents should be referred for in-depth dietary and health assessment.

    Adolescents with a BMI between the 85th and 95th percentiles are at risk for becoming overweight. A dietary and health assessment should be performed if:

    *   The BMI has increased by two or more units during the previous 12 months;

    *   There is a family history of premature heart disease, obesity, hypertension, or diabetes mellitus;

    *   The adolescent expresses concern about his or her weight; or

    *   The adolescent has elevated serum cholesterol levels or blood pressure.

    If this assessment is negative, the adolescent should be given general dietary and exercise counseling and should be monitored annually.

Assess adolescents with low BMIs (especially female adolescents) for eating disorders. If the eating pattern does not change promptly with intervention, referral is indicated.

Himes JH, Dietz WH. 1994. Guidelines for overweight in adolescent preventive services: Recommendations from an expert committee. *American Journal of Clinical Nutrition* 94(59):307–316.

4. Hyperlipidemia screening if any of the following risk factors are present:

   Parents or grandparents with a history of coronary or peripheral vascular disease before 55 years of age (obtain a fasting serum lipid profile that includes determination of the low-density lipoprotein [LDL] cholesterol value)

   Parents with a blood cholesterol level ≥240 mg/dL (obtain a nonfasting total blood cholesterol level; perform at least once)

   Hyperlipidemia screening at the discretion of the health professional if family history cannot be ascertained and any of the following risk factors are present in the family:

   > Smoking
   > Hypertension
   > Physical inactivity
   > Obesity
   > Diabetes mellitus
   > (obtain a nonfasting total blood cholesterol)

   Hyperlipidemia screening for adolescents over age 19 (perform once)

National Cholesterol Education Program (NCEP) Expert Panel on Blood Cholesterol Levels in Children and Adolescents. 1992. NCEP: Highlights of the report of the Expert Panel on Blood Cholesterol Levels in Children and Adolescents. *Pediatrics* 89(3):495–500.

American Academy of Pediatrics. 1989. Indications for cholesterol testing in children. *Pediatrics* 83(1):141–142

American Academy of Pediatrics, Committee on Nutrition. 1992. Statement on cholesterol. *Pediatrics* 90(3):469–473.

5. The Injury Prevention Program (TIPP) of the American Academy of Pediatrics produces parent information sheets that highlight injury prevention priorities at each age, as well as parent information sheets on specific issues such as water safety. Community-based prevention groups, such as SAFE KIDS, also produce injury prevention materials.

6. It is important to consider the sexual orientation of adolescents for psychosocial counseling reasons; however, it is sexual behavior, not sexual orientation, that should guide the health professional when discussing STD and HIV/AIDS prevention with the adolescent. When specific information is needed, questions such as "Do you have oral sex? Vaginal intercourse? Anal intercourse?" should be substituted for "do you have sex?" It should be noted that the vernacular may be needed in order for some teens to understand what these terms mean.

   Open-ended questions will encourage the adolescent to feel comfortable bringing up difficult topics such as sexual orientation and sexual behaviors. It is more likely that the health professional will obtain accurate information if it is not assumed that the adolescent is heterosexual. At times, it is helpful to introduce a sensitive question with an explanation of why it is being asked. Being open, nonjudgmental, and specific increases the likelihood that the adolescent will receive risk-reducing guidelines and psychosocial counseling.

   The health supervision visit is an excellent opportunity to educate adolescents about safer sex and pregnancy prevention. If, for example, the adolescent is using condoms for STD and HIV/AIDS and pregnancy prevention, make sure that they are being used correctly. Keep brochures about safer sex in the office.

# Bibliography

Alderman EM, Schonberg SK, Cohen MI. 1992. The pediatrician's role in the diagnosis and treatment of substance abuse. *Pediatrics in Review* 13(8):314–318.

American Academy of Pediatrics, Committee on Adolescence. 1993. Homosexuality and adolescence. *Pediatrics* 92(4):631–634.

American Academy of Pediatrics, Committee on School Health. 1992. *The Role of the Physician in School*. Elk Grove Village, IL: American Academy of Pediatrics.

American Academy of Pediatrics, Committee on Sports Medicine. 1988. Recommendations for participation in competitive sports. *Pediatrics* 81(5):737–739.

American College of Obstetricians and Gynecologists, Committee on Adolescent Health Care. 1993. *Adolescent Sexuality: Guides for Professional Involvement* (2nd ed.). Washington, DC: American College of Obstetricians and Gynecologists.

American Medical Association, Council on Scientific Affairs. 1989. *Recognition of Childhood Sexual Abuse as a Factor in Adolescent Health Issues*. Chicago, IL: American Medical Association.

American Medical Association, Council on Scientific Affairs. 1993. Adolescents as victims of family violence. *Journal of the American Medical Association* 270(15):1850–1856.

American Medical Association, Council on Scientific Affairs. 1993. Confidential health services for adolescents. *Journal of the American Medical Association* 269(11):1420–1421.

Anglin TM. 1987. Interviewing guidelines for the clinical evaluation of adolescent substance abuse. *Pediatric Clinics of North America* 34(2):381–399.

Blumenthal SJ. 1990. Youth suicide: The physician's role in suicide prevention. *Journal of the American Medical Association* 264(24):3194.

Brown RT, McIntosh SM, Seabolt VR, Daniel WA Jr. 1985. Iron status of adolescent female athletes. *Journal of Adolescent Health Care* 6(5):349–352.

Carnegie Council on Adolescent Development, Task Force on Education of Young Adolescents. 1989. *Turning Points: Preparing American Youth for the 21st Century*. Washington, DC: Carnegie Council on Adolescent Development.

Centers for Disease Control. 1991. Tobacco use among high school students—United States, 1990. *Journal of the American Medical Association* 266(13):1755–1756.

Comerci GD, Daniel WA Jr, eds. 1991. *Parenting the Adolescent: Practitioner Concerns*. Philadelphia, PA: Hanley and Belfus.

Comerci GD, Kilbourne KA, Harrison GG. Eating disorders: Obesity, anorexia nervosa, and bulimia. In AD Hofmann , DE Greydanus, eds., 1989. *Adolescent Medicine* (2nd ed., pp.441–461). East Norwalk, CT: Appleton and Lange.

Cromer BA, McLean CS, Heald FP. 1992. *A Critical Review of Comprehensive Health Screening in Adolescents*. New York, NY: Elsevier Science Publishing.

D'Angelo LJ, Farrow J. 1989. Clinical problems in adolescent medicine. *Journal of General Internal Medicine* 4(1):64–73.

Daniel WA Jr. 1973. Hematocrit:maturity relationship in adolesence. *Pediatrics* 52(3):388–394.

Deisher R, Remafedi G. Adolescent sexuality. In AD Hofmann, DE Greydanus, eds., 1989. *Adolescent Medicine* (2nd ed., pp. 337–346). Norwalk, CT: Appelton and Lange.

Dryfoos JG. 1990. *Adolescents at Risk: Prevalence and Prevention*. New York, NY: Oxford University Press.

Education Development Center. 1992. *Identification and Prevention of Youth Violence: A Protocol for Health Care Providers*. Boston, MA: Violence Prevention Project, Department of Health and Hospitals.

Elders MJ, Hui J. 1993. Making a difference in adolescent health. *Journal of the American Medical Association* 269(11):1425–1426.

Elster AR, Kuznets NJ. 1994. *American Medical Association Guidelines for Adolescent Preventive Services (GAPS): Recommendations and Rationale*. Baltimore, MD: Williams and Wilkins.

Espeland K. 1993. Inhalent abuse: Assessment guidelines. *Journal of Psychosocial Nursing* 31(3):11–14.

Friedman SB, Fisher M, Schonberg SK, eds. 1992. *Comprehensive Adolescent Health Care*. St. Louis, MO: Quality Medical Publishing.

Gaines E, Daniel WA Jr. 1974. Dietary iron intake of adolescents: Relationship of sex, race, and sex maturity ratings. *Journal of the American Dietetic Association* 65(3):275.

Glynn TJ, Anderson M, Schwarz L. 1991. Tobacco-use reduction among high-risk youth: Recommendations of a National Cancer Institute Expert Advisory Panel. *Preventive Medicine* 20(2):279–291.

Hechinger FM. 1992. *Fateful Choices: Healthy Youth for the 21st Century*. New York, NY: Carnegie Corporation of New York.

Himes JH, Dietz WH. 1994. Guidelines for overweight in adolescent preventive services: Recommendations from an expert committee. *American Journal of Clinical Nutrition* 59:307–316.

Hofmann AD, Greydanus DE, eds. 1989. *Adolescent Medicine* (2nd ed.). Norwalk, CT: Appelton and Lange.

Hoffman AE. Clinical assessment and management of health risk behaviors in adolescents. In VC Strasburger, DE Greydanus, eds., *Adolescent Medicine: State of the Art Reviews—The At-Risk Adolescent* (Vol. 1, No. 1, pp. 33–44). Philadelphia, PA: Hanley and Belfus, Inc.

Igra V, Millstein SG. 1993. Current status and approaches to improving preventive services for adolescents. *Journal of the American Medical Association* 269(11):1408–1412.

Jessor R. 1991. Risk behavior in adolescence: A psychosocial framework for understanding and action. *Journal of Adolescent Health* 12(8):597–605.

Joffe A, Radius SM. 1991. Health counseling of adolescents. *Pediatrics in Review* 12(11):344–351.

Klein JD, Brown JD, Childers KW, Oliveri J, Porter C, Dykers C. 1993. Adolescents' risky behavior and mass media use. *Pediatrics* 92(1):24–31.

Kreipe RE. Principles of office counseling: The healthy adolescent. In GD Comerci, WA Daniel Jr., eds. *Adolescent Medicine: State of the Art Reviews; Parenting the Adolescent, Practitioner Concerns* (Vol. 2, No. 2, pp. 277–290). Philadelphia, PA: Hanley and Belfus, Inc.

Liebman M, Kenney MA, Billon W, McCoy JH, Disney GW, Ercanli EG, Glover E, Lewis H, Clark AJ, Moak SW, Schilling P, Thye F, Wakefield T. 1983. The iron status of black and white female adolescents from eight southern states. *American Journal of Clinical Nutrition* 38:109–114.

Lloyd T, Andonk MB, Rollings N, Martel JK, Landis JR, Demers LM, Eggli D, Kieselhorst K, Kulin HE. 1993. Calcium supplementation and bone mineral density in adolescent girls. *Journal of the American Medical Association* 271(7):841–844.

Marks A. 1980. Aspects of biosocial screening and health maintenance in adolescents. *Pediatric Clinics of North America* 27(1):153–161.

Marks A, Fisher M. 1987. Health assessment and screening during adolescence. *Pediatrics* 80(1 Pt. 2):131–158.

Marsh JS. 1993. Screening for scoliosis. *Pediatrics in Review* 14(8): 297–298.

McAnarney ER, Hendee WR. 1989. The prevention of adolescent pregnancy. *Journal of the American Medical Association* 262(1):78–82.

McAnarney ER, Kriepe RE, Orr DP, Comerci GD. 1992. *Textbook of Adolescent Medicine*. Philadelphia, PA: WB Saunders Company.

Micheli LJ. 1984. *Pediatric and Adolescent Sports Medicine*. Boston, MA: Little, Brown and Company.

Millstein SG, Petersen AC, Nightingale EO, eds. 1993. *Promoting the Health of Adolescents: New Directions for the Twenty-first Century*. New York, NY: Oxford University Press.

Neinstein LS. 1991. *Adolescent Health Care* (2nd ed.). Baltimore, MD: Urban and Schwarzenberg.

Pelcovitz D, Kaplan S, Samit C, Krieger R, Cornelius D. 1984. Adolescent abuse: Family structure and implications for treatment. *Journal of the American Academy of Child Psychiatry* 23(1):85–90.

Peterson AC, Compas BE, Brooks-Gunn J, Stemmler M, Ey S, Grant K. 1993. Depression in adolescence. *American Psychologist* 48(2):155–168.

Raunikar RA, Sabio H. 1992. Anemia in the adolescent athlete. *American Journal of Diseases in Children* 146(10):1201–1205.

Reider B, ed. 1991. *Sports Medicine: The School-age Athlete*. Philadelphia, PA: WB Saunders Company.

Remafedi G, Farrow JA, Deisher RW. 1991. Risk factors for attempted suicide in gay and bisexual youth. *Pediatrics* 87(6):869–875.

Richardson JL, Radziszewska B, Dent CW, Flay BR. 1993. Relationship between after-school care of adolescents and substance use, risk taking, depressed mood, and academic achievement. *Pediatrics* 92(1):32–38.

Roye CF. 1993. Pap smear screening for adolescents: Rationale, technique, and follow-up. *Journal of Pediatric Health Care* 7(5):199–206.

Schonberg SK. 1988. *Substance Abuse: A Guide for Health Professionals*. Elk Grove Village, IL: American Academy of Pediatrics.

Schonfeld DJ. 1993. School-based crisis intervention services for adolescents: Position paper of the Committees on Adolescence and School Health, Connecticut Chapter of the American Academy of Pediatrics. *Pediatrics* 91(3):656–657.

Shearin RB, Jones RL. 1989. Drug and alcohol abuse: Medical and psychosocial aspects. In AD Hofmann, DE Greydanus, eds., *Adolescent Medicine* (2nd ed., pp. 463–498). Norwalk, CT: Appleton and Lange.

Slap GB. Youth in transition to adult health care. In ER McAnarney et al., eds. 1992. *Textbook of Adolescent Medicine* (pp. 245–248). Philadelphia, PA: WB Saunders Company.

Society for Adolescent Medicine. 1991. Position statements on reproductive health care for adolescents. *Journal of Adolescent Health* 12(8):657–661.

Society for Adolescent Medicine. 1992. Access to health care for adolescents: A position paper of the Society for Adolescent Medicine. *Journal of Adolescent Health* 13(2):162–170.

Stanton B, Romer D, Ricardo I, Black M, Feigelman S, Galbraith J. 1993. Early initiation of sex and its lack of association with risk behaviors among adolescent African-Americans. *Pediatrics* 92(1):13–19.

Strasburger VC, ed. 1990. *Basic Adolescent Gynecology: An Office Guide*. Baltimore, MD: Urban and Schwarzenberg.

Strasburger VC, Brown RT. 1991. *Adolescent Medicine: A Practical Guide*. Boston, MA: Little, Brown and Company.

Strasburger VC, Greydanus DE, eds. 1990. *The At-Risk Adolescent*. Philadelphia, PA: Hanley and Belfus.

Task Force on Pediatric AIDS. 1993. Adolescents and human immunodeficiency virus infection: The role of the pediatrician and intervention. *Pediatrics* 92(4):626–629.

US Congress, Office of Technology Assessment. 1991. *Adolescent Health: Volume II. Background and the Effectiveness of Selected Prevention and Treatment Services*. Washington, DC: U.S. Government Printing Office.

US Congress, Office of Technology Assessment. 1991. *Adolescent Health*. Washington, DC: Office of Technology Assessment, U.S. Congress.

US Preventive Services Task Force. 1993. Screening for adolescent idiopathic scoliosis: Policy statement. *Journal of the American Medical Association* 269(20):2664–2666.

US Preventive Services Task Force. 1993. Screening for adolescent idiopathic scoliosis: Review article. *Journal of the American Medical Association* 269(20):2667–2672.

West J, Remafedi G. 1989. Gay and lesbian youth: Their comprehensive care in pediatric practice. *Contemporary Pediatrics* 6(8):125–138.

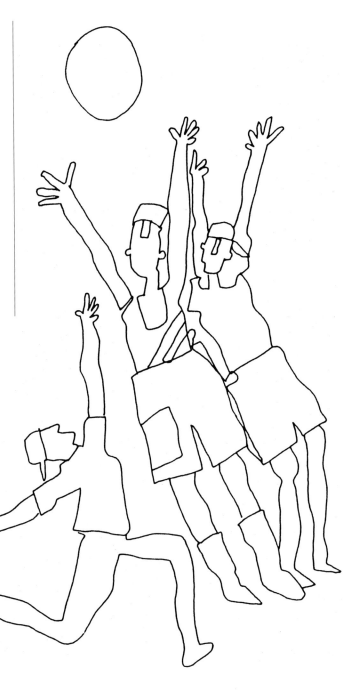

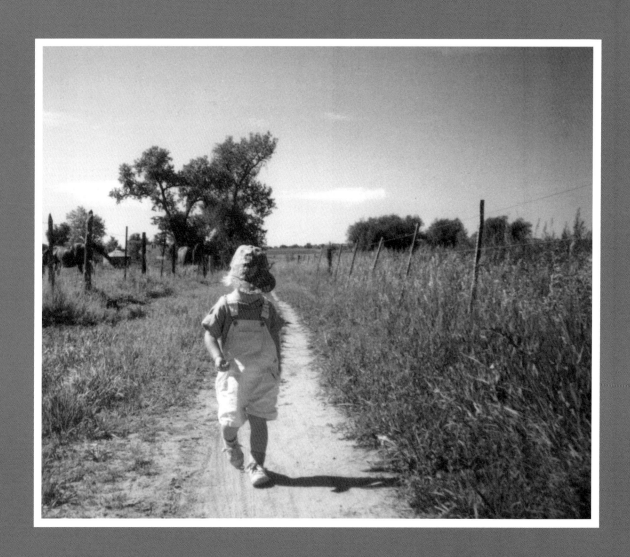

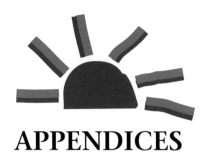

# APPENDICES

# Appendix A: Bright Futures Periodicity Schedule

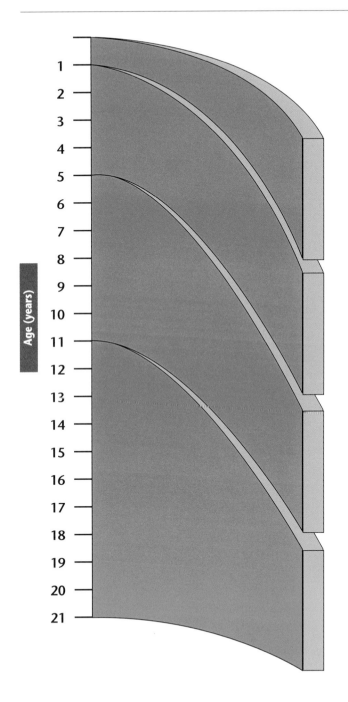

**Age (years)**

1
2
3
4
5
6
7
8
9
10
11
12
13
14
15
16
17
18
19
20
21

## INFANCY PERIODICITY SCHEDULE

| | |
|---|---|
| Prenatal | 2 Months |
| Newborn | 4 Months |
| First Week | 6 Months |
| 1 Month | 9 Months |

## EARLY CHILDHOOD PERIODICITY SCHEDULE

| | |
|---|---|
| 1 Year | 2 Years |
| 15 Months | 3 Years |
| 18 Months | 4 Years |

## MIDDLE CHILDHOOD PERIODICITY SCHEDULE

| | |
|---|---|
| 5 Years | 8 Years |
| 6 Years | 10 Years |

## ADOLESCENCE PERIODICITY SCHEDULE

| | |
|---|---|
| 11 Years | 17 Years |
| 12 Years | 18 Years |
| 13 Years | 19 Years |
| 14 Years | 20 Years |
| 15 Years | 21 Years |
| 16 Years | |

# Appendix B: Medical History

The medical history form is an important instrument for obtaining information relevant to health supervision. It is used to compile demographic information and chronicle past illnesses and present health concerns. While forms used by different health professionals vary, there are several key elements: contact information, a description of the family, and medical, developmental, and behavioral information on both the child and the family. Health professionals may supplement the form with additional questions to obtain a comprehensive history.

## Contact information

Contact information allows the health professional to follow up with the child and family and maintain continuity of health supervision.

| Child/adolescent | Parent/caregiver |
|---|---|
| Name | Name |
| Address | Address |
| Telephone number | Telephone number |
| Date of birth | Relationship to child (parent, step-parent, guardian) |
| | Employment status (company name, job title, address, telephone number) |
| | Marital status |

## Description of the family

The medical history form can provide the health professional with insight into the home environment of the child or adolescent. Questions about the people caring for the child or living in the child's home can help the health professional discover possible influences on the child's development, well-being, and general health. It is also important to obtain information on major changes in the family (e.g., new family members, family separation, chronic illnesses, or death). Ascertaining the parents' or caregivers' language preferences, education, and reading level helps the health professional communicate more effectively with the family.

## Medical, developmental, and behavioral information

The medical history form can identify important medical, developmental, and behavioral issues.

Documenting the medical history of the parents or caregivers can be particularly useful. Health conditions that have a genetic component or tend to occur among members of the same family should definitely be noted.

The form completed by the family should highlight key events in the child's medical history. By including questions on the frequency and occurrence of medical problems, health professionals can better identify and treat health concerns such as allergies, skin problems, neurological disorders, vision problems, bone or joint injuries, muscular ailments, infectious diseases, chronic illnesses, or other diseases or illnesses.

The medical history form assists health professionals in tracking interventions such as immunizations, hospitalizations, and surgeries. Questions about medications taken may be included as well.

Key milestones in the child's development (e.g., tooth eruption, walking, onset of female menses) can be documented through the medical history form.

The form can include questions about the health habits of the child and family. Seat belt use, smoking, participation in athletic or other exercise programs, and consumption of alcohol may be assessed. Questions on sexual activity may be included for adolescents. Seeking information about nutrition and diet can help reveal concerns such as poor eating habits and identify illnesses such as anorexia nervosa or bulimia.

Additional clues about health status may be gleaned from the child's academic and social performance. Questions that identify the strengths and vulnerabilities of the child and family can be particularly valuable.

Swander H, ed. 1992. *Preparticipation Physical Evaluation*. Elk Grove Village, IL: American Academy of Family Physicians, American Academy of Pediatrics, American Medical Society for Sports Medicine, American Orthopaedic Society for Sports Medicine, American Osteopathic Academy of Sports Medicine.

# Appendix C: AAP Recommended Immunization Schedule

The following *American Academy of Pediatrics Recommended Schedule for Immunization of Healthy Infants and Children* was revised and published in the Twenty-Third Edition of the Report of the Committee on Infectious Diseases, 1994 *Red Book* (see p. 23). The *Red Book* was introduced at the end of April at the Academy Spring Session in Denver. The recommended age for the third dose of OPV in the routine childhood immunization schedule has been expanded from 15–18 months to 6–18 months of age; and the recommended age for the first dose of MMR has been expanded from 15 months to 12–15 months of age. Please consult your 1994 *Red Book* for other changes in recommendations and related information. The Academy will publish an updated immunization schedule each year in the interval before the next edition of the *Red Book* is published.

| Recommended Age[a] | Immunization(s)[b] | Comments |
|---|---|---|
| Birth | HBV[c] | |
| 1 to 2 months | HBV[c] | |
| 2 months | DTP, Hib[d], OPV | DTP and OPV can be initiated as early as 4 weeks after birth in areas of high endemicity or during outbreaks. |
| 4 months | DTP, Hib[d], OPV | 2-month interval (minimum of 6 weeks) recommended for OPV to avoid interference from previous dose. |
| 6 months | DTP, (Hib[d,e]) | |
| 6 to 18 months | HBV[c], OPV | |
| 12 to 15 months | Hib[d], MMR | MMR should be given at 12 months of age in high-risk areas. If indicated, tuberculin testing may be done at the same visit. |
| 15 to 18 months | DTaP or DTP | The 4th dose of diphtheria-tetanus-pertussin vaccine should be given 6 to 12 months after the third dose of DTP and may be given as early as 12 months of age, provided that the interval between doses 3 and 4 is at least 6 months and DTP is given. DTaP is not currently licensed for use in children younger than 15 months of age. |
| 4 to 6 years | DTaP or DTP, OPV | DTaP or DTP and OPV should be given at or before school entry. DTP or DTaP should not be given after the 7th birthday. |
| 11 to 12 years | MMR | MMR should be given at entry to middle school or junior high school unless 2 doses were given at or after the 1st birthday. |
| 14 to 16 years | Td | Repeat every 10 years throughout life. |

[a]These recommended ages should not be construed as absolute. For example, 2 months can be 6 to 10 weeks. However, MMR usually should not be given to children younger than 12 months. If measles vaccination is indicated, monovalent measles vaccine is recommended, and MMR should be given subsequently, at 12 to 15 months.

[b]Vaccine abbreviations: HBV, hepatitus B virus vaccine; DTP, diphtheria and tetanus toxoids and pertussis vaccine, adsorbed; DTaP, diphtheria and tetanus toxoids and acellular pertussis vaccine, adsorbed; Hib, *Haemophilus influenzae* type b conjugate vaccine; OPV, oral poliovirus vaccine (containing attenuated poliovirus types 1, 2, and 3); MMR, live measles, mumps, and rubella viruses vaccine; Td, adult tetanus toxoid (full dose) and diphtheria toxoid (reduced dose), adsorbed, for children ≥ 7 years and adults.

[c]See 1994 *Red Book:* Report of the Committee on Infectious Diseases. Table 3.13 (p. 232). An acceptable alternative to minimize the number of visits for immunizing infants of HBsAg-negative mothers is to administer dose 1 at 0 to 2 months, dose 2 at 4 months, and dose 3 at 6 to 18 months.

[d]See 1994 *Red Book:* Report of the Committee on Infectious Diseases. Table 3.8 (p. 211).

[e](Hib: Dose 3 of Hib is not indicated if the product for doses 1 and 2 was Pedvax HIB [PRP-OMP], available from Merck & Co, West Point, PA.)

# Appendix D: ACIP Recommended Immunization Schedule

The following is the Advisory Committee on Immunization Practices (ACIP) Recommended Schedule for Immunization.

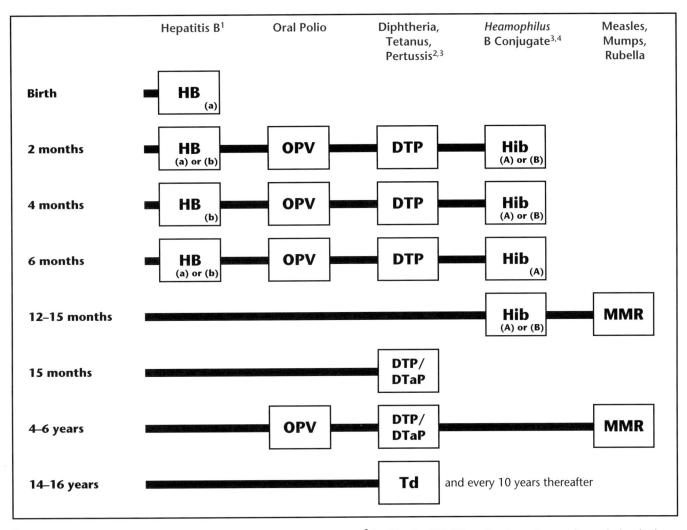

[1]Hepatitis B vaccine may be given in either of two schedules:
 (a) Birth. 1–2 months. 6–18 months.
 (b) 1–2 months. 4 months. 6–18 months.

[2]DTP preparation containing acellular pertussis vaccine (DTaP) is recommended for the fourth and fifth doses, but whole-cell DTP may still be used if DTaP is not available.

[3]Combination DTP/Hib conjugate vaccine may be used when both shots are scheduled simultaneously.

[4]There are two schedules for Hib conjugate vaccines:
 (a)HbOC (Hib TITER™), PRP-T (ActHib™), or DTP/HbOC
   (TETRAMUNE™): 2, 4, 6, and 12–15 months.
 (b)PRP-OMP (PedvaxHIB®): 2, 4, and 12–15 months.

Source: Centers for Disease Control and Prevention. November 1993.

# Appendix E: Lead Toxicity Screening

## Lead Toxicity Screening for Medicaid-Eligible Children

All children ages 6–72 months of age are considered at risk for lead poisoning and must be screened. A blood lead test must be used to screen Medicaid-eligible children for lead poisoning.

Beginning at six months of age, a verbal risk assessment must be performed at every visit. At a minimum, the following questions must be asked:

Does your child live in or regularly visit a house built before 1960? Was his or her child care center/preschool/babysitter's home built before 1960? Does the house have peeling or chipping paint?

Does your child live in a house built before 1960 with recent, ongoing, or planned renovation or remodeling?

Have any of your children or their playmates had lead poisoning?

Does your child frequently come in contact with an adult who works with lead? (Examples are construction, welding, pottery, or other trades practiced in your community.)

Does your child live near a lead smelter, battery recycling plant, or other industry likely to release lead? (Give examples in your community.)

Do you give your child any home or folk remedies that may contain lead?

Does your child live near a heavily traveled major highway where soil and dust may be contaminated with lead?

Does your home's plumbing have lead pipes or copper with lead solder joints?

If the answers to all questions are negative, a child is considered at low risk for high doses of lead exposure but must receive a blood lead test at 12 months and 24 months of age.

If the answer to any question is positive, a child is considered at high risk for high doses of lead exposure and a blood lead test must be obtained immediately.

If the initial blood lead test results are ≤ 10 µg/dL, the child must have a screening blood lead test at every visit prescribed in the state's EPSDT periodicity through 72 months of age, unless the child has already received a blood lead test within the six months preceding the periodic visit.

If a child is found to have blood lead levels ≥10 µg/dl, providers are to use their professional judgment with reference to CDC guidelines covering patient management and treatment, including follow-up blood tests.

# Appendix F: Vision Screening Guidelines (Ages 3 and Older)

## FUNCTION & RECOMMENDED TESTS

### Distance visual acuity

Snellen Letters
Snellen Numbers
Tumbling E
HOTV
Picture Tests
Allen Figures
LH Tests

### Ocular alignment

Unilateral Cover Test at 10 ft. or 3 m (or)

Random Dot E Stereotest at 40 cm
(630 secs of arc)

## REFERRAL CRITERIA

Any eye movement

Less than four of six correct

### Ages 3–5 years

1. Less than four of six correct on 20-ft. line with either eye tested at 10 ft. monocularly (i.e., less than 10/20 or 20/40)

2. Two-line difference between eyes, even within the passing range (i.e., 10/12.5 and 10/20 or 20/25 and 20/40)

### Ages 6 years and older

1. Less than four of six correct on 15-ft. line with either eye tested at 10 ft. monocularly (i.e., less than 10/15 or 20/30)

2. Two-line difference between eyes, even within the passing range (i.e., 10/10 and 10/15 or 20/20 and 20/30)

## COMMENTS

1. Tests listed in decreasing order of cognitive difficulty; the highest test that the child is capable of performing should be used; in general, the Tumbling E or the HOTV test should be used for ages 3–5 years and Snellen Letters or Numbers, for age 6 and older

2. Testing distance of 20 ft. is recommended for all visual acuity tests for ages 3–5 years

   Testing distance of 10 ft. is recommended for all visual acuity tests for age six and older

3. A line of figures is preferred over single figures

4. Nontested eye should be covered by occluder held by examiner or by adhesive occluder applied to eye; the examiner must ensure that it is not possible to peek with the nontested eye

Vision Screening Guidelines developed by the American Academy of Pediatrics, Section of Ophthalmology Committee, 1991–92: Robert Gross, M.D., Chairperson, Walter Fierson, M.D., Jane D. Kivlin, M.D., I. Matthew Rabinowicz, M.D., David R. Stager, M.D., Mark S. Ruttum, M.D., AAPOS, Earl R. Crouch, Jr., M.D., AAO.

The recommendations in this statement do not indicate an exclusive course of treatment or serve as a standard of medical care. Variations, taking into account individual circumstances, may be appropriate.

# Appendix G: Body Mass Index

The Body Mass Index (BMI) is defined as weight (kg)/height (m)$^2$. It can be used to evaluate the appropriate range of body weight by comparing the adolescent's BMI to age-based and sex-specific national norms. BMI should not be calculated if the adolescent has disabilities that confound measurements of height or weight.

After the adolescent's height and weight are measured, the BMI can be calculated [weight (kg)/height (m)$^2$] or determined using the Body Mass Index for Selected Statures and Weights Table on the next page. Once the BMI is determined, use the appropriate chart below to determine whether the adolescent needs further evaluation or counseling regarding his or her weight.

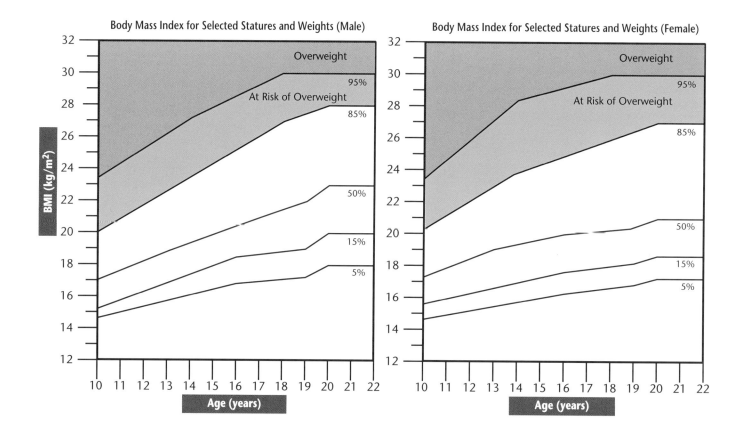

# Body Mass Index (BMI, in kg/m²) for Selected Statures and Weights

Height m (in)

| Weight kg (lb) | 1.24 (49) | 1.27 (50) | 1.30 (51) | 1.32 (52) | 1.35 (53) | 1.37 (54) | 1.40 (55) | 1.42 (56) | 1.45 (57) | 1.47 (58) | 1.50 (59) | 1.52 (60) | 1.55 (61) | 1.57 (62) | 1.60 (63) | 1.63 (64) | 1.65 (65) | 1.68 (66) | 1.70 (67) | 1.73 (68) | 1.75 (69) | 1.78 (70) | 1.80 (71) | 1.83 (72) | 1.85 (73) | 1.88 (74) | 1.90 (75) | 1.93 (76) |
|---|---|---|---|---|---|---|---|---|---|---|---|---|---|---|---|---|---|---|---|---|---|---|---|---|---|---|---|---|
| 20 (45) | 13 | 13 | 12 | 12 | 11 | 11 | 10 | 10 | 10 | 9 | 9 | 9 | 8 | | | | | | | | | | | | | | | |
| 23 (50) | 15 | 14 | 13 | 13 | 12 | 12 | 12 | 11 | 11 | 10 | 10 | 10 | 9 | 9 | 9 | 9 | 8 | | | | | | | | | | | |
| 25 (55) | 16 | 15 | 15 | 14 | 14 | 13 | 13 | 12 | 12 | 12 | 11 | 11 | 10 | 10 | 10 | 9 | 9 | 9 | | | | | | | | | | |
| 27 (60) | 18 | 17 | 16 | 16 | 15 | 15 | 14 | 13 | 13 | 13 | 12 | 12 | 11 | 11 | 11 | 10 | 10 | 10 | 9 | 9 | | | | | | | | |
| 29 (65) | 19 | 18 | 17 | 17 | 16 | 16 | 15 | 15 | 14 | 14 | 13 | 13 | 12 | 12 | 12 | 11 | 11 | 10 | 10 | 10 | 10 | | | | | | | |
| 32 (70) | 21 | 20 | 19 | 18 | 17 | 17 | 16 | 16 | 15 | 15 | 14 | 14 | 13 | 13 | 12 | 12 | 12 | 11 | 11 | 11 | 10 | 10 | | | | | | |
| 34 (75) | 22 | 21 | 20 | 20 | 19 | 18 | 17 | 17 | 16 | 16 | 15 | 15 | 14 | 14 | 13 | 13 | 12 | 12 | 12 | 11 | 11 | 11 | 10 | | | | | |
| 36 (80) | 24 | 22 | 21 | 21 | 20 | 19 | 19 | 18 | 17 | 17 | 16 | 16 | 15 | 15 | 14 | 14 | 13 | 13 | 13 | 12 | 12 | 11 | 11 | 11 | | | | |
| 39 (85) | 25 | 24 | 23 | 22 | 21 | 21 | 20 | 19 | 18 | 18 | 17 | 17 | 16 | 16 | 15 | 15 | 14 | 14 | 13 | 13 | 13 | 12 | 12 | 12 | 11 | | | |
| 41 (90) | 27 | 25 | 24 | 23 | 22 | 22 | 21 | 20 | 19 | 19 | 18 | 18 | 17 | 17 | 16 | 15 | 15 | 14 | 14 | 14 | 13 | 13 | 13 | 12 | 12 | 12 | | |
| 43 (95) | 28 | 27 | 25 | 25 | 24 | 23 | 22 | 21 | 20 | 20 | 19 | 19 | 18 | 17 | 17 | 16 | 16 | 15 | 15 | 14 | 14 | 14 | 13 | 13 | 12 | 12 | | |
| 45 (100) | 29 | 28 | 27 | 26 | 25 | 24 | 23 | 22 | 22 | 21 | 20 | 20 | 19 | 18 | 18 | 17 | 17 | 16 | 16 | 15 | 15 | 14 | 14 | 14 | 13 | 13 | 13 | 12 |
| 48 (105) | 31 | 30 | 28 | 27 | 26 | 25 | 24 | 24 | 23 | 22 | 21 | 21 | 20 | 19 | 19 | 18 | 17 | 17 | 16 | 16 | 16 | 15 | 15 | 14 | 14 | 13 | 13 | 13 |
| 50 (110) | 32 | 31 | 30 | 29 | 27 | 27 | 25 | 25 | 24 | 23 | 22 | 22 | 21 | 20 | 19 | 19 | 18 | 18 | 17 | 17 | 16 | 16 | 15 | 15 | 15 | 14 | 14 | 13 |
| 52 (115) | 34 | 32 | 31 | 30 | 29 | 28 | 27 | 26 | 25 | 24 | 23 | 23 | 22 | 21 | 20 | 20 | 19 | 18 | 18 | 17 | 17 | 16 | 16 | 16 | 15 | 15 | 14 | 14 |
| 54 (120) | 35 | 34 | 32 | 31 | 30 | 29 | 28 | 27 | 26 | 25 | 24 | 24 | 23 | 22 | 21 | 20 | 20 | 19 | 19 | 18 | 18 | 17 | 17 | 16 | 16 | 15 | 15 | 15 |
| 57 (125) | 37 | 35 | 34 | 33 | 31 | 30 | 29 | 28 | 27 | 26 | 25 | 25 | 24 | 23 | 22 | 21 | 21 | 20 | 20 | 19 | 19 | 18 | 17 | 17 | 17 | 16 | 16 | 15 |
| 59 (130) | 38 | 37 | 35 | 34 | 32 | 31 | 30 | 29 | 28 | 27 | 26 | 26 | 25 | 24 | 23 | 22 | 22 | 21 | 20 | 20 | 19 | 19 | 18 | 18 | 17 | 17 | 16 | 16 |
| 61 (135) | 40 | 38 | 36 | 35 | 34 | 33 | 31 | 30 | 29 | 28 | 27 | 27 | 25 | 25 | 24 | 23 | 22 | 22 | 21 | 20 | 20 | 19 | 19 | 18 | 18 | 17 | 17 | 16 |
| 64 (140) | 41 | 39 | 38 | 36 | 35 | 34 | 32 | 31 | 30 | 29 | 28 | 27 | 26 | 26 | 25 | 24 | 23 | 22 | 22 | 21 | 21 | 20 | 20 | 19 | 19 | 18 | 18 | 17 |
| 66 (145) | 43 | 41 | 39 | 38 | 36 | 35 | 34 | 33 | 31 | 30 | 29 | 28 | 27 | 27 | 26 | 25 | 24 | 23 | 23 | 22 | 21 | 21 | 20 | 20 | 19 | 19 | 18 | 18 |
| 68 (150) | 44 | 42 | 40 | 39 | 37 | 36 | 35 | 34 | 32 | 31 | 30 | 29 | 28 | 28 | 27 | 26 | 25 | 24 | 24 | 23 | 22 | 21 | 21 | 20 | 20 | 19 | 19 | 18 |
| 70 (155) | 46 | 44 | 42 | 40 | 39 | 37 | 36 | 35 | 33 | 33 | 31 | 30 | 29 | 29 | 27 | 26 | 26 | 25 | 24 | 23 | 23 | 22 | 22 | 21 | 21 | 20 | 19 | 19 |
| 73 (160) | 47 | 45 | 43 | 42 | 40 | 39 | 37 | 36 | 35 | 34 | 32 | 31 | 30 | 29 | 28 | 27 | 27 | 26 | 25 | 24 | 24 | 23 | 22 | 22 | 21 | 21 | 20 | 19 |
| 77 (170) | 50 | 48 | 46 | 44 | 42 | 41 | 39 | 38 | 37 | 36 | 34 | 33 | 32 | 31 | 30 | 29 | 28 | 27 | 27 | 26 | 25 | 24 | 24 | 23 | 23 | 22 | 21 | 21 |
| 79 (175) | | 49 | 47 | 46 | 44 | 42 | 40 | 39 | 38 | 37 | 35 | 34 | 33 | 32 | 31 | 30 | 29 | 28 | 27 | 27 | 26 | 25 | 24 | 24 | 23 | 22 | 22 | 21 |

267

# Body Mass Index (BMI, in kg/m²) for Selected Statures and Weights

Height m (in)

| Weight kg (lb) | 1.24 (49) | 1.27 (50) | 1.30 (51) | 1.32 (52) | 1.35 (53) | 1.37 (54) | 1.40 (55) | 1.42 (56) | 1.45 (57) | 1.47 (58) | 1.50 (59) | 1.52 (60) | 1.55 (61) | 1.57 (62) | 1.60 (63) | 1.63 (64) | 1.65 (65) | 1.68 (66) | 1.70 (67) | 1.73 (68) | 1.75 (69) | 1.78 (70) | 1.80 (71) | 1.83 (72) | 1.85 (73) | 1.88 (74) | 1.90 (75) | 1.93 (76) |
|---|---|---|---|---|---|---|---|---|---|---|---|---|---|---|---|---|---|---|---|---|---|---|---|---|---|---|---|---|
| 82 (180) |  | 51 | 48 | 47 | 45 | 44 | 42 | 40 | 39 | 38 | 36 | 35 | 34 | 33 | 32 | 31 | 30 | 29 | 28 | 27 | 27 | 26 | 25 | 24 | 24 | 23 | 23 | 22 |
| 84 (185) |  |  | 50 | 48 | 46 | 45 | 43 | 42 | 40 | 39 | 37 | 36 | 35 | 34 | 33 | 32 | 31 | 30 | 29 | 28 | 27 | 26 | 26 | 25 | 25 | 24 | 23 | 23 |
| 86 (190) |  |  |  | 49 | 47 | 46 | 44 | 43 | 41 | 40 | 38 | 37 | 36 | 35 | 34 | 32 | 32 | 31 | 30 | 29 | 28 | 27 | 27 | 26 | 25 | 24 | 24 | 23 |
| 88 (195) |  |  |  | 51 | 49 | 47 | 45 | 44 | 42 | 41 | 39 | 38 | 37 | 36 | 35 | 33 | 32 | 31 | 31 | 30 | 29 | 28 | 27 | 26 | 26 | 25 | 25 | 24 |
| 91 (200) |  |  |  |  | 50 | 48 | 46 | 45 | 43 | 42 | 40 | 39 | 38 | 37 | 35 | 34 | 33 | 32 | 31 | 30 | 30 | 29 | 28 | 27 | 27 | 26 | 25 | 24 |
| 93 (205) |  |  |  |  |  | 50 | 47 | 46 | 44 | 43 | 41 | 40 | 39 | 38 | 36 | 35 | 34 | 33 | 32 | 31 | 30 | 29 | 29 | 28 | 27 | 26 | 26 | 25 |
| 95 (210) |  |  |  |  |  |  | 49 | 47 | 45 | 44 | 42 | 41 | 40 | 39 | 37 | 36 | 35 | 34 | 33 | 32 | 31 | 30 | 29 | 28 | 28 | 27 | 26 | 26 |
| 98 (215) |  |  |  |  |  |  | 50 | 48 | 46 | 45 | 43 | 42 | 41 | 40 | 38 | 37 | 36 | 35 | 34 | 33 | 32 | 31 | 30 | 29 | 28 | 28 | 27 | 26 |
| 100 (220) |  |  |  |  |  |  |  | 49 | 47 | 46 | 44 | 43 | 42 | 40 | 39 | 38 | 37 | 35 | 35 | 33 | 33 | 31 | 31 | 30 | 29 | 28 | 28 | 27 |
| 102 (225) |  |  |  |  |  |  |  | 51 | 49 | 47 | 45 | 44 | 42 | 41 | 40 | 38 | 37 | 36 | 35 | 34 | 33 | 32 | 31 | 30 | 30 | 29 | 28 | 27 |
| 104 (230) |  |  |  |  |  |  |  |  | 50 | 48 | 46 | 45 | 43 | 42 | 41 | 39 | 38 | 37 | 36 | 35 | 34 | 33 | 32 | 31 | 30 | 30 | 29 | 28 |
| 107 (235) |  |  |  |  |  |  |  |  |  | 49 | 47 | 46 | 44 | 43 | 42 | 40 | 39 | 38 | 37 | 36 | 35 | 34 | 33 | 32 | 31 | 30 | 30 | 29 |
| 109 (240) |  |  |  |  |  |  |  |  |  | 50 | 48 | 47 | 45 | 44 | 43 | 41 | 40 | 39 | 38 | 36 | 36 | 34 | 34 | 33 | 32 | 31 | 30 | 29 |
| 111 (245) |  |  |  |  |  |  |  |  |  |  | 49 | 48 | 46 | 45 | 43 | 42 | 41 | 39 | 38 | 37 | 36 | 35 | 34 | 33 | 32 | 31 | 31 | 30 |
| 113 (250) |  |  |  |  |  |  |  |  |  |  | 50 | 49 | 47 | 46 | 44 | 43 | 42 | 40 | 39 | 38 | 37 | 36 | 35 | 34 | 33 | 32 | 31 | 30 |
| 116 (255) |  |  |  |  |  |  |  |  |  |  |  | 50 | 48 | 47 | 45 | 44 | 42 | 41 | 40 | 39 | 38 | 37 | 36 | 35 | 34 | 33 | 32 | 31 |
| 118 (260) |  |  |  |  |  |  |  |  |  |  |  |  | 49 | 48 | 46 | 44 | 43 | 42 | 41 | 39 | 39 | 37 | 36 | 35 | 34 | 33 | 33 | 32 |
| 120 (265) |  |  |  |  |  |  |  |  |  |  |  |  | 50 | 49 | 47 | 45 | 44 | 43 | 42 | 40 | 39 | 38 | 37 | 36 | 35 | 34 | 33 | 32 |
| 122 (270) |  |  |  |  |  |  |  |  |  |  |  |  |  | 50 | 48 | 46 | 45 | 43 | 42 | 41 | 40 | 39 | 38 | 37 | 36 | 35 | 34 | 33 |
| 125 (275) |  |  |  |  |  |  |  |  |  |  |  |  |  |  | 49 | 47 | 46 | 44 | 43 | 42 | 41 | 39 | 38 | 37 | 36 | 35 | 35 | 33 |
| 127 (280) |  |  |  |  |  |  |  |  |  |  |  |  |  |  | 50 | 48 | 47 | 45 | 44 | 42 | 41 | 40 | 39 | 38 | 37 | 36 | 35 | 34 |
| 129 (285) |  |  |  |  |  |  |  |  |  |  |  |  |  |  | 50 | 49 | 47 | 46 | 45 | 43 | 42 | 41 | 40 | 39 | 38 | 37 | 36 | 35 |
| 132 (290) |  |  |  |  |  |  |  |  |  |  |  |  |  |  |  | 50 | 48 | 47 | 46 | 44 | 43 | 42 | 41 | 39 | 38 | 37 | 36 | 35 |
| 134 (295) |  |  |  |  |  |  |  |  |  |  |  |  |  |  |  | 50 | 49 | 47 | 46 | 45 | 44 | 42 | 41 | 40 | 39 | 38 | 37 | 36 |
| 136 (300) |  |  |  |  |  |  |  |  |  |  |  |  |  |  |  |  | 50 | 48 | 47 | 45 | 44 | 43 | 42 | 41 | 40 | 39 | 38 | 37 |

# Appendix H: Bright Futures General Bibliography

American Academy of Ophthalmology. 1991. *Infant and Children's Vision Screening: Policy Statement.* San Francisco: American Academy of Ophthalmology.

American Academy of Pediatric Dentistry. 1994. Recommendations for preventive pediatric dental care (Revised May 1992). *Pediatric Dentistry* 15(7):39.

American Academy of Pediatrics. 1989. Indications for cholesterol testing in children. *Pediatrics* 83(1):141–142.

American Academy of Pediatrics. 1988. *TIPP: The Injury Prevention Program.* Elk Grove Village, IL: American Academy of Pediatrics.

American Academy of Pediatrics, Ad Hoc Task Force on Definition of the Medical Home. 1992. The medical home. *Pediatrics* 90(5):774.

American Academy of Pediatrics, Committee on Child Abuse and Neglect. 1991. Guidelines for the evaluation of sexual abuse of children. *Pediatrics* 87(2):254–260.

American Academy of Pediatrics, Committee on Early Childhood, Adoption and Dependent Care. 1991. Initial medical evaluation of an adopted child. *Pediatrics* 88(3):642–644.

American Academy of Pediatrics, Committee on Early Childhood, Adoption, and Dependent Care. 1987. *Health in Day Care: A Manual for Health Professionals.* Elk Grove Village, IL: American Academy of Pediatrics.

American Academy of Pediatrics, Committee on Environmental Health. 1993. Lead poisoning: From screening to primary prevention. *Pediatrics* 92(1):176–182.

American Academy of Pediatrics, Committee on Infectious Diseases. 1994. *1994 Red Book: Report of the Committee on Infectious Diseases* (23rd ed.). Elk Grove Village, IL: American Academy of Pediatrics.

American Academy of Pediatrics, Committee on Nutrition. 1992. Statement on cholesterol. *Pediatrics* 90(3):469–473.

American Academy of Pediatrics, Section of Ophthalmology Committee. 1992. *Vision Screening Guidelines.* Elk Grove Village, IL: American Academy of Pediatrics.

American Academy of Pediatrics, Committee on Practice and Ambulatory Medicine. 1986. Vision screening and eye examination in children. *Pediatrics* 77(6):918–919.

American Academy of Pediatrics, Committee on Practice and Ambulatory Medicine. 1988. Recommendations for preventive pediatric health care. *Pediatrics* 81(3):466.

American Academy of Pediatrics, Committee on Psychosocial Aspects of Child and Family Health. 1993. The pediatrician and the "new morbidity." *Pediatrics* 92(5):731–733.

American Academy of Pediatrics, Committee on Psychosocial Aspects of Child and Family Health. 1988. *Guidelines for Health Supervision II.* Elk Grove Village, IL: American Academy of Pediatrics.

American Academy of Pediatrics, Committee on Psychosocial Aspects of Child and Family Health. 1992. The pediatrician and childhood bereavement. *Pediatrics* 89(3):516–518.

American Academy of Pediatrics, Committee on School Health. 1991. School health assessments. *Pediatrics* 88(3):649–650.

American Academy of Pediatrics, Committee on School Health. 1993. *School Health: Policy and Practice* (5th ed.). Elk Grove Village, IL: American Academy of Pediatrics.

American Academy of Pediatrics, Committee on Sports Medicine and Fitness. 1991. *Sports Medicine: Health Care for Young Athletes* (2nd ed.). Evanston, IL: American Academy of Pediatrics.

American Association for Pediatric Ophthalmology and Strabismus Committee. 1991. Eye care for the children of America: The American association for pediatric ophthalmology and strabismus. *Journal of Pediatric Ophthalmology and Strabismus* 28(2):64–67.

Attie I, Brooks-Gunn J, Petersen AC. 1990. A developmental perspective on eating disorders and eating problems. In M Lewis, SM Miller, eds., *Handbook of Developmental Psychopathology* (pp. 409–420). New York: Plenum.

Barness LA, ed. 1993. *Pediatric Nutrition Handbook* (3rd ed.). Elk Grove Village, IL: American Academy of Pediatrics, Committee on Nutrition.

Bass JL, Christoffel KK, Widome M, Boyle W, Scheidt P, Stanwick R, Roberts K. 1993. Childhood injury prevention counseling in primary care settings: A critical review of the literature. *Pediatrics* 92(4):544–550.

Berenson GS. 1993. Cholesterol: Myth vs. reality in pediatric practice. *American Journal of Diseases in Children* 147(4):371–373.

Bernard B. 1992. Fostering resiliency in kids: Protective factors in the family, school, and community. *Prevention Forum* 12(3):1–16.

Boyle CA, Decouflé P, Yeargin-Allsopp M. 1994. Prevalence and health impact of developmental disabilities in US children. *Pediatrics* 93(3):399–403.

Bross D, Krugman R, Lenferr M, Rosenberg DA, Schmitt B. 1988. *The New Child Protection Team Handbook.* New York: Garland Publishing Company.

Casey P, Sharp M, Loda F. 1979. Child-health supervision for children under 2 years of age: A review of its content and effectiveness. *Journal of Pediatrics* 95(1):1–9.

Casey PH, Bradley RH, Caldwell BM, Edwards DR. 1986. Developmental intervention: A pediatric clinical review. *Pediatric Clinics of North America* 33(4):899–923.

Casey PH, Bradley RH, Nelson JY, and Whaley SA. 1988. The clinical assessment of a child's social and physical environment during health visits. *Journal of Developmental and Behavioral Pediatrics* 9(6):333–339.

Centers for Disease Control and Prevention. 1993. FDA approval of use of a new haemophilus b conjugate vaccine and a combined diphtheria-tentanus-pertussis and haemophilus b conjugate vaccine for infants and children. *Journal of the American Medical Association* 269(18):2359

Children's Safety Network. 1991. *A Data Book of Child and Adolescent Injury*. Washington, DC: National Center for Education in Maternal and Child Health.

Christner AM, ed. 1992. *Children's Self-Esteem: Tips to Promote Competence and Confidence*. Providence, RI: Manisses Communications Group, Inc.

Christoffel KK. 1990. Violent death and injury in US children and adolescents. *American Journal of Diseases in Children* 144(6):697–706.

Christoffel KK. 1992. Pediatric firearm injuries: Time to target a growing population. *Pediatric Annals* 21(7):430–436.

Clarke WR, Lauer RM. 1992. The predictive value of childhood cholesterol screening. *Journal of the American Medical Association* 267(1):101–102.

Costello EJ, Edolbrock C, Costello AJ, Dulcan MK, Burns BJ, Brent D. 1988. Psychopathology in pediatric primary care: The new hidden morbidity. *Pediatrics* 82(3):415–424.

Cross AW. 1985. Health screening in schools: Part I. *Journal of Pediatrics* 107(4):487–494.Cross AW. 1985. Health screening in schools: Part II. *Journal of Pediatrics* 107(5):653–661.

Crouch ER, Crouch ER. 1991. Pediatric vision screening: Why? When? What? How? *Contemporary Pediatrics* 8 [Special issue 8]:9–30.

Cullen KJ. 1976. A six-year controlled trial of prevention of children's behavior disorders. *Journal of Pediatrics* 88(4):662–666.

Darby PL, Garfinkel PE, Garner DM, Coscina DV, eds. 1983. *Anorexia Nervosa: Recent Developments in Research*. New York: Alan R. Liss.

Dixon SD, Stein MT. 1987. *Encounters with Children: Pediatric Behavior and Development* (2nd ed.). St. Louis, MO: Mosby Year Book.

Dworkin PH. 1989. Developmental screening: Expecting the impossible? *Pediatrics* 83(4):619–622.

Dworkin PH. 1989. British and American recommendations for developmental monitoring: The role of surveillance. *Pediatrics* 84(6):1000–1010.

Dworkin PH. 1992. Developmental screening: (Still) expecting the impossible? *Pediatrics* (89):1253–1255.

Elders MJ. 1993. Portrait of inequality. *Journal of Health Care for the Poor and Underserved* 4(3):153–162.

Elster AR, Kuznets NJ. 1994. *American Medical Association Guidelines for Adolescent Preventive Services (GAPS): Recommendations and Rationale*. Baltimore, MD: Williams and Wilkins.

Epps RP, Manley MW. 1991. A physicians' guide to preventing tobacco use during childhood and adolescence. *Pediatrics* 88(1):140–144.

Fine M. *Adolescent Health: Time for a Change—Volume II. Middle and Secondary School Environments as They Affect Adolescent Well-Being* (NTIS No. PB 91-154 328). Washington, DC: US Congress, Office of Technology Assessment. Springfield, VA: Distributed by National Technical Information Services.

Finelli EK. 1993. Changing the course. *Building Block for Life* 17(1):1–4.

Finelli EK. 1992, November. Hunger: More than a lack of food. *Harbinger*: 19.

Frankenburg WK, Dodds J, Archer P, Bresnick B, Maschka P, Edelman N, Shapiro H. 1990. *Denver II*. Denver, CO: Denver Developmental Materials.

Frankenburg WK. 1994. Preventing developmental delays: Is developmental screening sufficient? *Pediatrics* 93(4):586–589.

Gielen AC, Joffe A, Dannenberg AL, Wilson MEH, Beilenson PL, DeBoer M. 1994. Psychosocial factors associated with the use of bicycle helmets among children in counties with and without helmet use laws. *Journal of Pediatrics* 124(2):204–210.

Green M. 1986. Behavioral and developmental components of child health promotion: How can they be accomplished? *Pediatrics in Review* 8(5):133–140.

Green M. 1992. 20 interview questions that work. *Contemporary Pediatrics* 9(11):47–71.

Green M. 1992. *Pediatric Diagnosis: Interpretation of Symptoms and Signs in Infants, Children, and Adolescents* (5th ed.). Philadelphia, PA: WB Saunders.

Greene JC, Louie R, Wycoff SJ. 1989. Preventive dentistry: I. Dental caries. *Journal of the American Medical Association* 262(24):3459–3463.

Greenspan S, Greenspan NT. 1985. *First Feelings: Milestones in the Emotional Development of Your Baby and Child*. New York: Viking Penguin.

Griffen AL, Goepferd SJ. 1991. Preventive oral health care for the infant, child, and adolescent. *Pediatric Clinics of North America* 38(5): 1209–1226.

Guteluis MF, Kirsch AD, MacDonald S, Brooks MR, McErlean T. 1977. Controlled study of child health supervision: Behavioral results. *Pediatrics* 60(3):284–304.

Haber JS. 1992. Preventive health care for children and adolescents: A developmental prospective. Unpublished manuscript.

Halfon N, Berkowitz G, Klee L. 1992. Mental health service utilization by children in foster care in California. *Pediatrics* 89(6):1238–1244.

Hall DMB. 1989. *Health for All Children: A Programme for Child Health Surveillance*. Oxford, England: Oxford University Press.

Hamburg D. 1991. *The Family Crucible and Healthy Child Development*. New York: Carnegie Corporation of New York.

Hamburg D. 1992. *Today's Children: Creating a Future for a Generation in Crisis*. New York: Times Books.

Harvey B. 1994. Should blood lead screening recommendations be revised? *Pediatrics* 93(2):201–204.

Herdt G. 1989. *Gay and Lesbian Youth*. New York: Harrington Park Press.

Horwitz SM, Leaf PJ, Leventhal JM, Forsyth B, Speechley KN. 1992. Identification and management of psychosocial and developmental problems in community-based, primary care pediatric practices. *Pediatrics* 89(3):480–485.

Johnson K, Siegal M. 1990. Resources for improving the oral health of maternal and child populations. *Journal of Public Health Dentistry* 50(6):418–426.

Jordan EA, Duggan AK, Hardy JB. 1993. Injuries in children of adolescent mothers: Home safety education associated with decreased injury risk. *Pediatrics* 91(2):481–487.

Kelly B, Sein C, McCarthy PL. 1987. Safety education in a pediatric primary care setting. *Pediatrics* 79(5):818–824.

Kemper KJ. 1994. Follow-up of tuberculin skin tests. *Journal of Health Care for the Poor and Underserved* 5(1):1–4.

Kemper KJ. 1992. Self-administered questionnaire for structured psychosocial screening in pediatrics. *Pediatrics* 89(3):433.

Kemper KJ, Rivara FP. 1993. Parents in jail. *Pediatrics* 92(2):261–263.

Klerman LV, Reynolds DW. 1994. Interconception care: A new role for the pediatrician. *Pediatrics* 93(2):327–329.

Magramm I. 1992. Amblyopia: Etiology, detection, and treatment. *Pediatrics in Review* 13(1):7–14.

Merz B. 1989. New studies fuel controversy over universal cholesterol screening during childhood. *Journal of the American Medical Association* 261(6):814.

Murray RB, Zentner JP. 1993. *Nursing Assessment and Health Promotion; Strategies Through the Life Span*. Norwalk, CN: Appleton and Lange.

Nader PR. 1985. Improving the practice of pediatric patient education: A synthesis and selective review. *Preventive Medicine* 14:688–701.

Nader PR. 1990. The concept of "comprehensiveness" in the design and implementation of school health programs. *Journal of School Health* 60(4):133–138.

National Cholesterol Education Program (NCEP) Expert Panel on Blood Cholesterol Levels in Children and Adolescents 1992. NCEP: Highlights of the report of the Expert Panel on Blood Cholesterol Levels in Children and Adolescents. *Pediatrics* 89(3):495–500.

Newman TB, Browner WS, Hulley SB. 1992. Childhood cholesterol screening: Contraindicated. *Journal of the American Medical Association* 267(1):100–101.

Olds DL, Henderson CR, Tatelbaum R. 1994. Prevention of intellectual impairment in children of women who smoke cigarettes during pregnancy. *Pediatrics* 93(2):228–233.

Osborn LM, Woolley FR. 1981. Use of groups in well child care. *Pediatrics* 67(5):701–706.

Perry C, Silvis G. 1987. Smoking prevention: Behavioral prescriptions for the pediatrician. *Pediatrics* 79(5):790–799.

Peter G. 1992. Childhood immunizations. *New England Journal of Medicine* 327(25):1794–1800.

Piomelli S. 1994. Childhood lead poisoning in the '90's. *Pediatrics* 93(3):508–511.

Pipes P. 1989. *Nutrition in Infancy and Childhood* (4th ed.). St. Louis, MO: CV Mosby Company.

Reisinger KS, Bires JA. 1980. Anticipatory guidance in pediatric practice. *Pediatrics* 66(6):889–892.

Schmitt BD. 1992. *Instructions for Pediatric Patients*. Philadelphia, PA: WB Saunders Company.

Schmitt BD. 1991. *Your Child's Health: The Parents' Guide to Symptoms, Emergencies, Common Illnesses, Behavior, and School Problems*. New York: Bantam Books.

Senturia YD, Christoffel KK, Donovan M. 1994. Children's household exposure to guns: A pediatric practice-based survey. *Pediatrics* 93(3):469–475.

Sharp L, Pantell RH, Murphy LO, Lewis CC. 1992. Psychosocial problems during child health supervision visits: Eliciting, then what? *Pediatrics* 89(4):619–623.

271

Shelton TK, Jeppson ES, Johnson BH. 1987. *Family-Centered Care for Children with Special Health Care Needs*. Washington, DC: Association for the Care of Children's Health.

Sox HC, Woolf SH. 1993. Evidence-based practice guidelines from the US Preventive Services Task Force. *Journal of the American Medical Association* 269(20):2678.

Starfield B. 1991. Childhood morbidity: Comparisons, clusters, and trends. *Pediatrics* 88(3):519–526.

US Department of Health and Human Services, Alcohol, Drug Abuse, and Mental Health Administration, Office of Substance Abuse Prevention. 1992. *Parent Training Is Prevention: Preventing Alcohol and Other Drug Problems Among Youth in the Family*. Rockville, MD: US Department of Health and Human Services, Alcohol, Drug Abuse, and Mental Health Administration, Office of Substance Abuse Prevention.

US Department of Health and Human Services, Public Health Service, Centers for Disease Control. 1991. *Preventing Lead Poisoning in Young Children: A Statement by the Centers for Disease Control*. Atlanta, GA: US Department of Health and Human Services, Public Health Service, Centers for Disease Control.

US Department of Health and Human Services, Public Health Service, National Institutes of Health, National Heart, Lung and Blood Institute, National Cholesterol Education Program. 1991. *Report of the Expert Panel on Blood Cholesterol Levels in Children and Adolescents* (NIH Publication No. 91-2732).

US Department of Health and Human Services, Public Health Service. 1991. *Healthy People 2000: National Health Promotion and Disease Prevention Objectives*. Washington, DC: US Department of Health and Human Services, Public Health Service.

US Preventive Services Task Force. 1989. *Guide to Clinical Preventive Services: An Assessment of the Effectiveness of 169 Interventions*. Baltimore, MD: Williams and Wilkins.

Vaughan R, Litt I. 1989. *Child and Adolescent Development: Clinical Perspectives*. Philadelphia, PA: WB Saunders Company.

Wasserman RC. Screening tests in general pediatric practice. 1990. In Green M, Haggerty RJ, eds. *Ambulatory Pediatrics* (4th ed., pp. 83–87). Philadelphia, PA: WB Saunders Co.

Whaley LF, Wong DL. 1989. *Essentials of Pediatric Nursing* (3rd ed.). St. Louis, MO: CV Mosby Co.

Widome MD. 1992. Injury illiteracy. *Pediatrics* 89(6):1091–1093.

Wissow LS, Roter DL, Wilson MEH. 1994. Pediatrician interview style and mothers' disclosure of psychosocial issues. *Pediatrics* 93(2):289–295.

# Appendix I: Art Credits

Listed below are the photographers whose work appears in this volume. Additional photographs were contributed from personal collections.

Earl Zubkoff of Earl Zubkoff Photography in Silver Spring, Maryland, provided expertise not only in photography but also in photograph management.

Michael David Brown did the illustrations for the document, and Michael David Brown, Inc., of Rockville, Maryland, did part of the prepress production.

Marcos Ballestero of the National Center for Education in Maternal and Child Health designed and illustrated the cover of this publication.

| Photographer | Page Numbers |
| --- | --- |
| Elaine Blackman | xx, 56 |
| Pam Hallum | 181 |
| Harvey Finkle | 46 |
| Marie Hanak | 220, 236 |
| Peggy Harrison | xviii, 143 |
| Rick Reinhard | 1, 40, 48, 80, 114, 132, 144, 152, 161, 166, 197, 223 |
| Martha Tabor | 12 |
| Fred Wright | 2, 52, 75, 162 |
| Earl Zubkoff | 34, 79, 124, 195, 196, 204, 227, 238, 241, 243, 251 |

# Evaluation Form

Please help us improve future editions and create implementation materials. Please copy this form, take a few minutes to share your comments about Bright Futures, and return the form to the address or fax number given below.

1. What is your occupation?
   - ○ Dentist
   - ○ Early Childhood Educator
   - ○ Family Physician
   - ○ Health Care Administrator
   - ○ Health Educator
   - ○ Mental Health Professional
   - ○ Nurse
   - ○ Nurse Practitioner
   - ○ Nurse-Midwife
   - ○ Nutritionist
   - ○ Parent
   - ○ Pediatrician
   - ○ Policymaker
   - ○ Program Director
   - ○ Social Worker
   - ○ Teacher/Professor
   - ○ Other (specify) _____
   _____

2. What type of agency or facility do you work in?
   - ○ Child Care Facility
   - ○ Community Health Center
   - ○ Head Start Center
   - ○ Health Professional Schools
   - ○ Hospital
   - ○ Managed Care Organization
   - ○ National MCH Organization
   - ○ Private Practice
   - ○ Public Health Clinic
   - ○ School, College, or University
   - ○ State Health Department
   - ○ WIC Clinic
   - ○ Other (specify) _____
   _____

3. Do you find this book useful?
   - ○ More useful than most     ○ Average     ○ Less useful than most
   - ○ Parts of it are useful (specify) _____
   _____

4. How do you plan to use this book?
   - ○ Educate policymakers
   - ○ Recommend it to colleagues
   - ○ Other (specify) _____
   - ○ Train staff, other professionals or students
   - ○ Use the information in my work setting
   - ○ Develop an action plan for my organization
   _____

5. What is the most helpful part of this book? _____
   _____
   _____

6. What would make it more helpful? _____
   _____
   _____

7. What types of implementation materials would be helpful? (e.g., cue cards, curriculum, parent guides, videotapes) _____
   _____
   _____

8. Additional comments: _____
   _____
   _____

SEND TO:  Evaluator, *Bright Futures*, NCEMCH
          2000 15th Street North, Suite 701
          Arlington, VA  22201-2617
          (703) 524-7802
          (703) 524-9335 fax